The Consultant Dietitian
Developing Marketable Skills in
Health Care

The Consultant Dietitian
Developing Marketable Skills in Health Care

Carolyn Breeding

Donna M. Foster

Marianne Smith Edge

 VAN NOSTRAND REINHOLD
New York

Library of Congress Catalog Card Number 90-42628
ISBN 0-442-31884-7

Printed in the United States of America.

Van Nostrand Reinhold
115 Fifth Avenue
New York, New York 10003

Chapman and Hall
2-6 Boundary Row
London, SE1 8HN, England

Thomas Nelson Australia
102 Dodds Street
South Melbourne 3205
Victoria, Australia

Nelson Canada
1120 Birchmount Road
Scarborough, Ontario MIK 5G4, Canada

16   15   14   13   12   11   10   9   8   7   6   5   4   3   2   1

Library of Congress Cataloging in Publication Data
Breeding, Carolyn, 1949–
    The consultant dietitian : developing marketable skills in health
care / Carolyn Breeding, Donna M. Foster, Marianne Smith Edge.
        p.   cm.
    Includes bibliographical references and index.
    ISBN 0-442-31884-7
    1. Dietetics—Practice.   I. Foster, Donna, 1940–   . II. Smith
Edge, Marianne.   III. Title.
RM218.5.B74   1991
613.2'023—dc20   90-42628
                                                              CIP

Contents

Preface

Dietary consulting, like the long-term care market it often serves, has come into its own in the last 20 years. Increased demand for expertise in this area, flexible hours, and unlimited opportunity has lured many dietitians into the field.

Unfortunately dietary consulting requires a great deal of knowledge in many areas sometimes not adequately addressed by academics. The beginning dietary consultant is often at a loss in determining where to begin and how to proceed to develop a career as a consultant to the health care market. There are few job descriptions available to answer the many questions concerning what areas to address and how to evaluate needs in these areas.

Although each health care facility is unique and has special needs, there is a common denominator, so to speak, of areas that should be evaluated and addressed in order to assess these needs. The purpose of this book is to define these basic areas and to assist the dietary consultant in appropriate evaluation of each one. Once evaluation is accomplished, an individualized plan can be developed for each facility.

As consultants in this market for a number of years we have watched the profession of dietary consulting develop and mature and have found it regrettable that so few references exist to guide the beginning consultant or aid the established practitioner. In this book we hope to provide information that will increase the consultant's expertise and provide guidance for development and definition of the role of the dietary consultant. In addition, we wish to provide good reference information, examples of forms that may be used in many different areas, and practical suggestions that will by useful to the consultant on a day-to-day basis. This material is designed to be individualized by the consultant to fill a variety of needs.

Dietary consulting has produced some of the most innovative, creative dietitians we know, yet working independently as a consultant sometimes fails to produce adequate support systems and networking. We encourage all dietary consultants to work closely with their state practice group of Consultant Dietitians in Health Care Facilities. This organization, a practice group of the American Dietetic Association, can provide opportunities to meet and work with other consulting dietitians and can be a source of useful contacts and continuing education in the field.

In the meantime, we wish to share the knowledge and expertise we have acquired over the years working in a variety of health care settings with an equally wide variety of administrators and dietary managers.

It takes a special personality to work effectively with people in many different situations. Each facility has unique needs and concerns and requires an individual approach by the dietary consultant. Appropriate resources provide invaluable insight into the assessment and resolution of these needs and concerns. We hope to be one of these resources!

ACKNOWLEDGMENTS

Writing a book is a long, sometimes difficult process. The authors wish to acknowledge the contributions and support of several individuals who have made the process easier and the book better.

First and foremost, we would like to express our gratitude to Jim Foster for his tireless efforts on our behalf and for his devotion to the project. His endless hours in front of the computer have not gone unnoticed or unappreciated.

Special thanks are extended to Willena Beagle, Ph.D., for her work on the section of nutrition assessment relating to tube feeding. Her enthusiasm and professionalism are much appreciated.

Thanks also to Deborah Sutherlin, M.S., R.D., for her authorship of the chapter on equipment. Her knowledge of the impact of equipment on the many aspects of food production and service is a valuable addition to the book.

In addition, we would like to acknowledge the efforts of Jeffrey Arnold, R.Ph., who graciously allowed us to include his table on drug/nutrient interactions.

Last and certainly not least, we wish to express gratitude to our families for their love and support during the last two years and for their faith in us and the project.

The Consultant Dietitian
Developing Marketable Skills in
Health Care

1

Developing and Marketing a Consultant Business

The information in this chapter is designed to provide an overview of the dietary consultant's role in the health care setting to help aspiring dietitians determine whether consulting in health care is a good career choice.

WHAT IS A CONSULTANT?

In 1975, 90 percent of skilled nursing facilities used the services of a dietitian (DHEW 1975). Approximately 20 years ago, less than 1 percent of the nursing homes in the United States employed professional dietitians (Cashman 1967). Consulting has become big business in the last two decades and is projected to become even more important as the number of long-term care facilities continues to multiply. The growth of the extended care industry, paralleling the growth of the aging population of the United States, will provide even more opportunities for the consultant dietitian in the future.

Although dietary consultants are employed in many sectors of business and industry, the term "dietary consultant" still often implies association with the health care industry. More than half of all dietitians today work in hospitals and nursing homes (Job Market Shines for Dietitians 1989). Before making the decision to become a consultant dietitian in health care it is important to understand who a consultant dietitian is, what duties he or she is expected to perform, and what personality traits are helpful.

The consultant dietitian is a health care professional who is qualified through education and experience in both administrative and clinical skills (Consultant Dietitians in Health Care Facilities 1981), a self-employed specialist hired by the administrator to improve the function of the department (Gilbert 1984). The required education is generally a formal course of study in nutrition or dietetics that qualifies the individual for registration by the American Dietetic Association. Experience can be defined as a minimum of two to three years of professional work in foodservice or clinical dietetics. The wider the range of experience in various aspects of the field the better since the dietary consultant must

1

be knowledgeable and able to claim expertise in a variety of administrative and clinical settings.

The consultant dietitian usually does not assume staff or line responsibility but does observe, evaluate, instruct, and recommend (Consultant Dietitians in Health Care Facilities 1981). This approach to achieving change is more indirect than that of a full-time dietitian; the consultant's role is to motivate and train rather than to command (Gilbert 1984).

The Consultant Dietitian: How To Consult—A Guide to Success (1981), a publication by Consultant Dietitians in Health Care Facilities, a practice group of the American Dietetic Association, lists the following responsibilities of the consultant dietitian:

1. Plan and implement nutritional care for all patients/residents
   a. Perform initial and continued nutritional assessments of individuals with appropriate documentation
   b. Update patient nutritional care plans regularly and document appropriately
   c. Integrate recommendations into the total health care plan
   d. Provide nutritional counseling with patients/residents and/or family and significant others
   e. Bring to the physician's attention any individual nutritional inadequacies with appropriate suggestions for correction of problems
   f. Communicate with the health care team to integrate specific goals and approaches into the total health care plan
   g. Provide individual counseling regarding food choices and intake to meet optimal nutritional needs
   h. Participate in discharge planning
   i. Serve as a liaison with all other health professionals, including the nurse, physician, physical therapist, pharmacist, and occupational therapist
2. Evaluate the food delivery system on a regular basis
   a. Monitor foodservice for efficiency, economy, and quality
   b. Make realistic recommendations regarding the dietary department
   c. Assure presence of well-defined written policies and procedures for all foodservice activities: food purchasing, handling and storage, food preparation and service, energy conservation, sanitation, and safety
   d. Review and revise policies and procedures regularly
   e. Approve all menus and diet modifications
   f. Assure availability of standardized recipes for regular and modified diets
   g. Review system of receiving and implementing diet prescriptions
   h. Assist in developing budget proposals and cost control procedures consistent with facility policies
   i. Evaluate equipment needs for new or existing foodservice facilities and assist in planning layout design

3. Assist in planning, organizing, implementing, and evaluating staff development programs
4. Participate in appropriate facility committees and conferences
5. Promote effective communications within the facility and the community

The preceding list gives specific duties but does not indicate how consultants in the field divide their time. In a study recently conducted by Southern Illinois University, consultants reported spending an average of 37 percent of their time in foodservice management, 33 percent in nutrition care, 16 percent in staff education and training, and 14 percent in interdepartmental communication (Welch et al. 1988). It must be emphasized, however, that each facility or account will have different needs and require different aspects of the consultant's expertise. Much depends on the strengths and weaknesses of the dietary manager with whom the consultant works.

TRAITS OF SUCCESSFUL CONSULTANTS

Success in the field of consulting depends on skills and personal traits that enable a professional to adapt to self-employment easily. Successful consultant dietitians are

- *Self-motivated:* Consultants must be motivated to obtain new accounts to develop and adhere to a schedule, and to do their best even in the absence of a supervisor. The drive to excel must come from within.
- *Able to prioritize:* It is a rare consultant who has time to do everything that needs to be done at each account. Successful consultants are able to determine what needs to be done and in what order.
- *Good at motivating others:* As professionals working in an advisory rather than a line capacity, consultants must be able to motivate others to follow directions.
- *Flexible:* Consultants are often called upon to perform a wide range of duties and must often work within someone else's time frame. Successful consultants develop the ability to adapt to new situations and people.
- *Knowledgeable:* It goes without saying that the best consultant dietitians are knowledgeable about all aspects of dietary services and seek to update this knowledge through continuing education.
- *Self-confident:* Consultant dietitians must maintain self-confidence even in the face of rejection. Self-confidence is also necessary to motivate others.
- *Disciplined:* Without a high degree of self-discipline it is difficult to develop and adhere to the schedules and work plans that self-employment demands.
- *Enthusiastic:* Successful consultants radiate enthusiasm for the job and truly enjoy their work.
- *Good communicators:* It is important to be able to communicate effectively in order to motivate others. The consultant dietitian must be able to communicate with a wide range of health care professionals, including physicians,

nurses, administrators, and pharmacists. To be a part of the health care team, good communication skills are a must.
- *Innovative:* Successful consultants have the ability to assess problems and develop innovative solutions. This is particularly important in view of the cost constraints imposed on the health care industry today and in the foreseeable future.

If, after reading through this introductory section on consulting, you still think consulting is the career for you, it is time to deal with the specifics of starting a dietary consulting business.

DEVELOPING AND MARKETING DIETARY CONSULTING AS A BUSINESS

Consulting dietetics is a business. Whether you consult with five or fifty accounts, it should be perceived as a bona fide business rather than merely a source of a second income. When a decision is made to initiate a business, details abound! Suddenly, all the things taken for granted while working for someone else are now your responsibility.

Do not be overwhelmed. By putting things into perspective it is possible to develop an action plan that can be implemented step by step. It may be helpful to list what decisions and actions are necessary to begin. A general "Business Start-up Checklist" (Kentucky Commerce Cabinet 1986) includes the following basic steps:

- Choose the product or service.
- Develop a business plan.
- Present the business plan to finance sources (financial institution or investors).
- Obtain adequate finance commitments.
- Choose the business name.
- Open a business checking account.
- Obtain necessary licenses and permits including tax accounts with state and federal governments.
- Secure a lease for your place of business (if applicable).
- Obtain adequate insurance—liability, disability, and medical.
- Secure equipment, machinery, and furniture necessary to the operation of the business.
- Hire appropriate employees and/or support services.
- Plan a target date to begin business.
- You're in business!

When reviewing the business checklist, you will notice that the first item has been accomplished: Consulting dietetics has been chosen as the service to be provided. By writing out the business plan, however, more specific direction can be given to the service.

BUSINESS PLANS

What is a business plan? A business plan is defined as "a series of coordinated plans that spells out in considerable detail where a business currently is and where the business is headed" (Seigel 1987). It is a map and a guideline to profitability, the real objective of any business. A business plan can be broad, covering the entire consulting service, or limited to one specific component of the company. When writing a business plan, addressing specific questions can be helpful in developing an organized, well-planned business statement. These questions encompass four major areas: description of the business, a marketing plan, an organization plan, and a financial plan (Kentucky Commerce Cabinet 1986).

1. Writing a description of the business
    a. What type of business are you planning?
    b. What products or services will you sell?
    c. What type of opportunity is it (part-time, expansion, year-round)?
    d. What are the growth opportunities?
    e. Why does it promise to be successful?
2. Developing a marketing plan
    a. Who are the potential customers?
    b. How will you attract and hold your share of the market?
    c. Who are your competitors? How are their businesses prospering?
    d. How will you promote your services?
    e. Who will be your best customers?
    f. Where will the business be located?
    g. What factors will influence your choice of location?
3. Developing an organization plan
    a. Who will manage the business?
    b. How many employees will be needed? What will they do?
    c. What are your plans for employee hiring, salaries and wages, benefits, training, and supervision?
    d. How will you manage finances?
    e. How will you manage record keeping?
    f. What consultants or specialists will you need? Why will you need them?
    g. What legal form of ownership will you choose? Why?
    h. What licenses and permits will you need?
    i. What regulations will affect your business?
4. Developing a financial plan
    a. What is the total estimated business income for the first year? Monthly for the first year? Quarterly for the second and third years?
    b. What will it cost to open the business and sustain it for eighteen months of operation?
    c. What is the estimated monthly cash flow during the first year?
    d. What will your personal financial needs be?
    e. What volume of business will be needed to make a profit the first three years?

     f. What is the break-even point?

    g. What are the projected assets, liabilities, and net worth prior to initiating the business?

    h. What will the capital value of the equipment be?

    i. What are your total financial needs?

    j. What are your potential funding sources?

    k. How will the money from lenders or investors be used?

    l. How will the loan be secured?

The written business plan develops logically out of the responses to these questions, as the following example illustrates. (Note that the plan also includes personal data and credit information on the prospective proprietor.)

EXAMPLE 1: BUSINESS PLAN OF DIETARY MANAGEMENT SYSTEMS

Overview

The company.   Dietary Management Systems (DMS) will be a business that offers dietary consultation services to hospitals and long-term care facilities in the tri-state area.

The market.   DMS will provide services to those facilities that are financially unable to provide a position for a full-time dietitian.

Competition.   At the present time there are 16 registered dietitians in the tri-state area: ten employed full-time by larger hospitals, three at the area health department and one in private practice with a physician; two retired practitioners maintain one or two long-term care accounts. DMS is the only independent dietary consulting service in this area.

Location.   The business will be conducted out of the owner's residence. An office has been established within the residence for the sole purpose of conducting DMS business.

Management.   The owner has a B.S. degree in dietetics from the University of Rhode Island and an M.S., in public health/nutrition from Southern State University. She has worked as a health care marketing representative with Nordstrom Foods and a corporate dietitian with Naldon Medical Centers.

Personnel.   During the first stage of operation the owner will be the only consultant. After accounts are established, other dietitians will be used in a subcontractual arrangement.

Financial

First Year	
Consulting fees	$25,000.00
Speakers fees	$300.00
Operating expenses (plus tax)	$4,000.00
Net Profit	$21,300.00

I. The Company and Its Business

Dietary Management Systems (DMS) will be a computerized dietary consulting business that provides foodservice management assistance, nutrition assessments, inservice programs, and sanitation audits to small hospitals and long-term care facilities in the tri-state area.

DMS will start in October of this year and will be a sole proprietorship. The probability of success is very high because of professional and experienced management, a wide open market, and an excellent location.

Appointments will be made one or two weeks prior to visitation at the facility.

II. The Market

Small to medium-sized hospitals and long-term care facilities are required to employ the service of a qualified dietitian in order to meet state regulations. In most cases they are unable financially to support a full-time dietitian. The need for a consultant dietitian has grown due to the increased number of long-term care facilities in the tri-state area.

DMS will pull business from a 150-mile radius. This would include:

State 1	State 2
1. Lewisburg	1. Rock Springs
2. Centralia	2. Harstfield
3. Gainsville	3. Christian
4. Mooresville	4. Tall City
5. Lafayette	5. Norrisville
6. Hartland	6. Ebersville
7. Buchannon	7. Morrissey
8. Bakersville	
9. Corinth	

The above market will be the primary target area.

The growth potential is very high because of the increase in population of elderly, long-term care residents.

III. Competition

At the present time there is no other private dietary consulting business in the tri-state area. There are 16 registered dietitians:

Area General Hospital—3
St. Michael's Hospital—3
Guenther Memorial Hospital—4
Maude Lester, R.D.—retired
Sara Phipps, R.D.—retired
Peggy Peters, R.D.—private practice with George M. Cox, M.D.
Hart County Public Health Department—3

IV. Location

DMS will be located in the owner's residence. A separate room will be designated as the office space for Dietary Management Systems.

Equipment will include: desk, chair, phone (private line for business), storage cabinets, calculators, copier, FAX machine, and computer (leased).

Estimated cost of office equipment: $5,000.00.

V. Management

For the last five years, I have been a healthcare marketing representative with Nordstrom Foods, which has its headquarters in St. Paul, Minnesota. My duties include working with nursing home corporations on product approvals and presentations of seminars for the company's health care accounts.

Prior to my employment at Nordstrom, I was a corporate dietitian with Naldon Medical Centers, Little Rock, Arkansas. My duties included introducing employee meal programs in 29 facilities, supervising the implementation of dining service marketing programs and food cost control systems, conducting dietary audits, and developing annual standardized menu cycles.

I graduated from the University of Rhode Island with a B.S. degree in dietetics and from Southern State University with an M.S. public health/nutrition.

I am a registered dietitian.

VI. Personnel

Joe Smith will be the legal representative and Mead Associates will be the accountants. Secretarial services will be subcontracted.

I will be the sole consulting dietitian until such time as it is necessary to hire other dietitians on a subcontractual basis.

VII. Financial

The financial requirements are:

1. Initial start-up from equity we have built in our home. This amount is estimated at $10,000.00

2. A line of credit to be used for unexpected expenses which may occur in the first year of operation. Application is being made for $2,500.00.

VIII. Personal Data

Name: Jane R. Smith
Address: 1700 Old Town Road, Richland, Arkansas 72205
Phone: 702-686-1882
Family status: Married
Husband's employment: Teacher, Pulaski County Public School System
Education:
    B.S. in dietetics from the University of Rhode Island
    M.S. in public health/nutrition from Southern State University
    Registered dietitian
Career development:
Present employment: Healthcare Marketing representative; Nordstrom Foods, St. Paul, MN; Brad Spencer, supervisor
Prior employment: Corporate dietitian; Naldon Medical Centers, Little Rock, AR; John House, supervisor
Professional Organizations:
    Consultant Dietitians in Health Care Facilities, board member
    American Dietetic Association, board member
    Interests: Computers, needlework
    Hobbies: Running, tennis

IX. Credit Inquiry

Name: Jane R. Smith   Social Security No. 222-55-8888
State of financial condition as of July 28, 1987.

Assets		Liabilities	
Cash	$3,500.00	Accounts and bills due	$1,123.00
Real Estate (residence)	$79,900.00	Notes payable to banks (secured)	$1,904.00
Auto Maxima 1986	$4,000.00	Mortgages on real estate	$59,200.00
Auto Ford 1978	$3,000.00		
Cash value of Insurance	$5,000.00		
Total assets	$95,400.00	Total Liabilities	$62,227.00
Net worth	$33,173.00		

Combined income for year ended 1988: $46,000.00

Credit References:

1. Credit Thrift	6. VISA
2. Daviess County Teachers FCU	7. American Express
3. Citizens State Bank	8. Master Card
4. First Nationwide Bank	9. Chevron Oil Corp.
5. Whirlpool Employees FCU	

A business plan actually consists of two main components: the strategic plan and the annual business plan (Rose 1987).

The Annual Business Plan

The annual business plan focuses on two major parts: the operating plan and the financial plan. The operating plan is a one-year plan for producing a product or service, selling and marketing it effectively, and accounting for the administrative requirements of the service. The operating plan would be beneficial if one decided to launch a one-time project such as a weight management program or distribution of an inservice manual. Prior to initiating one of these projects, profitability needs to be analyzed. A good idea does not always prove to be beneficial financially (Rose 1987).

The second component of the annual business plan is the financial plan. It shows how much cash the business expects to use and how it will finance cash requirements. The general components of the financial plan include the balance sheet, the income statement, cash flow estimates, supporting schedules for analyses, and performance ratios and statistics. The assistance of a CPA or bookkeeper is highly recommended when developing this area.

The Strategic Business Plan

Strategic planning is a thought-provoking, time-intensive project initially but can provide significant benefits in the long term. The preceding questions (pages 5–6) will assist you in writing the strategic plan since this plan spans more than one year and establishes broad goals for the organization as related to marketability, organizational structure, growth expectations, and profitability. In the strategic plan, the organization's strengths, weaknesses, opportunities, and threats (SWOT) are also identified (Rose 1987). Strengths and weaknesses are internal (personal) characteristics, whereas opportunities and threats generally come from external forces and environments. Identifying SWOTs will be discussed in more detail in the section devoted to the marketing plan.

The Business Description

The first major area of the strategic plan deals with the business description. However, prior to developing the section on services and/or products the company will provide, one must evaluate the SWOT.

Strengths should focus on individual talents and areas of expertise.

Brainstorm and develop a list of every area of dietetics and foodservice management of which you have expertise and knowledge. How will these strengths improve your marketability? Most successful business owners have these strengths in common: self-motivation, endurance (long work hours with limited amount of rest), goal orientation, and self-direction.

As you identify your strengths also identify your weaknesses. Be honest with yourself and list those areas of dietetics in which you have little knowledge or work situations in which you lack confidence. A work opportunity is not always a good opportunity if it involves areas in which you possess the least amount of expertise and knowledge. Consider an example: a free-standing clinic contacts you regarding the availability of a position for a consultant renal dietitian. The hourly fee and benefits are excellent but your knowledge in renal dialysis is limited. Is it advantageous for the company to accept this opportunity, realizing the additional hours that would be required to increase the knowledge base? Would it be detrimental accepting a consultant (expert) role and not being able to provide the expertise needed by the clinic? A good initial impresssion of you and your company are vital in establishing a sound business within the community. By evaluating strengths and weaknesses prior to accepting a business opportunity, you can prevent both professional and financial disaster.

Once strengths and weaknesses have been established, list the opportunities and possibilities available in your area. Become familiar with the local business community. Read the business sections of local newspapers, identify business and health care leaders in the area, and become a member of the local chamber of commerce. Establishing yourself as a business in the community provides the opportunity to network with influential community leaders as well as to gain "inside" information on pending projects that may be of interest to the company. Health care is an aggressive, competitive business, and consultant dietitians must be aggressive to address the needs of those financially involved with these projects.

In addition to available opportunities, "threats" must be identified. Who are your competitors? Are they other privately owned dietary consulting firms? Hospital-based dietary consultant services? Corporate food management companies? Corporate-owned health care facilities? Self-styled nutrition experts?

By identifying potential threats or competition, a business plan can be developed that will make the most of your strengths and personal qualities, giving you a unique and fresh approach that distinguishes you from the competition.

Completing the SWOT analysis gives one the information and text needed to complete the first major area of the business plan, the description of the business.

Marketing Plan

The SWOT analysis also initiates your marketing plan by identifying your competition, which provides insight into how to obtain and keep a share of the market. This insight is essential in developing marketing tools.

How are you going to "sell" your business? If one is established in a particular aspect of dietary consulting, "word of mouth" is an excellent advertising tool. However, if the company seeks to move into new areas, effective marketing tools are essential.

First, establish a name for the business. Consider whether you will name the business after yourself or establish a name that will identify the type of business. It may be disadvantageous to name a business after yourself in the event serious problems arise. Be creative and choose an alternative name in case you find, when filing corporation papers, that a similar business name is already established.

Second, design a logo. Logos should be unique, creative, and representative of the company. Utilize support services with this project. Most printing companies have graphic artists who can assist you with design ideas. Obtain their ideas on effective logos, including colors to be used. They are the experts in this area—use them! Once the business name and logo are established, business cards and professional stationery can be developed. Using the same color palette for the business cards and stationery will give your company a professional look. It is more economical to purchase these items in quantity (250 to 500 lots) even if they last for several years. Professionally printed stationery, envelopes, and statements are highly recommended and contribute to the perception of an established business. It makes good marketing sense to design a brochure that describes your services. A brochure is an excellent way to "sell" a multi-faceted business. Again, a professionally designed and printed brochure is a factor in establishing the company in the business and health care community. Utilizing the talents of a marketing or advertising firm to assist in brochure design is a good financial investment. By providing the advertising personnel with the goals and objectives of the company, personal brochure design ideas, and the target audience, marketing materials can be developed to meet your needs with a creative, fresh approach. Again, continue to use the same color palette when printing brochures as the one selected for your business cards and stationery. Make sure the marketing materials cite your professional credentials, degrees, honors, training, and experience in areas connected with services offered. Do not sell yourself short!

Another consideration in developing the marketing plan is how you will promote services in addition to the word-of-mouth route. Since commercial advertising is not inexpensive, it is important to consider avenues that will yield the best financial results for the initial dollar investment. If you are a chamber of commerce member, consider advertising in the monthly newsletter, especially if your company boasts a corporate wellness component. Usually newsletters of this kind are distributed to and read by contact persons in a company. Another possibility for exposure is a letter with a brochure sent to key businesses or health care institutions. Addressing the letter to the president or administrator of an identified business can sometimes help "open the door" more quickly for your company than general newspaper advertising. Dietary consulting is a specialized yet varied business, so advertising dollars need to be spent wisely.

In addition to investing in printed materials and advertising, it is important to establish yourself as a business owner and entrepreneur within the community. Become involved in civic organizations outside the dietetic/foodservice profession. Through these organizations, one can establish working relationships with key business leaders and associates that can promote business growth. Whether we believe it or not, the old saying, "It's not what you know, but who you know" is true in the business world.

In completing the marketing plan, consider whether office location will affect the growth of your business. If your business deals primarily with consultant contracts with nursing homes, hospitals, or even corporate wellness programs, the location of the office is not an essential part of the total marketing program. A home-based office may therefore be feasible and more economical. If the focus of your business is with the medical community (physician referrals), it may be advantageous to establish your business within a medical office building complex. The increased accessibility of your services would compensate for the financial expense.

Business Structure

After establishing the purpose and marketing plan of the business, the dietary consultant must determine which legal structure will be right for the business. The three major variables to consider when choosing the legal form of a business are liability, control, and taxes. The legal structures from which to choose for organizing a business are sole proprietorships, partnerships, and corporations. Before choosing a particular structure, one should ask the following questions:

1. Will the entrepreneur (dietitian) be the sole owner? If not, how many other people will have ownership interest? How much control will each owner have? In what manner will the risks and rewards of the business be shared?
2. How important is it for all owners to limit personal liability for debts or claims against the business?
3. Which form of business organization will result in the most advantageous tax treatment for both the business and the individual owner?
4. What legal form will be the simplest and least expensive, both to establish and maintain?
5. What are the buiness's long term plans? (Siegel 1987)

Professional assistance by attorneys and CPAs will be helpful to sort out the conflicting answers that may arise from these questions. Remember the option chosen initially is not forever binding and can be changed if the business needs and conditions change.

The three basic business structures are: sole proprietorship, partnership, and corporation (Kentucky Commerce Cabinet 1986).

1. *Sole proprietorship:* This is the simplest form of business organization. The business has no existence apart from the individual owner. Its liabilities are one's personal liabilities, and one's proprietary interest ends at death. One undertakes the risks of business to the extent of all assets, whether used in the business or personally owned. In some states, filing with the secretary of state or the county clerk under the Fictitious Name Act is not required to form a sole proprietorship, unless the business is under an assumed name. On the federal level, the business owner needs to keep accurate accounting records and file a Schedule C (profit or loss from a business or profession) with Form 1040 by the tax filing deadline. Sole proprietorships must operate on a calendar year, choosing either the cash or accrual method of accounting. From the tax-saving standpoint, it is now more advantageous to operate as a sole proprietor due to the higher corporate tax rates created by the Tax Reform Act of 1986.

2. *Partnership:* This is the relationship existing between two or more persons who join together to carry on a trade or business with each person contributing money, property, labor, or skill and each expecting to share in the profits or losses of the business. Any number of persons may join in a partnership. Each partner is personally liable for all business debts and to a certain extent liable for certain acts of each partner. Each partner can incur debts, sign contracts, and make business obligations.

A limited partnership has one or more general partners who are responsible for managing the business and are liable for the total debts incurred. This type of partnership also includes one or more limited partners who are liable only to the extent of their investment. If two or more persons decide to share profits and losses from a business and each contributes cash, other property, labor, or skill to the business, there is usually a partnership whether or not a formal partnership agreement is made. However, it is recommended that you consult an attorney when drawing up a partnership agreement so that each partner clearly understands what rights and obligations each partner has to the business.

Since partners do not take a salary, each partner must include a statement of the partnership's income, losses, deductions, and/or credits on his or her federal income tax (Form 1040) (Seigel 1987). Partners must pay self-employment taxes as if they were sole proprietors.

3. *Corporation:* This is the most complex form of business structure and, in reality, only a small percentage of American business is formally incorporated (Seigel 1987). Incorporation can be a costly and time-consuming process.

A corporation is an entity by law. A corporation has a life separate from its owners and has its own rights and duties. It is owned by stockholders but not necessarily managed by one. It is organized according to both state and federal statutes. A corporation is liable for its own debts and taxes and is free to distribute or retain its income as it sees fit. Even though incorporation offers a number of income tax advantages, the federal government frowns on incorporation solely for acquiring tax advantages.

A subchapter S corporation can offer entrepreneurs advantages available to both a partnership and corporation. It is basically a small business corporation, the type most dietary consulting businesses form if incorporation is deemed necessary. The advantage is forming this type of corporation is that income is usually taxed in a manner similar to a partnership. The small business corporation usually pays no tax itself, because the earnings are divided among the owners according to each owner's share in the company. Taxes are paid on the individual's share of the corporation's income. Although the formation of a subchapter S corporation may sound enticing, the legal and accounting cost of starting and maintaining it could overshadow some of the tax advantages.

Table 1-1 summarizes the advantages and disadvantages of each structure discussed. In addition to determining the legal structure of a business, one must be aware of licenses or permits needed to operate a business. In order to register a business with the Internal Revenue Service, a form SS-4 should be submitted. This form requests a federal identification number that should be used instead of your social security number when filing taxes and receiving

Table 1-1. Forms of Business Organization

Form of Business Organization	Advantages	Disadvantages
Sole proprietorship	Low start-up costs Greatest freedom from regulation Direct control by owner Minimal working capital requirements Tax advantage to small owner All profits to owner	Unlimited liability Lack of continuity Difficult to raise capital
Partnership	Ease of formation Low start-up costs Additional sources of venture capital Broader management base Possible tax advantage Limited outside regulation	Unlimited liability Lack of continuity Divided authority Difficulty in raising additional capital Difficulty in finding suitable partners
Corporation	Limited liability Specialized management Transferable ownership Continuous existence Legal entity Possible tax advantages Lack of restrictions in raising capital	Extensive outside regulation Expensive organizing Charter restrictions Extensive record keeping Double taxation

Source: Reprinted by permission from U.S. Small Business Administration, *Starting and Managing a Small Business of Your Own,* Washington, D.C.

payment from contractors. Forms can be obtained from your accountant or local IRS office.

In some areas or cities, business permits, sales tax licenses, and other documents may be required. Permit requirement information can be obtained through personnel at city hall or the county courthouse.

Even though the three basic forms of business structures have been defined and the necessity of permits discussed, it is still sound business judgment to seek business and legal advice from an accountant, an attorney, and a banker before deciding on the particular legal structure to form.

An attorney, especially one knowledgeable in the area of incorporation, can provide guidance in developing a business structure advantageous for one's individual business plans. Attorneys, while not inexpensive, can be valuable members of the business team, if you involve them from the initial conception of your business. Attorneys can assist in developing and reviewing contracts and letters of agreement received from potential clients, interpret state and federal regulations related to your business, and assist with obtaining copyrights for materials developed. An attorney can offer advice for determining the most beneficial type of employment structure for your company. Attorney fees range from $50 to $150 per hour or more for specialized work. These fees also apply for phone calls and other services provided on your behalf.

Another valuable member of the business team is the accountant or CPA. This team member can offer assistance in setting up a bookkeeping or records system to suit your needs. If the system is set up correctly and simply, the dietary consultant should be able to perform the bookkeeping functions during the year, needing only income tax assistance. A good accountant should also provide tax advantage information to structure the practice to the best advantage. The hourly fee for an accountant or CPA usually ranges from $30 to $125 per hour. Obtaining an accountant who has experience in business, especially individually owned business, is a sound financial investment.

The business team would not be complete without the involvement of a banker or business planner. Whether you initially need financial assistance or not, establishing a working relationship with a banker knowledgeable in the small business area is important. Investigate the services available from each lending institution prior to establishing a business account. Obtain information pertaining to loan requirements and interest-bearing checking accounts. Inquire whether basic financial counseling and credit analysis is available to all customers. A good relationship with your financial institution can be helpful in obtaining future loans for business expansion.

The Small Business Administration of the U.S. government is another alternative for obtaining financial advice as well as a business loan. The law stipulates, however, that SBA loans can be made only to businesses that are unable to obtain funds from banks or other private sources. This usually occurs when the personal assets of the business owner or the type of business will not qualify for a regular loan, not because the owner is a poor risk. Securing an SBA loan is a competitive and time-consuming task, but can be attractive since the interest rates are usually lower than rates quoted by commercial lending institutions. Even if you are not seeking financial assistance, the SBA can be a valuable resource for writing business plans and clarifying current business laws and regulations.

The Financial Plan

To complete your business plan, one must establish financial goals. The primary goal of any business is profit. Developing a business plan should make one realize starting a business is not for the person seeking a hobby or an avenue for philanthropic work. A business is for profit! Consultant Dietitians in Health Care Facilities (CDHCF 1988) has outlined factors that affect a company's profitability:

Fees: When pricing services, establish income needs and follow the "rule of three": one third salary, one third overhead, and one third profit. Final fee structure, however, is subject to competition, economic conditions, and the amount the market will bear.

Overhead expense: Is rental office space essential to the growth of your business? If not, overhead expenses can be reduced by establishing an in-home office. Home offices are also tax deductible, but be aware of the requirements. Are daily secretarial services required? Some dietary consultants may regard doing their own secretarial work as a savings, but consider the hourly rate for secretarial services versus your own established hourly fee. It seldom pays to do your own typing. Different types of secretarial services are available, including those with complete computer and word processing capabilities that charge by the hour. Other services may require a contracted number of hours. Seeking secretarial assistance through business colleges or vocational schools is another possibility. Is it necessary to purchase your own computer, word processor, and copier? Only if you have mastered the use of computers, would it be advisable to purchase one. Initially, working with a secretarial service that can provide these services may be less expensive. Buying or leasing a copier may be beneficial to the operation of your business. Investigate leasing options prior to purchasing one. Since copiers often require expensive maintenance, a lease that includes a maintenance agreement may prove a better bargain initially.

Employee expenses: Will hiring full-time employees initially help your business or create a financial drain? Subcontracting accounts to qualified individuals may be one way to expand your business initially without substantially decreasing profitability. Recent tax law changes have made hiring workers as contractors rather than employees even more cost effective (Vierling 1989). Dietitians using subcontractors instead of employees can save substantial amounts of money in taxes, insurance, and benefits. The consulting business hiring contractors is not liable for

1. *Social security taxes:* Social security taxes are now assessed at 7.51

percent rate on the first $48,000.00 of income for a possible tax savings of $3,604.80.

2. *Unemployment taxes:* The federal unemployment tax rate is now 6.2 percent on the first $7,000.00 of income for a potential savings of $434.00.

3. *Workmen's compensation:* Using contractors eliminates workmen's compensation premiums, resulting in considerable savings.

4. *Benefit plan payments:* Payments to pension, profit sharing, or health insurance plans are not required for contractors, but would be necessary if workers were employees.

Use of contractors rather than employees can result in a significant cash savings. Reporting requirements are minimal. The total amount paid to each subcontractor in a calendar year is reported on Form 1099 when filing annual federal tax returns. Even though the use of a subcontractor can be more economically feasible for the company, be aware of the guidelines issued by the IRS in Revenue Ruling 87-41 defining the difference between an independent contractor and an employee. These guidelines are summarized below.

- *Instructions:* A worker who must comply with instructions about when, where, and how to work, is ordinarily an employee.
- *Training:* If the worker is required to receive training in order to perform services, an employment relationship is probable.
- *Integration:* Integration of the worker's services into the business operation generally shows that the worker is subject to direction and control and usually considered an employee.
- *Services rendered personally:* If services must be rendered personally, this indicates interest in the methods used as well as the result, and thus an employment relationship.
- *Hiring, supervising, and paying assistants:* If the worker hires, supervises, and pays other assistants pursuant to a contract in which the worker agrees to provide materials and labor, and under which the worker is responsible for the attainment of results, an independent contractor status is indicated.
- *Continuing relationship:* A continuing or recurring nature of work suggests an employment relationship.
- *Set hours of work:* The establishment of set hours of work by the company tends to indicate an employment relationship.
- *Full time required:* An independent contractor has more freedom as to when and for whom he will work than a worker who is required to devote substantially full time to the business.
- *Doing work on business premises:* If the work must be performed on the company's premises, it suggests control by the company and an employment relationship.
- *Order or sequence set:* The more the company controls this factor, the more employment is suggested.
- *Reporting:* The more the worker must report, the greater the control, indicating employment.

- *Payment made by jobs or on a straight commission:* Generally indicates the worker is an independent contractor. Payment made by the hour, week, or month generally points to an employment relationship.
- *Payment of traveling expenses:* An employer generally retains the right to regulate the employee's business activities.
- *Furnishing of tools, equipment, and materials:* Independent contractors more often than not furnish their own tools, equipment, and materials.
- *Significant investment:* Independent contractors more often invest in facilities that are used in performing services.
- *Realization of profit or loss:* A worker who can realize profit or loss from the services is generally an independent contractor.
- *Worker for more than one firm at a time:* An independent contractor will often perform services for more than one firm at a time.
- *Making service available to public:* This factor indicates the status of an independent contractor.
- *Right to discharge:* An independent contractor cannot be fired so long as he produces a result that meets contract specifications.
- *Right to terminate:* If a worker can terminate services without liability, an employment relationship is indicated. (Vierling 1989)

No one factor determines whether a worker is a contractor or an employee. The main point to remember is that the company must be consistent, and treat all individuals who are not employees as independent contractors on all federal tax returns and correspondence. It is also recommended that companies have independent contractors sign agreements stating their position as independent contractors responsible for self-payment of income and social security taxes (Vierling 1989).

Personal insurance and professional expenses: Remember your business is yours! There is no longer an employer to pay insurance premiums, professional dues, or traveling expenses. These are now your responsibility. Despite the cost, insurance is important—particularly health, liability, and disability insurance. Business owners, especially in the dietary consulting area, usually seek health and liability insurance coverage but often forget the importance of disability insurance. Disability insurance plans provide a percentage of income if an extended illness or accident occurs preventing the insured from fulfilling the normal workload. Car and travel expenses need to be included if business requires one to travel extensively to accounts. It is a good idea to include a mileage reimbursement clause in your contracts.

Professional dues and continuing education workshops and seminars are expenses that are necessary to remain competitive and need to be planned for in the annual budget.

Retirement plans: One does not plan to work forever! Goals must be set to enable the consultant to retire when the time comes and be financially secure during retirement.

The above factors are the major expenditures to consider when establishing financial goals. Tools of the dietary consultant's business include more than a briefcase, reference books, calculator, and a resume in hand. Consulting dietetics is a business, an exciting business but much work and planning are necessary to make it profitable.

REFERENCES

Ashmore, M. Catherine, and Pritz, Sandra G. 1982. *Developing the business plan.* Level 2 Research & Development series no. 240 BBS. (PACE). Columbus, Ohio: Ohio State University.

Cashman, J. 1967. Nutritionists, dietitians, and Medicare: An overview of Medicare. *Journal of the American Dietetic Association* (50):17.

Consultant Dietitians in Health Care Facilities. 1981. *The consultant dietitian: How to consult—A guide to success.* Columbus, Ohio: Ross Laboratories.

———. 1988. *How to consult manual.* Columbus, Ohio: Ross Laboratories.

Gilbert, Jayne H. 1984. The effective employment of a consultant dietitian. *Handbook for health care food service management.* Rockville, Md.: Aspen Publishing.

Helm, Kathy K. 1987. *The entrepreneurial nutritionist.* New York: Harper & Row.

Job market shines for dietitians. 1989. *Food Service Director* 2, no. 2 (February).

Kentucky Commerce Cabinet. 1986. *Small business development guide.* Frankfort.

Rose, James, 1987. *Hospital Food & Nutrition Focus.* 4, nos. 9, 11.

Seigel, Eric S. 1987. *The Arthur Young business plan guide.* New York: John Wiley & Sons.

U.S. Department of Health, Education and Welfare, Office of Nursing Home Affairs. 1975. *Long term care improvement study.* Publication no. (05)76-50021.

Vierling, A. Sue. 1989. Contract labor or employees—What's the difference? *Kentucky Business Advisor.* Kentucky Society of CPAs. Louisville, Kentucky.

Vogel, Gerry, and Nancy Doleysh. 1988. *Entrepreneuring: A nurse's guide to starting a business.* New York: National League of Nursing.

Welch, P., E. Oelrich, J. Endies, and Siu-wan Poor. 1988. Consulting dietitians in nursing homes: Time in role functions and perceived problems. *Journal of the American Dietetic Association* 88, no. 1:29–34.

2

Standards of Practice for the Dietary Consultant

What is a standard of practice? What does it mean to us as professionals? How can we bring this term to a level that is understandable and usable in our own practice? Reviewing definitions, historical background, intended applications and use of standards will help answer these questions.

A standard is "an agreed upon level of excellence" (ANA 1975, 30). Webster's New Collegiate Dictionary (1981) defines it as "something established by authority, custom, or general consent as a model or example." These definitions point out two important aspects of a standard. First, a standard is established by an authority. Second, it has to do with excellence.

Every professional needs a set of standards for the practice of that profession. In these days of accountability, liability, and legislation, standards of practice serve not only as a set of values, but also as guides or references by which the dietetic practitioner can evaluate his or her practice. The end result of written standards of practice is to upgrade the profession by clarifying what is expected of the practitioner and perhaps defining the profession as a whole. Standards are the basis for accountability as a professional group to the client. They delineate what dietitians can do for their clients and define their unique contributions. As a result, dietitians can achieve a degree of excellence that insures their role in health care today.

AMERICAN DIETETIC ASSOCIATION PRACTICE STANDARDS

The American Dietetic Association took a giant step forward in 1986 when it published six generic practice standards. These standards evolved over a four-year period from much hard work by the Quality Assurance Committee of the American Dietetic Association (ADA). The following general standards of practice are official statements made by the profession regarding the kind of practice expected of a dietitian (ADA 1986).

1. The dietetic practitioner establishes performance criteria, compares actual performance with expected performance, documents results, and takes appropriate action.

2. The dietetic practitioner develops, implements, and evaluates an individual plan for practice based on assessment of consumer needs, current knowledge, and clinical experience.
3. The dietetic practitioner, utilizing unique knowledge of nutrition, collaborates with other professionals, personnel, and/or consumers in integrating, interpreting, and communicating nutrition care principles.
4. The dietetic practitioner engages in life-long self-development to improve knowledge and skills.
5. The dietetic practitioner generates, interprets, and uses research to enhance dietetic practice.
6. The dietetic practitioner identifies, monitors, analyzes, and justifies the use of resources.

Implementing the Standards of Practice requires a monitoring of each individual's current practice. Each dietitian is accountable for the patient care services he or she provides and therefore must have a systematic mechanism for achieving acceptable standards of care. An organized plan of practice is the most efficient means of accomplishing this complex task.

Guidelines for Implementing Standards of Practice

In the spring 1989 issue of *The Consultant Dietitian,* the Quality Assurance Committee of the Consultant Dietitians in Health Care Facilities (CD-HCF) practice group of ADA published the following criteria based on the ADA Standards of Practice.[1]

STANDARD 1. The dietetic practitioner establishes performance criteria, compares actual performance with expected performance, documents results, and takes appropriate action.

Sample Outcome Criteria	*Suggested Documentation*
1.1 Studies show that the administrative/professional staff feel the CD is functioning according to his/her performance criteria.	1.1 The CD annually prepares a written document listing his/her plan of work, methods of accomplishment and the desired date of completion.
1.2 Consultation reports are acknowledged by the administration and dietary manager. Follow-up is evident by time lines and completion dates met on recommendations.	1.2 CD reports are available and acknowledged by administrator and dietary manager.
1.3 The Dietetics Department complies with all applicable state and federal regulations.	1.3 Copies of recent surveys indicate compliance with regulations. Problem areas are noted and actions initiated by the CD to correct.

[1] These guidelines have been reviewed by The Council on Practice Quality Assurance Committee and must be field tested before they are considered valid. The guidelines are therefore a draft.

1.4 The facility's Dietetics Department uses forms in the efficient operation of the department.

1.4 The CD periodically evaluates food service forms as completed by the dietary manager including employee evaluation, food cost records, temperature records, etc.

1.5 Food quality is evident by measurements conducted in the food service department.

1.5 The CD observes the meal as prepared and served, monitors temperatures, tastes the food and makes comments in the monthly report regarding the quality of the meal.

STANDARD 2. The dietetic practitioner develops, implements, and evaluates an individual plan for practice based on assessment of consumer needs, current knowledge, and clinical experience.

Sample Criteria

Suggested Documentation

2.1 A contract between the CD and the facility specifies a plan for services.

2.1 CD contract specifies responsibilities of the CD and of the Facility.

2.2 A nutritional assessment is completed for every resident.

2.2 Facility dietetics department policy and procedure manual details system, and patient care adults determine the system has been implemented.

2.3 The menus are coordinated, implemented and evaluated.

2.3 Menus prepared and evaluated for nutritional adequacy, resident acceptance, therapeutic diets and costs. The CD will provide analysis of menus for nutritional adequacy.

2.4 Products/services are coordinated and evaluated.

2.4 Evidence in CD reports or other documentation that the CD evaluates the meal delivery system, current products/services used and products considered for purchase.

2.5 A system for environmental sanitation is developed, implemented and evaluated.

2.5 Written reports of periodic sanitation and maintenance reports are prepared or evaluated by the CD as per the facility dietetics department policy and procedure manual.

STANDARD 3. The dietetics practitioner, utilizing unique knowledge of nutrition, collaborates with other professionals, personnel, and/or consumers, in [integrating,] interpreting, and [communicating] nutrition care principles.

Sample Criteria

Suggested Documentation

3.1 Resident is evaluated for physical condition and food acceptance.

3.1 Resident visits are recorded in the weekly/monthly report.

3.2 Nutritional care is evaluated and documented in the residents' medical record.

3.2 The CD makes pertinent notations in residents' charts at regular intervals. Documentation of conferences with appropriate staff concerning nutrional problems appears in monthly report.

3.3 Inter/intra departmental communications are developed, coordinated and monitored.

3.3 Facility dietetics department policy and procedure manual details the method of communication within and outside of the dietary department.

3.4 The facility's dietetics operations manual is developed, implemented and reviewed annually.

3.4 Facility dietetics department policy and procedure manual states by whom the manual was prepared and details schedule for review and revision. Manual will contain the organization chart, job descriptions, work schedules, department policies, samples of forms used and other information as deemed necessary.

3.5 Nutrition resources are available to resident/family, dietary staff, facility staff and administration.

3.5 Nutrition counseling sessions and recommendations for appropriate activities are documented in the monthly report.

3.6 Unique knowledge of nutrition principles [is] demonstrated by on-going community service projects.

3.6 The CD will be available for participation in the local chapter of such organizations as American Heart Association, American Diabetes Association, and American Red Cross.

3.7 Facility/staff education and dietetics department in-service education are developed, implemented and evaluated.

3.7 Facility dietetics department policy and procedure manual details the facility's plan for education of the dietetics staff and the facility staff and there are documented reports of staff education dietetic department in-services given.

STANDARD 4. The dietetic practitioner engages in life-long self-development to improve knowledge and skills.

Sample Criteria

Suggested Documentation

4.1 Standards for membership are met in professional organizations.

4.1 Provides evidence of membership in the American Dietetic Association and CD-HCF Dietetic Practice Group. Provides evidence of maintaining status as a Registered Dietitian.

4.2 Practice is enhanced by improving competency and learning related skills.

4.2 The CD meets continuing education requirements as established by the Commission on Dietetic Registration of the American Dietetic Association, attends workshops, professional meetings, seminars, and college classes on dietetic as well as related skills (e.g. writing, speaking, computers, media, time management, etc.).

4.3 Self-assessment to identify professional strengths and weaknesses is conducted.

4.3 The CD has a written specific plan for professional development, including completion dates.

4.4 A personal development style is adopted to enhance his/her professional image.
4.5 High standards of ethics are adhered to both personally and professionally.

4.4 The CD will, as much as possible, adopt a regular exercise program, and consume an adequate diet.
4.5 The CD will personally compare his/her professional conduct with the Code of Ethics for Profession of Dietetics.

STANDARD 5. The dietetic practitioner generates, interprets, and uses research to enhance dietetic practice.

Sample Criteria

5.1 Daily practice standards reflect current nutrition and management research and implement results.

5.2 Resident oriented research will be initiated and evaluated.

5.3 New products and current trends will be evaluated and implemented.

Suggested Documentation

5.1 Reference material on nutrition, food systems management and equipment will be on file. Evaluation of menus, meal service systems, and nutritional assessments will justify implementation of research.

5.2 CD will initiate and evaluate research of the nutritional status of residents. Surveys reflecting resident acceptance of programs will be on file.

5.3 Information on new items and trends will be on file. Any surveys/questionnaires justifying the implementation of these items and results (i.e. increased efficiency) will be available.

STANDARD 6. The dietetic practitioner identifies, monitors, analyzes, and justifies the use of resources.

Sample Criteria

6.1 Tangible resources in the operation of the department are identified and justified.

6.2 Current management practices of the facility are analyzed.
6.3 Department costs are monitored and evaluated.

Suggested Documentation

6.1 Diet manuals and Policy and Procedure Manuals will be on file and in use. Documentation of recommendations will be in CD report.

6.2 CD reports will document management studies conducted.
6.3 CD reports may include average care costs from the long term care industry and recommend plans of action to control departmental cost.

STANDARDS OF PRACTICE QUESTIONNAIRE

Another tool to assist the consultant dietitian in writing a plan of practice is the following list of questions consultant dietitians need to ask themselves, published by the Quality Assurance Committee (CD-HCF 1988).

212124

1. Do you annually prepare a written document listing your plan of work at each facility, the methods of accomplishment and the desired date of completion?
2. Do you provide a written consultation report after each visit to the client which evaluates actual current performance of the facility's dietary department and suggests actions to improve performance as necessary?
3. Do you have copies and are knowledgeable of all city, county, state and federal legislation and regulations regarding your client?
4. Do you have copies of or have read recent surveys and noted items of noncompliance regarding your clients?
5. Do you provide forms or help develop forms to be used in the operation of the facility food service department?
6. Do you observe meal preparation and service and document comments in your written reports?
7. Do you monitor temperatures and taste the food and document comments in your written reports?
8. Does your contract with each facility specify your responsibilities and those of the facility?
9. Have you developed and do you implement a system for nutritional assessment of residents?
10. Is the nutritional assessment procedure explained in the policy and procedure manual?
11. Are the menus prepared and evaluated for patient acceptance, therapeutic diets and cost?
12. Have you provided an analysis of at least three days' menus for nutritional adequacy?
13. Do your written reports include regular documentation of your evaluation of the meal delivery system, current products/services used and products considered for purchase?
14. Do you include in your written reports regular evaluation of the sanitation and maintenance procedures of the facility?
15. Does your written report include records of patient visits, observations of their physical condition and evaluations of their food acceptance?
16. Do you make pertinent notations in patient charts at regular intervals?
17. Do you document in the patient's charts conferences with appropriate staff concerning nutritional problems of the patients?
18. Do you assist each facility in the development, implementation and annual review of the Policy and Procedure Manual for that facility's dietary department?
19. Do you document in your written reports your counseling sessions and recommendations for appropriate activities regarding facility staff, patients, their families and the dietary staff?
20. Do you participate in local community service projects where your expertise is used?
21. Do you document in your written report staff education and dietary department in-services given?

22. Are you an active member of your professional associations and practice groups?
23. Do you maintain your RD status and LD status if appropriate?
24. Do you regularly attend workshops, meetings, seminars, and/or college classes to improve competency in your practice or to improve your skills in related areas such as writing, speaking, computers, media, time management, etc.?
25. Do you have a written specific plan for professional development, including completion dates?
26. Have you adopted a personal development style which includes a regular exercise program, consumption of an adequate diet and on-the-job dress that will enhance your professional appearance?
27. Have you compared and evaluated your personal conduct standards of ethics with the Standards of Professional Responsibilities of the American Dietetic Association?
28. Do you have available and are you using current reference materials?
29. Do you initiate and evaluate research of the nutritional status of the clients?
30. Is there documented evidence of patient acceptance of nutrition programs in the facility?
31. Do you evaluate and facilitate the implementation of new products and trends in nutrition care?
32. Do you have a current, approved Diet Manual?
33. Do you analyze current management practices of the facility and document your findings?
34. Do your reports include average care costs from the long term care industry and recommend plans of action to control departmental costs?

For each question answered *"no,"* list your plan for change and dates for completion and for revaluation. You may find the format shown in Figure 2-1 helpful.

You may find help in addressing these questions in the newly revised (1988) *How to Consult* manual published by the Consultant Dietitians in Health Care Facilities, practice group of the American Dietetic Association.

How do you measure up? You may not want to confront some of these questions. Unless someone is monitoring you, it takes motivation to carry through a plan for change, but the results are rewarding. How can you accomplish objectives without knowing what you want? This personal quality assurance program provides guidelines for setting personal goals. Increased pride and self-confidence in the job setting will be the result.

AMERICAN DIETETIC ASSOCIATION CODE OF ETHICS

While the ADA Standards of Practice provide a means to evaluate the practice, the code of ethics of the American Dietetic Association provides a set of moral rules of conduct. Specifically, the code of ethics defines ethical behavior for the

Question Answered "No"	Plan for Change	Completion Date	Reevaluation Date
	Example		
#1: Do you annually prepare a written document listing your plan of work at each facility, the method of accomplishment and the desired date of completion?	Will develop annual plan of work with input from the dietary manager and administrator.	Dec. 31	6 months

Figure 2-1. Format to use with the standards of practice questionnaire.

dietitian. This code is included below as an additional checklist to gauge performance.

Rules of Professional Conduct and Ethics

1. Responsibility to the Profession and the Association
   - To serve the common good without regard for personal advantage.
   - To continue to read, study, and apply the principles of nutrition in the service of humanity.
   - To be enthusiastic about the profession and to give full loyalty and support to its ideas.
   - To deport myself in accordance with the principles and goals of the profession.
   - To refuse personal identification or tacit approval in commercial advertising or promotion except under certain conditions indicated by Association policy.
   - To promote good nutrition, but never to prescribe dietary treatment except under direction of a physician.
2. Responsibility to Employer or Organization
   - To serve loyally the organization by whom employed.
   - To strive to fulfill the objectives of the organization, cooperating fully with all associates and other departments.
   - To refuse compensation or gifts, directly or indirectly from suppliers or others dealing with employer or organization by whom employed.
   - To use personal talents, time, and efforts for those tasks which cannot be assigned to others, delegating responsibility where it can be assumed.

- To maintain free communication with employer, employees and associates.
- To respond positively to opportunities to accept greater responsibility.
3. Responsibility to Related Professional Groups
    - To understand the aims and ideals of related professions.
    - To cooperate with related professional groups in working toward common goals.
4. Responsibility to the Community
    - To try to protect the public against fraud, misrepresentation, misinformation or unethical practices in matters concerned with food, nutrition and diet therapy.
    - To use specialized knowledge in service to the community and to assist other professions in meeting health needs everywhere.
    - To be interested in the welfare of the people of the community and participate in community activities.
    - To recognize and perform the duties of citizenship.
5. Responsibility for Personal Ethics
    - To observe the Golden Rule.
    - To practice good nutrition and be a worthy person.
    - To hold in confidence all personal information acquired in the performance of professional duties.
    - To be frank in acknowledgment of errors, omissions, and limitations of knowledge.
    - To be honest, and honorable in word, thought and deed.

AMERICAN DIETETIC ASSOCIATION STANDARDS OF PROFESSIONAL RESPONSIBILITY

Similar to the rules of conduct are the following Standards of Professional Responsibility (ADA 1982).

1. The American Dietetic Association member provides professional service with objectivity and with respect for the unique values of individuals.
    - The member avoids discrimination on the basis of factors that are irrelevant to the provision of professional services, including, but not limited to, race, creed, sex, and age.
    - The member provides sufficient information to enable clients to make their own informed decisions.
2. The American Dietetic Association member accurately presents professional qualifications and credentials.
    - The member uses "R.D." or "registered dietitian" only when registration is current and authorized by the Commission on Dietetic Registration.
    - The member permits use of his/her name for the purpose of certifying

that dietetic services have been rendered only if he/she has provided or supervised the provision of those services.

3. The American Dietetic Association member remains free of conflict of interest while fulfilling the objectives and maintaining the integrity of the dietetic profession.

   - The member advances and promotes the profession while maintaining professional judgment, honesty, integrity, loyalty, and trust to colleagues, clients, and the public.
   - The member promotes or endorses products only in a manner that is neither false nor misleading.

4. The American Dietetic Association member assumes responsibility and accountability for personal competence in practice.

   - The member maintains knowledge and skills required for continuing professional competence.
   - The member recognizes the limits of his/her qualifications and seeks counsel or makes referrals as appropriate.
   - The member adheres to accepted standards for his/her area of practice.

5. The American Dietetic Association member complies with all applicable laws and regulations concerning the profession, but seeks to change them if they are inconsistent with the best interests of the public and the profession.

6. The American Dietetic Association member presents substantiated information and interprets controversial information without personal bias, recognizing that legitimate differences of opinion exist.

7. The American Dietetic Association member maintains the confidentiality of information.

8. The American Dietetic Association member conducts him/herself with honesty, integrity, and fairness.

   - The member makes and fulfills professional commitments in good faith.
   - The member who wishes to inform the public and colleagues of his/her services does so by using factual information. The member does not advertise in a misleading manner.
   - The member makes all reasonable effort to avoid bias in any kind of professional evaluation.
   - The member provides objective evaluation of candidates for professional association memberships, awards, scholarships, or job advancements.

9. The American Dietetic Association member accepts the obligation to protect society and the profession by upholding the Standards of Professional Responsibility and by reporting alleged violations of the Standards through the defined review process of The American Dietetic Association.

REFERENCES

American Dietetic Association (ADA). 1982. *Standards of professional responsibility.* Chicago, Ill.: American Dietetic Association.

————. 1986. *Standards of practice*. Chicago, Ill.: American Dietetic Association.

American Nurses' Association (ANA). 1975. *A plan for implementation of the standards of nursing practice*. Kansas City, Mo.: American Nurses' Association.

Consultant Dietitians in Health Care Facilities (CD-HCF). 1988. *How to consult manual*. Columbus, Ohio: Ross Laboratories.

————. 1989. Quality assurance guidelines criteria for consultant dietitians in health care facilities. *The Consultant Dietitian* (Spring): 21–24.

Webster's new collegiate dictionary. 1981. Springfield, Mass.: G. & C. Merriam Co.

3

Facility Needs Assessment

Once an account is obtained it is important to make an accurate assessment of the status and needs of the dietary department and related areas of concern. This assessment, if done correctly, can be a marketing tool for the consultant as well as an opportunity to prove one's expertise and cost effective skills.

The dietary department is a multi-faceted operation with many interrelated areas. The consultant must divide the department into service categories and assess each area thoroughly. These areas can be divided as follows: preassessment reviews, physical plant, food preparation, therapeutic diets and tray service, staffing, sanitation and infection control, administrative records, and clinical records. Each area will be discussed individually and checklist questions covering all areas will be provided for quick and thorough assessment.

PREASSESSMENT REVIEW

Before beginning the assessment process, review two records—recent survey reports from the local health department and state and federal licensure survey reports.

The local health department survey report should reveal any recent sanitation problems or violations. The manager should have made notations on the back of the form concerning each violation, noting both when it was corrected and how. If problems have been identified, pay special attention to these areas to determine if corrections have been followed through.

The state and federal licensure survey report should reveal any areas in the department, or related to the department, which have been cited for deficiencies. It is important that the dietary department be in compliance with all state and federal regulations at all times. If the dietary department of a facility incurs violations year after year, the consultant should question the integrity of both the dietary manager and the administrator. Do not accept an account if it appears you are being hired in name only. Your reputation as a competent consultant can be affected by the survey results received by each of your facilities. It is best to establish in the beginning whether a consultant's recommendations are likely to be followed and to forgo those accounts not concerned with quality or with correction of any problems identified by surveying agencies.

PHYSICAL PLANT

Although there is often little that can be done to the physical plant of a facility, it is still necessary to study it with several things in mind.

First, is there adequate equipment for the size of the facility and the type of menu in use? If so, is the equipment arranged in the best, most efficient way? Look at the department with an open mind and ask whether the current arrangement works well or whether, by rearranging a few items, the department could be made more efficient. Observe the preparation and service of a meal to determine how employees use each area in the kitchen and to evaluate work flow.

Also check current storage areas to assess adequacy of space and ventilation. Check thermometers in these areas.

Note each piece of equipment. Is it in good repair? Are dietary employees using each piece correctly and in a manner that makes the best use of all equipment? Sometimes employees will not use a particular piece of equipment because it is new and they do not have a good understanding of the operation. A good inservice by the manufacturer can correct this.

SANITATION AND INFECTION CONTROL

Sanitation is the cornerstone of a good dietary department and its importance cannot be overemphasized. Health care facilities have a particular interest in the area since many residents are already debilitated and may suffer irreparable harm from poor food-handling techniques or unsanitary conditions.

To evaluate sanitation properly, it is necessary to be familiar with the state foodservice code. Copies of this are usually available from the local health department and should be reviewed thoroughly. Obtain one for the dietary manager as well. This code will provide specific information about all areas of the foodservice department. Since specifications vary somewhat from state to state, more general areas will be discussed in this section.

When reviewing sanitation, observe dietary employees for proper hand-washing techniques. You may even quiz one or two to determine the level of knowledge in this area. Check for proper food-handling techniques—the use of tongs, gloves, and so forth. Employees should not eat, smoke, or chew gum in the department and should have clean uniforms, proper shoes, and hairnets. In addition, they should not wear nail polish or elaborate jewelry. Aprons should be cleaned daily or should be disposable. Dietary employees should have yearly TB tests or chest X-rays to rule out tuberculosis infection.

In the dishroom, clean and soiled areas should be separate to prevent contamination of clean dishes. Hand-washed items should always be washed, rinsed, and sanitized. Check the dishmachine for proper temperatures—150°F for the wash cycle and 180°F for the rinse cycle—and verify the use of a sanitizing agent for hand-washed items and food contact surfaces. Low temperature dishmachines should reach at least 120°F and should be used with a sanitizing agent.

Check refrigerators and freezers for proper temperatures: 32°F or lower for freezers and 38°F for refrigerators. Employees should ideally check and record these temperatures twice daily, once early in the morning and again before the department is closed for the evening. This double check assures that any fluctuation in temperatures would be noticed quickly. All items in these units should be labeled and dated to allow use of older items first. Leftovers should be checked daily and any items too old for safe use should be discarded.

If roaches or signs of rodents are observed, verify the presence of a pest control program.

Mopheads, dishrags, and potholders should be washed frequently and stored in a covered container to await cleaning. It is not acceptable simply to soak these items in bleach in lieu of washing them.

A cleaning schedule should be posted, with evidence available that it is being followed. Employees should have training in proper cleaning procedures for each piece of equipment as well as the floor and walls. Cleaning procedures should be available, written and specific, for all areas of the department. In general the dietary department and related areas should give the overall appearance of being clean, neat, and organized.

FOOD PREPARATION

During the initial observation, food preparation skills should be observed.

Check the menu for the day of observation. The cook should be following the menu exactly or have an acceptable reason for making a substitution. The person in charge of meal preparation should be familiar with the menus and capable of discussing appropriate substitutes for therapeutic diets listed on the menu.

Any menu substitutions should be recorded, dated, and filed to provide an accurate record of meals served. Review this record, if available, to evaluate adherence to the menu and the cooks' ability to determine appropriate substitutions. Cooks should be able to choose substitutions that are nutritionally equivalent to the food being replaced.

At the end of the meal note the amount of food left over. Leftovers should be minimal. If a significant amount of food is left, however, evaluate how it is handled. Is it to be reused or discarded? If it is to be reused, is it removed from the steamtable as quickly as possible, labeled, dated, and chilled quickly to an appropriate temperature?

A file or collection of standardized recipes should be available and should be calculated for common amounts necessary for the size of the facility. In a 75-bed facility a recipe that yields 20 servings may be difficult to use. A poor quality product may result or the recipe may be ignored for one the cook prefers. To achieve consistent quality in foodservice, recipes standardized for amounts commonly needed are a must.

Note the ingredients used. All ingredients should be of good quality and obtained from approved sources, particularly meats. Food should be appropriately seasoned unless a particular seasoning is restricted by a physician's order. Because making one large batch of food for everyone is easier than making several smaller batches with seasoning variations, many cooks will try to eliminate seasoning altogether. This approach often results in bland, unappetizing food that is not well accepted by residents.

Food should be prepared as close to serving time as possible. If prepared too early, many foods break down and become mushy and colorless or dry and tough. Nutrients are lost. French fries prepared at 9:30 for lunch at 12:00 will not retain a quality appearance or taste for that extended period of time. Few foods will.

After food has been prepared it should be held on the steamtable at an appropriate temperature of 140°F or above. The cook should check the temperature at each meal. Recording temperatures can increase the likelihood of regular checks. Temperatures of cold foods should be monitored as well. Foods served chilled should be 45°F or below.

During service of the meal good food-handling and portioning techniques should be evidenced. Tongs and gloves should be used to avoid touching food with bare hands. Proper portioning utensils should be used as specified on the menu or by the manager. Scoops and dippers yield consistent portions. Meat should be sliced on a commercial slicer and slices should be weighed periodically to verify standardized portions.

All equipment should be used efficiently with no one piece overloaded. For instance, if a steamer is available, vegetables should be prepared in it rather than on the range so there will be variety in preparation and all equipment will be used effectively.

If employee meals are served, check whether dietary employees follow established facility procedures (such as using meal tickets, and not taking partial meals or making substitutions). Do dietary employees adhere to these procedures or are they "just eating this piece of chicken because it is going to be thrown away"? If this practice is tolerated, cooks may unconsciously prepare more food than is necessary in order to have some left to eat. How this situation is handled, however, depends on the policy of the administration. The consultant can only inform the administrator that it is happening and describe the possible financial impact.

If a snack program is in place, note preparation of the snacks. Are standardized recipes used? Are snacks prepared in appropriate amounts and labeled, if necessary, for special diets?

THERAPEUTIC DIETS

It is an important part of the dietary consultant's job to evaluate preparation and service of therapeutic diets.

Diet orders should be obtained from the physician at the time of admission and recorded in the physician's orders section of the chart. The order should be clearly written and easy to understand. For instance, instead of "gallbladder diet," the order should state "low fat"; instead of "salt free," "3 g sodium." The consultant should work with the physician and with the nursing department to clarify and standardize diet orders as much as possible. During the needs assessment phase, problems in this area should be identified.

All diets should be on the menu. There may be an exception made in a situation where the facility has only one patient on the diet. In this case a written description of the diet and necessary restrictions should be posted in the dietary department for easy referral. Diets should be prepared according to instructions on the menu or according to posted instructions.

The consultant should observe preparation techniques of therapeutic diets and verify correct service by spot-checking trays for accuracy according to menu directions.

Dietary personnel should appear knowledgeable concerning dietary principles for therapeutic diets as evidenced by correct preparation of the food, correct condiments on the tray, and accurate service.

Tray cards should match the physician's diet order from the chart and should be clearly written and easily understood.

TRAY SERVICE

Observe trays for correct food items, condiments, and flatware. The food should be attractively and neatly served. One food item should not run into the other, nor should bread be placed on top of food causing bread to become soggy and unpalatable.

Food preferences and dislikes should be noted on the diet cards and dietary employees should substitute for items listed as dislikes.

Check temperatures of some food items at the point of service and record. The facility should have developed standards for temperatures of both hot and cold foods at point of service. Evaluate the temperature range by these standards.

Trays should be filled as efficiently as possible, using the ratio of four trays per minute as a guideline. Trays should be delivered as quickly as possible and not allowed to remain on food carts for long periods of time. This can be a problem for trays going to residents. Temperatures taken from items on these trays will be helpful in defining what time frame is too long. The facility may also have a policy developed to define what the time frame should be. For instance, a policy might read, "All trays will be passed within 20 minutes of leaving the dietary department." If the facility has such a policy, evaluate the service by these standards.

Residents should appear ready to receive the meal. Servers should assist residents as necessary, cutting meat, opening cartons, and so on. Patients who eat in bed should appear to be comfortable. Bedside trays should be properly positioned—not too high or too far away.

Interview residents about the quality of the meals and meal service. Note the amount of food returned to the kitchen to determine the level of acceptance of the meal.

If snacks are served, evaluate how quickly they are passed and whether they are delivered to the appropriate residents. Observe whether part of the snacks are consumed by employees. What types of controls are in place for the snack and nourishment system? Snacks and supplements can be a substantial part of total food cost and should be carefully controlled.

ADMINISTRATIVE RECORDS

Administrative records will vary facility by facility. The following records are generally standard and in use in most facilities:

Monthly Consultant Reports

Most facilities require at least a monthly report by the consultant dietitian. The reports should contain information concerning work done during the month and recommendations for improvements. Reports should provide insight into previous problems in the department and how they were resolved as well as evidence that the facility is aware of certain problems or working toward established goals. Through the monthly report, the dietary consultant documents his or her visits to the facility and input to each department.

Policies and Procedures

Dietary policies and procedures should provide an up-to-date record of policies established by the department and how they are implemented. The dietary departments should be operating as specified in this manual or the manual should be revised. The policy and procedure manual is an excellent orientation tool for new employees as well as an excellent reference for long-term employees. It should be clearly and simply written and be readily available to dietary employees. All major aspects of the department operation should be covered.

Inservice Records

A record of all inservices available to the department should be available. Since inservice requirements may vary, it is important to be familiar with requirements in your area. Inservice topics should include subjects important to the department such as therapeutic diets and sanitation as well as any required by surveying agencies.

Food Cost Records

It is extremely important that the dietary manager keep records of food purchased, number of meals served, and monthly inventory so that food cost per patient per day can be calculated. This figure provides feedback to the manager for evaluating compliance with the budget as designated by the administrator. It also allows the manager to project expenses and thus have input in the budget planning process. Monthly food cost records are a check on employee preparation and service practices and will reflect the presence or absence of good control in these areas.

Work Schedules

The work schedule for all dietary employees should be posted. Hours scheduled need to be adequate to produce the menu as written and to maintain proper sanitary conditions. Further information on evaluation of staffing patterns is addressed in Chapter 4.

CLINICAL RECORDS

Clinical records required will vary by level of care and state and federal requirements. During the needs assessment process, evaluate whether the facility keeps appropriate clinical records. Some of the more common records required by intermediate and skilled care facilities are discussed below.

In intermediate and skilled care facilities the dietary consultant should do an initial nutrition assessment on all new admissions as soon after admission as possible. The assessment form should contain appropriate information on weight, eating habits, diagnosis, diet therapy, lab data, medications, physical condition, and so on. It is necessary to be familiar with state and federal requirements in this area. An example of a nutrition assessment form is provided in Appendix A.

Progress notes may be made by the dietitian, in some states, or by the dietary manager. Both regulation and the amount of dietary consulting time allotted will be a factor in deciding who is responsible for this documentation. Progress notes should reflect the patient's current nutrition status and should assess the patient's response to goals and approaches established by the dietitian in the assessment or by the interdisciplinary care plan committee.

The interdisciplinary care plan should reflect awareness of nutritional problems and needs and should provide an integrated approach by all disciplines toward resolution of these problems.

A method should be established to monitor accuracy of diet orders transmitted to the dietary department. A periodic random check may be made by the dietary manager or a monthly list compiled by the person in charge of medical records listing each patient and the current diet order as specified in the physician's orders. The manager can then use this list to check diet cards for accuracy. Diet cards should match the physician's most recent diet order.

There should be a system in place for the consultant to make recommendations to the medical staff by direct phone call, a written note on the chart, or by using the charge nurse as an intermediary. This system will vary by facility and will be determined in fact by the physician's wishes.

The weight of each patient should be monitored at least monthly and more frequently if necessary. Both nursing and dietary should show evidence through progress notes and monthly summaries that weights are being monitored and any significant deviations in weight noted.

Intake should be observed and recorded on all patients whose condition requires it. This may include patients with a history of poor intake, diabetic patients, or patients with a history of weight loss.

Assessments for patients fed by tube should be more detailed and include the dietitian's evaluation of the current regimen, including total calories, protein, and fluid received and any recommendations for change in these areas.

The facility diet manual should be current—not more than five years old— and relevant to diets served by the facility. Dietary employees should demonstrate familiarity with the manual.

Evaluation of the preceding factors will give a good overview of the status of the department and any areas in need of attention. The consultant should take the time to do a thorough assessment and use the subsequent report to market his or her professional expertise. Make sure the report is well organized, clearly written, and accurate. It is important to turn in professional looking reports— typed if possible—that reflect the image you wish to project.

NEEDS ASSESSMENT CHECKLIST

The following list of questions can serve as a guideline for the needs assessment process.

Physical Plant

1. Is equipment adequate for menus and facility size?
2. Is the department layout efficient?
3. Are storage areas adequate and properly ventilated?
4. Is equipment clean and in good repair?

Sanitation

1. Do employees exhibit correct food-handling techniques?
2. Is the dishroom separated into clean and soiled areas?
3. Are dishmachine temperatures appropriate and monitored?
4. Are freezer and cooler temperatures appropriate and monitored?
5. Is a pest control program in place and effective?
6. Are items in the cooler and freezer labeled and dated?
7. Are mops, dishrags, and potholders cleaned regularly?
8. Is a cleaning schedule posted and followed?
9. Are employees taught proper cleaning procedures?
10. Are employees appropriately dressed?

Food Preparation

1. Are menus followed?
2. Are standardized recipes in use?
3. Is food fresh and obtained from approved sources?
4. Is food appropriately seasoned?
5. Are meals prepared as close to serving time as possible?
6. Are steamtable temperatures appropriate?
7. Are chilled food temperatures appropriate?
8. Are good portioning techniques observed?
9. Are substitutions recorded?
10. Are leftovers kept to a minimum?
11. Are employees' meals served according to company policy?
12. Are snacks prepared according to appropriate procedure?

Therapeutic Diets

1. Do diet cards match physician's orders?
2. Are diet orders specific and clear?
3. Are all diets covered on the menu?
4. Are therapeutic diets prepared and served correctly?
5. Are dietary personnel knowledgeable concerning therapeutic diets?

Tray Service

1. Do trays contain appropriate condiments?
2. Are trays set with appropriate flatware?
3. Is food attractively and neatly served?
4. Are resident food preferences and dislikes observed?
5. Are temperatures correct at the point of service?
6. Are trays passed quickly?
7. Do aides provide appropriate service to residents?
8. Do residents appear ready for the meal?
9. Do residents express satisfaction with the meal service?
10. Are the amounts of food returned to the kitchen not excessive?
11. Are snacks prepared at appropriate times in appropriate amounts?

Administrative Records

1. Are monthly consultant reports present?
2. Are policies and procedures up to date?
3. Are inservices regularly scheduled and appropriate?
4. Are accurate food cost records kept by the dietary manager?
5. Is staffing appropriate for the size of the facility?

Clinical Records

1. Are there assessments on each chart? Are they appropriate?
2. Are progress notes current?
3. Is the dietary input on care plans appropriate?
4. Are monthly weights available on all residents?
5. Are food intake records available on appropriate residents?
6. Are diet cards checked regularly against physician's orders?
7. Does the consultant have a system for making recommendations to medical staff?
8. Do assessments of tube-fed residents appear appropriate?
9. Was the facility diet manual published within last five years?

4

Department Management

STAFFING THE DIETARY DEPARTMENT

Next to food costs, labor costs represent one of the two largest categories of operating expenses and account for 50 to 60 percent of most foodservice budgets. When census falls and budget cuts are necessary, labor is therefore the first area that administrators review. Dietary managers need to consider minimum quality standards for work to be accomplished and incorporate these standards into a staffing guide. Labor costs must be controlled, but not at the expense of quality.

Unfortunately, at this time there are no staffing standards for various kinds of health care facilities, only "rules of thumb." Very often current staffing is based on opinions of employees doing the work or statistics from a previous year, both of which can be unrealistic. How, then, can labor costs be effectively controlled? Before looking at methods of determining staffing needs, consider the number of variables that can affect staffing.

- How competent is the dietary manager?
- Are employees well-trained?
- How complicated is the menu?
- What types of special services are provided?
- Are convenience foods used?
- What is the size of the food preparation area, tray line, and dishwashing area? How conveniently are these areas arranged?
- How many modified diets are served?
- What is the seating capacity of the dining room?
- What is the rate of labor turnover and what is the nature of the local labor market? Is labor plentiful in the area? Are there colleges or schools nearby that would increase the availability of persons interested in part time work?

1. How competent is the dietary manager? The more highly trained and experienced a supervisor is, the better able he or she is to provide accurate forecasts of staffing problems and needs. It is important for the dietary manager to be able to define minimum quality requirements for work to be done and to schedule labor as efficiently as possible. Are written performance standards followed as employees work? Performance standards are an example of criteria-based performance evaluations. They set forth evaluative criteria by which a job duty is measured.

2. Are employees well-trained? Are there written job descriptions that define the duties and responsibilities of a specific job? A well-written job description gives employees a clear understanding of what they are supposed to do, how and when to do it, and what the desired result should be (see "Job descriptions" below). A clear definition of duties helps both employees and the supervisor to work toward the same objective. Effective training is the best tool for increasing productivity. Too often new employees are placed with other untrained employees and subsequently pick up their poor work habits. It is wiser to take the time to train people at the beginning of employment and ensure a job well done, rather than try to undo bad work habits later. Food quality, patient satisfaction, and orientation of the dietary employee are to be discussed in more depth in another section.

3. How complicated is the menu? The nature of a cook's position will depend on the needs of the clients, the complexity of the menu, and the number of items to be prepared. A simple-to-prepare cycle menu can be used to ease the workload on a dietary department. A complex menu can put an unnecessary burden on the cooks. The consulting dietitian should always consider staffing when writing menus.

4. What types of special services are provided? How much catering is done by the facility? Are special birthday and anniversary meals prepared for residents? How much does the recreation department involve dietary in activities? Extra functions may be expected with no increase in labor hours.

5. Are convenience foods used? The cost of convenience items such as frozen entrées may make them prohibitive in many health care settings. There is a tradeoff, however. The amount of production labor required to produce meals in a facility that utilizes an extensive amount of prepared convenience foods will be less than in a facility where all items are prepared "from scratch." For example: A dietary consultant is writing a set of cycle menus and plans to include lasagna in the cycle. The consultant must determine whether it is less expensive to staff enough labor to prepare the lasagna from scatch or to purchase the frozen, ready-to-eat version.

The raw ingredients for 48 servings of lasagna from scratch cost $22.10. Labor at $4.50 per hour for 1.5 hours preparation time contributes an additional $6.75 to the cost. By this method of preparation, the lasagna will cost $0.61 per serving.

On the other hand, four 6-pound trays of frozen lasagna cost $45.50 or $0.71 per serving. In this example the lasagna from scratch is the most economical to serve despite the labor required in preparation.

6. What is the size of the food preparation area, tray line, and dishwashing area? How conveniently are these areas arranged? The size and arrangement of the various areas will affect staffing. If an area such as the dishwashing area is conveniently arranged, labor needs may be reduced. If the areas are very small, as they are in some older kitchens, it may be necessary to limit staffing due to

lack of space. There are some older kitchens in existence where a tray line is impossible due to lack of space and improper arrangement of equipment.

7. What is the seating capacity of the dining room? This would affect staffing needs if, as is sometimes the case, dietary is responsible for passing trays to the dining room area or if dietary were selling meals to the staff and public, such as in a hospital cafeteria. If meals are sold, the number of seats in the dining room will have a bearing on the number of meals that need to be produced and therefore influence staffing.

8. What is the rate of labor turnover and what is the nature of the local labor market? Is labor plentiful in the area? Are there colleges or schools nearby that would increase the availability of persons interested in part-time work? In most foodservice operations there are "peak" periods and "down" periods. Economically, it is usually best to schedule lightly during "down" periods and heaviest during "peak" periods. This is most easily done in areas where part-time labor is plentiful. If this type of labor is not available, it is sometimes necessary to staff heavier than is actually necessary in order to keep staff.

How Many Modified Diets Are Served?

In facilities with a large number of therapeutic diets and limited use of convenience foods, more labor minutes per meal are necessary. Facilities with a relatively stable census and a majority of regular diets can do the job with fewer labor hours.

Determining Staffing Needs

As you can see, the great number of variables makes it difficult to use a standard staffing pattern for all facilities. If the number of variables can be kept to a minimum, it is easier to standardize staffing guidelines. One of the simplest methods to determine accurate staffing is to calculate labor minutes per meal. This system provides a guideline for evaluating understaffing or overstaffing, both of which may adversely affect a foodservice department. If the number of variables previously mentioned is kept to a minimum, the standard of 8–10 minutes per meal has proven to be a simple and workable guideline. The larger the facility the lower the figure should be. For example, an 80–90 bed facility can operate on less than 10 minutes per meal, while a facility with more than 90 beds should staff at less than 9 minutes per meal.

In order to arrive at minutes per meal served, the following formula can be used. This calculation does not include employee meals. The number of kitchen labor hours in one day is multiplied by 60 to determine labor minutes per day. Divide this figure by the number of patient meals served in one day. Consider the example of a 100-bed facility with a census of 90; the facility utilizes 42 dietary labor hours per day, or 2,520 minutes. Patient meals served per day (90 × 3) equal 270; 2,520 minutes per day divided by 270 meals per day equals 9.3 minutes per meal.

For the minutes per meal figure to be most accurate, the current two-week dietary schedule should be used. Many facilities do not have a constant daily number of dietary labor hours. The number may be lower on weekends and peak during the week when there is more activity. Total the dietary labor hours each day for a two-week period, divide this figure by 14, and calculate the minutes per meal based on this average.

The minutes per meal formula is a measurement tool for the administrator and dietary manager to analyze current staffing. It does not indicate how much the staffing hours should be changed, however, if an increase or decrease in census occurs. Because some facilities are set up for long-term care, a census variation of five patients would indicate a trend, and dietary staffing may need to be revaluated and new needs determined. To do this, use the decimal equivalent formula with the standards illustrated below:

$$\frac{\text{Hours actually worked} \times \text{days worked}}{\text{Meals served during the period}} = \text{labor hours per meal}$$

Labor hours per meal $\times$ 60 minutes = labor minutes per meal

EXAMPLE 1

If 10 dietary personnel work 8 hours for 7 days in a 100-bed facility (100% census) serving 3 meals a day for 7 days, the formula would look like this:

$$\frac{10 \text{ dietary personnel} \times 8 \text{ hours} \times 7 \text{ days}}{100 \text{ patients} \times 3 \text{ meals} \times 7 \text{ days}} = 0.27 \text{ labor hours per meal}$$

0.27 labor hours per meal $\times$ 6 minutes = 16.2 labor minutes per meal

EXAMPLE 2

If 8 dietary personnel work 8 hours for 7 days in a 60-bed facility (100 percent census) serving 3 meals a day for 7 days plus 10 employees eating, the formula would look like this;

$$\frac{8 \text{ dietary personnel} \times 8 \text{ hours} \times 7 \text{ days}}{60 \text{ patients} + 10 \text{ employees} \times 3 \text{ meals} \times 7 \text{ days}} = \frac{0.30 \text{ labor hours}}{\text{per meal}}$$

0.30 labor hours per meal $\times$ 60 minutes = 18.3 labor minutes per meal

The dietary manager's hours are included in the stated formulas. This may be misleading when the manager is a full-time supervisor and does not actually work in the kitchen. In light of this, the consultant and dietary manager may need to evaluate whether it is appropriate to include the manager's hours when using a formula such as minutes per meal.

Another method of evaluating staffing is to calculate dietary labor hours per patient per day. Since many other costs, such as food, chemicals, and paper supplies, are calculated in this manner, this method is familiar to and can easily be understood by administrators.

To calculate dietary labor hours per patient per day, take the average number of dietary labor hours per day and divide by the average patient census per day.

EXAMPLE 3

A 100-bed nursing facility with an average daily census of 98 for the month utilizes 40 dietary labor hours per day.

$$\frac{40 \text{ dietary labor hours}}{98 \text{ patients}} = \frac{0.41 \text{ dietary labor hours per patient}}{\text{per day for this monthly period}}$$

WORK SCHEDULES

Although the consultant dietitian is not usually responsible for planning work schedules, it is important to understand basic facts about scheduling in order to be of assistance to the dietary manager if the need arises.

A work schedule designates each employee's name and position and indicates the hours the employee is assigned to work. The schedule should state the times the employee is to start and finish, and days off should be designated (see Fig 4-1). Valuable additional information that can be included on the schedule is total labor hours scheduled per day, per week, or per employee. A good dietary manager should know the exact number of labor hours being utilized by the dietary department for a given period of time. In some companies, labor hours are allotted on a per patient per day ratio and so fluctuate according to patient census.

When developing a work schedule, decisions need to be made concerning when the work week will begin and end, when overtime will be paid, what guidelines will be followed for days off, and which type of schedule to implement.

The Work Week

A work week usually runs from Sunday through Saturday or from Monday through Sunday. The position of the weekend days in the work week will affect scheduling flexibility. By positioning one free Saturday and one free Sunday into different work weeks, the other days off (weekdays) may be assigned individually in each work week. The Monday through Sunday work week positions the free Saturday and Sunday (weekend) into a single work week, thus forcing assignment of the other two days off during one week. This plan drastically reduces scheduling flexibility by creating an extended stretch of consecutive work days that occur before the free weekend; that is, such schedules frequently call for employees to work seven-day stretches without a day off (Rose 1984, 158). Long stretches without a day off frequently result in employee fatigue and low morale. Quantity and quality of work may suffer.

Another scheduling option is a combination of a "week staff" and a "weekend staff." In this instance, the week staff works Monday through Friday while the weekend staff works Saturdays and Sundays.

The primary advantage of this scheduling procedure is that a Monday-through-Friday schedule is very attractive to many employees and may make filling these positions easier.

The first disadvantage is obvious. Since most employees do not like to work weekends—especially *every* weekend, these positions may be difficult to fill. Another disadvantage is the lack of supervision on weekends. If the dietary manager works Monday through Friday, the weekend shifts will not be well supervised, and organization and quality may suffer.

Although neither the consultant dietitian nor the dietary manager usually makes the decision of how the work week will run, it is good to understand how the work week affects the scheduling process.

Overtime

Persons responsible for scheduling need to be knowledgeable about state and federal regulations governing overtime. Federal law mandates that any hours in excess of 40 in a week constitute overtime. For example, in a typical two-week pay period an employee may work 38 hours one week and 42 hours the next. The employer will have to pay 2 hours overtime because the 40-hour limit has been exceeded in the second week. It does not matter that the previous week was under 40 hours. This must be considered in order to avoid scheduling an employee for hours beyond the normal work week and thus incurring the expense of overtime.

The dietitian should work with the manager to ascertain whether the manager's understanding in this area is such that overtime is avoided whenever possible. This is particularly important when the manager is trying to cover a call-in and must decide who is the best choice to cover the position.

Establishing Scheduling Guidelines

Before a schedule can be developed, guidelines must be established in the following areas:

1. Type of scheduling to be done
2. Length of the schedule
3. Number of employees (based on the job) on each shift
4. Number of free weekends each employee will receive
5. Number of consecutive days (both minimum and maximum) each employee will work before receiving a day off.

A schedule may be stacked or staggered. A stacked schedule is one in which the employees work the same hours each day. For example, in the dietary

Fourteen-Day Work Schedule

	Sun	Mon	Tue	Wed	Thu	Fri	Sat	Sun	Mon	Tue	Wed	Thu	Fri	Sat	Notes
1st Cook	—	5	5	5	5	—	5	5	5	—	5	5	5	—	
2nd Cook	5	5	5	—	5	5	—	—	5	5	5	5	—	5	
PM Cook	10:30	—	10:30	10:30	10:30	10:30	10:30	—	10:30	10:30	—	10:30	10:30	10:30	
Relief	—	10:30	5	5	—	5	10:30	10:30	—	5	10:30	5	5	—	
FSW	—	7	7	7	—	7	5	5	—	7	7	7	7	—	
Salad	5	5	—	5	5	5	—	—	5	5	5	—	5	5	
Dish	—	7	7	7	—	7	7	7	—	7	7	7	7	—	

Dish-Pot	—	10:30	10:30	10:30	10:30	—	10:30	10:30	—	10:30	10:30	10:30	10:30	—
Relief	7	—	—	7	10:30	10:30	7	10:30	—	—	—	—	—	7
Relief	10:30	—	3	3	3–7	3	3	—	3–7	—	—	—	—	10:30
Cashier	6:30	—	6:30	6:30	6:30	—	6:30	6:30	6:30	6:30	—	6:30	6:30	6:30
PM Cashier	3	3	—	—	6:30	6:30	—	—	—	3	3	3	3	—
PM Cashier	—	6:30	—	11:30	3	—	—	3	3	—	6:30	11:30	3	3

11:30–4:00 - Extra assigned to clean, do paperwork, etc.

Note: This is a 60-bed pediatric orthopedic hospital that operates a cafeteria serving 500 meals a day. Shifts: 1st and 2nd cook, 5:00 a.m.–1:30 p.m.; PM cook, relief dishwasher, 10:30 a.m.–7:00 p.m.; dishwasher, 7:00 a.m.–10:30 a.m.; 2nd relief dishwasher, 3:00 p.m.–7:00 p.m.; cashier, 6:30 a.m.–3:00 p.m.; PM cashier, 3:00 p.m.–7:00 p.m.

Figure 4-1. Sample work schedule.

department common stacked scheduling hours may be 6 A.M. to 2 P.M. and 12 P.M. to 8 P.M. These hours are established and do not vary.

In the example given the two shifts overlap. In some stacked schedules the shifts may be separate: for example, a 6 A.M. to 2 P.M. early shift and a 2 P.M. to 8 P.M. evening shift. In this instance employees have little contact with one another.

A staggered schedule is planned around peak periods and concentrates more labor hours during the busiest times. Employees are scheduled to arrive and leave at various times depending on need. This type of scheduling minimizes idle time and improves efficiency and flexibility, but may be more difficult to implement than the stacked schedule. Depending on the facility locale, part-time employees may be difficult to find and some employees may find fluctuating hours difficult to accommodate. The person responsible for scheduling must evaluate the area labor market. If, for example, the area is a college town, part-time positions may be easy to fill. In large cities part-time positions may be very difficult to fill and may have a high turnover rate.

Length of the schedule may be determined by history. What has the procedure been in the past? If possible, for employee convenience, it is good to plan the schedule a month in advance. This also reduces the time the manager must spend scheduling and allows employees to plan for days off.

The number of employees to be scheduled for each shift is determined by the number of labor hours allowed by management and by the amount and kind of work to be done on the shift. For instance, it has often been common practice in the dietary departments of long-term care facilities to schedule more labor hours on the early shift than on the late shift. This is because the early shift usually prepares two meals and the late shift only one.

Before the scheduling process can begin, the manager must also consider the number of free weekends to which each employee is entitled. This may be every other weekend or perhaps every third weekend. It is impossible to schedule every weekend free unless an entire weekend staff is available for weekends only. Reducing staff coverage on the weekend is usually not advisable since the same amount of work is usually required on the weekends as during the week. Good scheduling ensures the same quality of meals seven days per week.

Another consideration facing the person preparing the work schedule is the number of days (both minimum and maximum) each employee can expect to work before a day off. For example, the schedule may establish the following rule: an employee will work a maximum of five days without a day off and a minimum of two.

Cyclical versus "Random" Scheduling

Scheduling can often be done according to a pattern established by the manager. This pattern is repeated continuously for each employee. One example of this type of scheduling is the "four-two" scheduling illustrated in Figure 4-2. Each employee works four consecutive days and is off two.

Employee	Sun	Mon	Tue	Wed	Thu	Fri	Sat	Sun	Mon	Tue	Wed	Thu	Fri	Sat
1	X	X	X	X	O	O	x	X	X	X	O	O	X	X
2	O	O	X	X	X	X	O	O	X	X	X	X	O	O
3	X	X	O	O	X	X	X	X	O	O	X	X	X	X

Figure 4-2. "Four-two" scheduling scheme.

Cyclical scheduling is quick and easy to do. One particular advantage of the four-two pattern is that there are always several employees who will be scheduled for a "short" week during any given week. These employees can be utilized to cover call-ins without incurring overtime.

Random scheduling, on the other hand, does not make use of a pattern and is different for each employee every time the schedule is prepared. This type of scheduling is more time consuming for the manager but may be more flexible. An example of random scheduling is shown in Figure 4-3.

Proper scheduling is very important and the person responsible must thoroughly understand all the restrictions that apply before beginning. Poor scheduling can result in low employee morale and decreased efficiency related to fatigue or improper use of employees in positions to which they are unaccustomed.

POLICIES AND PROCEDURES

Effective, well-written policies are essential to effective management of a department. Policies are "guidelines for developing the principles or plans of the organization; a course of action designed to influence decisions" (Jernigan 1989). Policies are statements of conduct while procedures describe the method by which the policies are carried out. In short, policies state *what* is done and procedures tell *how* to do it. This is an often neglected area that should be addressed by the consultant dietitian on an initial visit. It is not unusual to find dietary policies either inaccurate or out of date because it is not an area that administrators understand and may be too difficult for the dietary manager to develop.

Not only do policies define the operation of dietary services offered, but also define interdepartmental procedures. Some dietary policies must be coordinated with the medical director, as well as with the nursing, housekeeping, and maintenance departments. It is imperative for cooperation between departments and to provide a high level of patient care that all department heads work together to achieve policies and procedures that maximize efficiency of operations within the health care facility.

It is important that policies be written as briefly and clearly as possible. They must reflect the philosophy of the facility and be approved by the administrator. The number and kinds of policies written will be determined by the type of

Employee	Sun	Mon	Tue	Wed	Thu	Fri	Sat	Sun	Mon	Tue	Wed	Thu	Fri	Sat
1	X	X	O	O	X	X	X	O	X	X	X	O	X	X
2	X	O	X	X	O	X	O	X	X	O	O	X	X	X
3	X	X	X	X	X	O	O	X	O	X	X	X	O	X

Figure 4-3. "Random" scheduling scheme.

facility and its size. The policies should reflect current standards of nutrition care. The policy manual is reviewed annually and signed by the consultant dietitian. At that time, all policies that are not being followed should be eliminated. Keep in mind that any discrepancy between a written policy and actual practice can be used as evidence of malpractice; therefore, policies must be enforced.

A well-prepared dietary policy manual serves many purposes other than meeting requirements established by various regulatory agencies. One main purpose is improvement in communication between the dietary manager and staff. The policy manual can be used during employee orientation and also as an inservice tool to prevent conflicting interpretations of standards and methods within the department. For example, a specific policy and procedure outlining how food is prepared and delivered will eliminate inconsistencies among the staff who are doing the work. Nutrition policies relating to patient care are also performance guidelines for the consultant dietitian in providing an acceptable standard of care for patients.

The following outline can be used as a guide when reviewing or writing a dietary policy manual to ensure that all important areas are addressed.

1. Statement of purpose and scope of the dietary department
    a. Resident foodservice
    b. Employee foodservice
    c. Guest meals
    d. Food for special events
2. Organization chart
    a. Facility organization chart
    b. Dietary organization chart
3. Purchasing and budget
    a. Responsibility for writing specifications, selecting vendors, inventory control, and ordering and receiving of food and other dietary supplies
    b. Meal census records
    c. Allocation of patient meals, employee meals, and nonfood items
    d. Responsibility for maintaining cost records
4. Menus
    a. Responsibility for writing, reviewing, and approving menus
    b. Pattern for regular and therapeutic patient menus
    c. Method of recording menu substitutions
5. Nutritional care
    a. Diet manual used and location of manuals in the facility
    b. Transmission of diet orders for new admissions, NPO or hold trays, diet changes, and room changes
    c. Between-meal nourishment including nutritional supplements
    d. Nutritional screening and assessment
    e. Dietary and interdisciplinary care plans
    f. Responsibility for visiting and/or instructing patients about diets

6. Meal and nourishment service
    a. Time schedule for meals and nourishments
    b. Responsibility for dining room service, tray delivery to patient rooms, tray return to dietary, and delivery of nourishments
7. Meal preparation
    a. Portion control
    b. Standardized recipes
    c. Responsibilities for meal supervision
8. Sanitation and infection control
    a. Cleaning schedule
    b. Personnel health
    c. Personal hygiene
    d. Equipment care and cleaning
    e. Responsibilities of housekeeping and maintenance
    f. Isolation
    g. Proper food handling procedures
    h. Food storage
    i. Kitchen safety
    j. Disaster plan
9. Inservice and orientation
    a. Plan for dietary orientation to facility and department
    b. Responsibility for ongoing employee training; scheduling, and subject matter

An example of policy guidelines is given below.

EXAMPLE 4. RESIDENT FOODSERVICE

Purpose: To establish a policy and procedure for providing foodservice to residents of this health facility.

Policy: To provide foodservice to residents every day in sufficient quantity and quality according to the orders of the physician and under the direction of a consulting dietitian who has met the qualifications of the American Dietetic Association.

Procedure for serving food:
1. Residents will be encouraged to eat in the dining room.
2. Residents who are able to be out of bed but are physically, mentally, or emotionally unable to go to the dining areas will be provided tray stands for table service in their rooms. Each tray will be identified with the resident's name, location, and kind of diet.
3. For bedfast residents, individual tray service will be provided.
4. Each resident will be provided with a napkin, flatware, and dishes and glassware, free of cracks and chips, necessary to eat the meals served, unless there are physician's orders to the contrary.
5. All food will be served neatly, attractively and at the proper temperature.

6. All meals will be prepared according to the planned weekly menu assuring that each resident receives an adequate nutritious diet.
7. Attention to individual food preferences that are reasonable will be given, consistent with diet and menu plans.
8. At least three well-balanced meals will be served at regularly scheduled hours. The evening meal and the succeeding breakfast will be served no more than 14 hours apart.
9. Adequate kitchen staff will be on duty each day according to the posted work schedule.

JOB DESCRIPTIONS

Job descriptions are a necessary part of the organization of a dietary department. The job description is an important communication and training tool. It not only enables the departmental staff to understand clearly the specific responsibilities involved in each of their jobs, it also allows the prospective employee to understand working conditions and job requirements before beginning a job. Since each facility or dietary operation is unique, job descriptions must be written to suit that particular operation. As jobs change, job descriptions must be updated.

The criteria-based performance appraisal (CBPA) is currently replacing the traditional job description, which simply lists tasks performed and not the quality or quantity of work. A criteria-based job description not only lists the major job tasks, but also performance standards by which those tasks are measured. The traditional job description relied heavily on personal judgment, but the goal of the CBPA is to set forth objective criteria by which an employee's performance is evaluated. Equal opportunity legislation has mandated that employers show that criteria are valid and nondiscriminatory toward race, sex, or religion.

From the list of tasks, the manager can formulate the major responsibilities for each job and the accepted standard of performance for those responsibilities. It is a good idea to review the finished job description with the employee to find out whether he or she understands and agrees or disagrees with the criteria. If there is not mutual understanding of the goals of the job description, the desired results will not be achieved.

When changing the performance appraisal system to be more objective, where should you start? Employees need and want to have their voices heard. An important way to involve personnel as a part of the process is with a job analysis, which breaks down the job into individual tasks. Ask employees to go through a week with a diary and write down everything that they do, when it is done, and how much time is required to do the job. This information provides valuable input from those people who know the most about their responsibilities—namely, the people doing the work. Once this has been done, you can combine the various tasks into major task categories for each position in the department, and formulate the accepted standard of performance for those tasks. It is a good idea to review the finished job description after doing the job analysis.

Performance standards are the acceptable level of task completion required to perform the job. Performance standards usually measure such issues as quantity, quality, time frame, motives, skills, and knowledge. It is the performance standard against which employees are evaluated and largely removes subjectivity from the appraisal process. In this system, one is evaluating behavior instead of the person. Employees' work either excels, meets the standard, or falls below expectations. Examples of criteria-based performance appraisals can be found in Figures 4-4 and 4-5.

When you review job descriptions, ask yourself the following questions:

1. Are the criteria specific and measurable?
2. Are they practical or achievable? Are there adequate resources such as people, time, and money?
3. Are they outcome-oriented?
4. Are the results measurable?

A criteria-based performance appraisal system offers many advantages. It has already been stated that, as an appraisal tool, it is more objective and does not require judgments, but rather observations of an employee's work. The terminology used describes behaviors and is not a personal attack on the employee. Ideally, this appraisal is developed with input from both management and staff. As a coaching tool, it can show what behaviors would lead to improved performance. The primary advantage of this type of job description for employees is that it gives them clear knowledge of what is expected. It provides a means of giving recognition for their work efforts or specific information on how they can improve if work does not measure up to standard. Because management and staff have worked on developing the tool together, staff feel they have participated in decisions that affect them. Benefits to managers using the CBPA are better control of the work, greater confidence in directing a department, and usually better relationships with their employees.

Employers need to realize the self-fulfilling prophecy that influences the behavior of our employees. Positive expectations breed positive results while negative expectations breed negative results. When performance expectations are worded positively and are measurable, it will result in motivating employees to want to do a better job and a means of providing recognition for their efforts.

INSERVICE TRAINING

Effective inservice training is an important part of the consultant dietitian's duties in the facility. Since most foodservice workers lack formal training in the field and are simply hired on as cooks or dishwashers without exhibiting actual skills, it is easy to see why so many departments are not able to provide quality services. Probably the most common form of so-called "training" is placing a new employee with the person already in the position in order to observe and/or learn the job from someone who may not be performing the job correctly in the

JOB DESCRIPTION/PERFORMANCE APPRAISAL
Name: _____

Type of Appraisal: ( ) Probationary ( ) Annual
( ) Other
Department: Dietary
Date Hired: _____
Date Evaluation Due _____

Position Title: Cook
Position Summary
1) Prepares all foods on regular and modified diet menu.
2) Serves foods to patients and employees as assigned.
3) Portions food accurately as specified in recipe.
4) Cleans as assigned by Foodservice Supervisor.
Machines, Tools, Equipment, and Work Aids
1) Must be able to operate various kinds of kitchen equipment.
2) Written resources include recipe books, menus, and diet manual.
Qualifications
1) High school education desirable, but must be able to read, write, and follow oral and written directions.
2) Must have some knowledge of foods and methods of preparation, also ability to plan work in order to meet established deadlines.
3) Experience in food preparation and service preferred.

On-The-Job-Training
1) On-the-job training under close supervision is provided.
2) Hospital orientation is provided to all new employees. Additional training shall be provided.
Knowledge, Skills, Aptitudes, and Physical Requirements
1) Must have some knowledge of foods and method of preparation.
2) Stands and walks short distances.
3) Lifts, bends, and handles various pieces of kitchen equipment.
Working Conditions
1) Works in clean, well-lighted kitchen that is well ventilated.
2) Atmosphere could be warm and humid on occasion.
3) Is exposed to sudden temperature changes when entering refrigerator and freezer.
4) Subject to burns from hot foods or utensils and cuts from knives and other sharp kitchen utensils.
Job Relationships
1) Responsible to: Director of Dietary
2) Interrelationships: Effective working relationships must be established with other dietary employees, nursing service, and others to promote customer satisfaction.

(Continued)

Figure 4-4. Job description and performance appraisal form for the position of cook.

Position Title: Cook		DNMS	MS	ES	Employee's Name:
Major Responsibilities	Performance Standards				Comments
DNMS = Does not meet standards MS = Meets standards ES = Exceeds standards					
To Department 1) Reviews menus to determine types and quantities of meats vegetables, soups, salads, and desserts to be prepared in accordance with meal preparation procedures	**1a)** Consistently sets up cook's area for preparing current days entrees and hot items, organizes work area before production begins by obtaining food items and necessary equipment beforehand **1b)** Consistently follows standardized recipes accurately **1c)** Consistently checks holding temperatures of hot food to ensure safety and keep within sanitation guidelines **1d)** Maintains a neat, orderly work area **1e)** Always keeps waste and overproduction to a minimum				
2) Always prepares the breakfast menu and hot foods at lunch in accordance with menu	**2a)** Hot foods are prepared using sanitary methods of food preparation **2b)** Hot foods are placed on the steamtable no more than 30 minutes prior to meal times				
3) Plans cooking schedule in conjunction with supervisor and/or dietitican to ensure food will be ready at specified time	**3a)** Always checks menu and diet sheet for amounts to prepare for patients **3b)** Always checks menu for necessary prepreparation (e.g., pulling frozen meat for cooking the next day)				

Figure 4-4. (*Continued*)

Position Title: Cook		DNMS	MS	ES	Employee's Name:
Major Responsibilities	**Performance Standards**				**Comments**
4) Confers with dietitian regarding modified diet preparation in order to ensure accuracy in patient diet prescription	**4a)** Asks questions if diet is not understood **4b)** Prepares modified diets according to written menus **4c)** Informs dietitian of any menu items that need to be substituted				
5) Confers with supervisor regarding the use of leftovers to avoid waste	**5a)** Always utilizes leftovers when possible **5b)** Always covers and dates all leftover food items				
6) Cleans the reach-in refrigerator in accordance with correct sanitation procedures	**6a)** Discards outdated foods **6b)** Wipes the inside and outside of refrigerator with sanitizing solution				
7) Observes and tastes food being cooked and adds ingredients or seasoning to improve flavor or texture as needed in order to serve quality products	**7a)** Uses proper tasting techniques **7b)** Closely observes cooking meals in order to prevent overcooking				
8) Carves portions of meat, fish, and fowl for individual servings and prepares or directs distribution of food to serving units. Apportions servings according to menu combinations or orders for patients in accordance with standardlized recipes	**8a)** Uses portion control equipment (tools) to portion menu items **8b)** Is accurate in portioning modified diets				
9) Maintains cooking area in a neat, clean, and orderly manner in accordance with departmental standards	**9a)** Sanitizes work counters at least three times during work shift **9b)** Cleans equipment and puts equipment and ingredients away as used **9c)** Cleans own work				

(Continued)

					Employee's Name:
Position Title: Cook		**DNMS**	**MS**	**ES**	
Major Responsibilities	**Performance Standards**				**Comments**
	station after each meal is prepared				
10) Cleans the kitchen area according to duties as assigned on cleaning schedule using correct cleaning and sanitizing procedures in Policy and Procedure Manual	**10a)** Knows regulations in the Kentucky State Food Service Code **10b)** Performs daily sanitation inspection and keeps monthly records confirming cleaning regularity				
11) Knows safe methods of using cooking equipment such as blenders, mixers, grills, etc.	**11a)** Uses equipment according to proper procedures in Policy and Procedure Manual or instructions **11b)** Avoids accidents while using equipment				
12) Sets up all hot foods for cafeteria according to established policy	**12a)** Plans cafeteria steamtable line setup to maximize color and texture variations and ease of service **12b)** Uses appropriate size pans for items to look most appetizing **12c)** Replenishes salads and desserts to ensure variety throughout the meal service **12d)** Always has a back-up of hot food items in the pass-through				
To Patient **1)** Serves tasty, well-prepared food according to sanitation requirements and proper cooking methods	**1a)** To preserve nutrition value, avoids overcooking or undercooking foods **1b)** Serves meals that are colorful and aesthetically pleasing				
2) Serves modified diets according to diet prescription ordered by physician	**2a)** Serves modified diets that are accurately served **2b)** Is familiar with the				

Figure 4-4. (*Continued*)

COOK				
Employee name: _____				
DNMS = Does not meet standards				
MS = Meets standards				
ES = Exceeds standards	**DNMS**	**MS**	**ES**	**Comments**
Quality of Work				
1. Food preparation				
a. Prepares quality foods in correct amounts needed for patients and employees according to menu				
b. Uses standardized recipes				
c. Incorporates basic food preparation skills to assure retention of nutritive value, palatabilty, and appetizing appearance of food				
d. Tastes food during preparation and adds ingredients or seasoning to improve flavor, color, or texture				
e. Follows menus provided, making changes only with the consent of dietitian				
f. Apportions food in accordance with yield in standardized recipes				
g. Prepares therapeutic diets according to instructions of dietitian				
2. Dishwashing and pot and pan washing				
a. Operates dishwasher following established policy and procedures				
b. Washes and sanitizes pots, pans, and food preparation utensils following established policy and procedures				
3. Foodservice to patients and employees				
a. Follows established policy and procedures for cafeteria service				
b. Follows established policy and procedures for patient cart service				
c. Checks temperature of food before serving to ascertain that it is acceptable				
4. Cleaning and sanitation				
a. Maintains kitchen equipment, food preparation areas, and dishwashing area in clean, sanitary condition				
b. Reports equipment breakdown or maintenance problems to dietitian				
5. Inventory control and purchasing				
a. Checks deliveries from vendors				
b. Assists with storeroom duties when needed				
6. Kitchen equipment and utensil operation and maintenance				
a. Reads and frequently reviews operations manuals for all equipment				
b. Maintains high safety standards while operating all equipment				

Figure 4-5. Form for criteria-based performance appraisal.

COOK	DNMS	MS	ES	Comments
Quality control 1. Plans cooking schedule so that food will be served as soon as possible after cooking 2. Tastes all food to insure optimum flavor				

Other behavioral factors
1. Attendance and reliability
  a. Does not abuse or take advantage of sick time or personal days absent
  b. Takes corrective action to prevent recurring absences
  c. Provides notification for absences and tardiness
2. Appearance and physical fitness
  a. Observes hospital personal appearance standards and uniform regulations policy
  b. Physically capable of performing position responsibilities without interruption due to short- or long-term illness or injury
3. Understanding of emergency procedures, and internal/external disaster procedures
4. Attitude and conduct
  a. Accountable for own conduct
  b. Promotes good working relationships among staff and with other departments				

Comments: _____ _____ _____ _____ _____				
_____ Employee signature				
_____ Department head signature				

Figure 4-5. (*Continued*)

first place. Not only is training necessary to ensure a safe work environment, it is important in ensuring the safety of the food we serve.

There are many benefits of training that have been identified (Rose 1987a):

- Better job performance
- Increased productivity
- Increased job satisfaction, morale, and cooperation

- Improved understanding of duties and responsibilities
- Decreased absenteeism
- Decreased turnover
- Decreased waste
- Improved safety awareness (prevention and reduction of accidents)
- Improved communications
- Increased clientele satisfaction

Certainly there are costs involved in training, but in the long run, the benefits far outweigh the costs in terms of job satisfaction, stability, and reduced rate of employee turnover.

Not everyone is an effective trainer. In addition to the ability to instruct others, an instructor must have extensive knowledge of job requirements, an ability to communicate effectively, objectivity and patience, a sense of humor, adequate time for training, the respect of the trainees, and an enthusiasm for the training assignment (Ninemeier 1985).

A good inservice program does not have to be costly, but does require planning. The content of the lesson should be directly related to the work performed. Shorter sessions (20 minutes) have been shown to be more effective than longer ones since you are more likely to retain the trainee's attention. It is important to use a variety of teaching methods and instructional materials, keeping in mind that most people retain 10 percent of what they read, 20 percent of what they hear, 30 percent of what they see, 50 percent of what they hear and see, 70 percent of what they say, and 90 percent of what they say and do (Drummond 1989).

The three main teaching activities are telling, showing, and doing (Rose 1987c). Trainers who use a combination of teaching techniques usually get the best results. For example, using visual aids along with a lecture or a demonstration following a lecture has more impact than lecturing by itself. Since people learn by doing, the most effective inservices involve the employee in the presentation. Lecturing, as a primary teaching technique, is not an effective means of learning because it is passive and does not involve the student. Question and answer, role playing, demonstrations, visual aids such as slides or videos, games or contests, and on-the-job training promote employee involvement and result in retention of information. Remember that the subject matter of inservice training must be pertinent to the employees' everyday job or it is wasted time.

It is unrealistic to expect perfection after one training session since individuals learn at different rates. Repetition is the key to success as a trainer. Learning is reinforced when the same material is presented in different ways.

Evaluation and documentation are important aspects of the inservice process. A trainer does not know if an employee has mastered a skill unless learning is evaluated. Pre- and posttests are the most commonly used forms of evaluation. Employees may also demonstrate that skills have been mastered. In any learning situation be sure to give feedback. People have a need to know how they are doing. The importance of documentation cannot be overly stressed because in a business context, if a task has not been documented, it is not considered to have been done.

Even with careful planning and inservice training, failure to master skills can be highly visible in a foodservice department. The following are the reasons that employees fail to learn (Rose 1989).

- Lack of commitment to education by the management staff
- Unrealistic, unrelated content, or material not pertinent to job
- Teachers who are ineffective and not perceived as being current and knowledgeable
- Techniques that are ineffective and complicate the learning process for the average student

Motivating and teaching foodservice employees is a challenge that confronts every dietitian in the field. The rewards are great when training is effective and successful.

ORIENTATION PROGRAM FOR DIETARY EMPLOYEES

Many health care facilities have orientation programs for new employees, but not all of these programs include orientation to specific departments. A program designed for dietary employees can have a positive effect on the new employee in many ways. A good orientation program can result in better performance, since the employee is given specific personal instruction in all areas relating to the job, as well as a broad overview of the dietary department's policies and procedures. Other benefits of a specific orientation program for dietary employees include

1. Increased employee confidence and morale (The employee knows precisely what is expected by the employer.)
2. Decreased likelihood of accidents resulting from inadequate employee training with equipment
3. Decreased employee turnover rate
4. Decreased likelihood of an employee's collecting unemployment benefits related to poor or inadequate job knowledge

Content of the Program

The orientation program for each facility will be different depending on the policies and procedures of the facility, as well as equipment and resources available. Orientation to the dietary department should include, but not be limited to, the following areas:

1. Introduction to the written dietary policies and procedures manual

2. Specific job descriptions for each position in the department
3. Orientation to the diet manual and procedures to follow for therapeutic diets
4. Familiarization with the menu
5. Training in the proper use and cleaning of all equipment
6. Review of dietary procedures for disaster plans, such as fire and tornadoes
7. Review of sanitation policies and procedures
8. Review of routine records to be kept by the dietary department
9. Miscellaneous information relating to dietary employees, such as where to store purses, how meals are purchased, and so on

Developing the Program

Before developing a dietary orientation program, make an outline list of all items that need to be included in it.

Decide what time frame is reasonable for accomplishing the orientation and, if the training is to last several days, how the topics will be divided. For example, day one may include orientation to written policies and procedures and to job descriptions and work schedules. Day two may deal with different topics as the employee becomes more oriented to the department. These topics may include therapeutic diets, operation and cleaning of equipment, and information on other job duties.

It is necessary to consider what resources are available as well. Does the facility have slides or films that can be incorporated into the program? Many facilities have a selection of audiovisual materials on pertinent topics, such as basic handwashing techniques or infection control. These resources can be valuable additions to the program and provide some welcome variety in the learning process.

Once the material for the program is organized, decide who will be responsible for each section. The dietary manager may do the majority of the training but may assign the new employee to an experienced employee for instruction in such areas as equipment operation or foodservice procedures.

In order to have a comprehensive program, it is important to develop the materials carefully. It is also imperative to have a place on the forms where each employee can sign in order to document proper training and orientation. This protects the employer in the event a conflict arises where proper training is in question. Examples of orientation materials are shown in Figures 4-6 and 4-7.

It is also important that the program be presented to and approved by the administrator of the facility before it is implemented since time spent orienting the new employee carries a price tag to the employer. A successful program, however, will reduce dietary expenses in the long run. Here again, development of a dietary orientation program by the dietary consultant can be an excellent opportunity for marketing the skills of the consultant. Be innovative. If the facility lacks an orientation program targeted for dietary employees, approach the administrator with the advantages of developing one. Improvements in the department reflect well on both the consultant and the administrator.

Foodservice Employee Orientation					
	Read	Demo	Practice	Review	Rating
Tour of facility					
Food carts					
Dress code					
Menus and special diets					
Dishwashing machine					
Garbage disposal					
Meat slicer					
Mixer and grinder					
Isolation procedures					
Inventory and stock rotation					
Proper refrigeration					
Proper storage of food					
Cleaning of vents and stove					
Fire drill and disaster plan					
Milk box					
Cleaning schedule					
Work schedule					
Can opener					
Serving of food					
Cleaning supplies					
Kitchen janitor closet					
3-Compartment sink: Wash, rinse, sterilize					

Figure 4-6. Sample form for foodservice employee orientation.

I have completed the above orientation program and have reviewed my ratings. I agree to adhere to the best of my ability to these policies and procedures, realizing that if I do not the Management has the right to terminate my employment.

_____   _____
Date   Signature of Employee

Rating Code: S-Satisfactory
                 U-Unsatisfactory
                 X-Phase Completion

Figure 4-6. (*Continued*)

Orientation Program for Dietary Employees

Purpose: The purpose of the orientation program is to provide an organized plan of orientation for all new dietary staff.

Policy: It is the policy of this facility to prepare each new member of the dietary staff for the position they will be assuming through a specifically outlined program of orientation. This program should provide the new employee with facts relevant to his or her position and a basic understanding of the types of resident care provided in this facility.

Responsibility: The responsibility for adherence to the following procedures shall rest with the Dietary Manager.

Procedures: On the first day of employment the Dietary Manager will take the employee on a brief tour of the facility and make introductions to other staff members and coworkers. After a tour of the facility, the employee will be given a tour of the dietary department to include both storage and dishroom areas. Following these tours, the Dietary Manager will review policies in the following areas:

1. Pay periods
2. Absence procedure
3. Coffee/lunch breaks/meal tickets
4. Time clock/cards
5. Telephone/intercom usage
6. PPD test
7. Parking rules
8. Location of fire alarms, extinguishers
9. Fire and disaster plan
10. Uniforms and appearance
11. Conduct/professionalism
12. Patient/family communications
13. Job description
14. Work schedule and hours
15. Infection control

Figure 4-7. Form for orientation of dietary employees.

Any time remaining can be spent observing or assisting coworkers. The second day of employment will be used to train the employee in the following areas:

1. Isolation procedures
2. Inventory and stock rotation
3. Proper storage of food
4. Reading and interpreting the menu
5. Portion sizes
6. Correct serving procedures
7. Checking food temperatures
8. Proper dishroom procedures, use of garbage disposal
9. Care and cleaning of the dishroom
10. Washing pots and pans
11. Cleaning schedule: (a) food carts; (b) meat slicer, (c) can opener, (d) ovens and ranges, (e) steam tables, (f) mixer, (g) walk-ins, (h) coffee machine, (i) food processor, (j) steamer, (k) hand sink, (l) floors, (m) any other area or equipment in the department
12. Review of therapeutic and modified diets

The remainder of the day will be spent demonstrating the operation of all equipment with which the employee is unfamiliar and allowing him or her to practice.

I have completed the orientation program for the dietary department as outlined above and understand the policies and procedures reviewed.

_____   _____
Date   Signature of employee

Figure 4-7. (*Continued*)

Employers need to realize the self-fulfilling prophecy that influences the behavior of our employees. Positive expectations breed positive results while negative expectations breed negative results. Performance expectations that are worded positively and are measurable will result in motivating employees to want to do a better job and will provide recognition for their efforts.

REFERENCES

Buchanan, Robert D. 1977. How to determine staffing needs. Part I. *Food Service Marketing* (July): 45–49.
———. 1976. How to determine staffing needs. Part 2. January. *Food Service Marketing.*
Consultant Dietitians in Health Care Facilities. 1981. *How to consult manual.* Columbus, Ohio: Ross Laboratories.
Clinical Management. 1987. 3, no. 8 (August): 30.

Drummond, Karen, MS, RD. 1989. In-service Training: How Do Employees Learn Best? *Hospital Food & Nutrition Focus* 6, no. 4:1–3.

Haimann, Theo, and Raymond Hilgert. 1977. *Supervision: Concepts and practices of management.* Cincinnati.

Henderson, P. 1976. Labor staffing guidelines for long-term care facilities. *Journal of the American Hospital Association* 50: 79–82.

Jernigan, Anna K. 1989. *The effective food service supervisor.* Rockville, Md: Aspen Publishers Inc.

Mahaffey, Mary, Mary Mennes, and Bonnie Miller. 1981. *Food service manual for health care institutions.* Chicago: American Hospital Association.

Ninemeier, Jack. 1985. Managing foodservice operations: A systems approach for healthcare and institutions. West Lafayette, Ind.: Purdue Research Foundation.

Rose, James C. 1988. Monitrend and your FTEs. *Hospital Food Nutrition Focus* 5, no. 4: 1, 7.

————. 1987a. Inservice Education and Orientation: Part 1. *Hospital Food & Nutrition Focus* 3, no. 11: 1–3.

————. 1987b. Inservice Education and Orientation: Part 2. *Hospital Food & Nutrition Focus* 3, no. 12:1–2.

————. 1987c. Inservice training: how do employees learn best? *Hospital Food & Nutrition Focus* 6, no. 4:1–3.

————. 1984. *Handbook for health care foodservice management.* Aspen Systems Inc.

Schwegel, Richard, MBA, RD, DHCFA. 1987. Criteria-based performance review. *Hospital Food & Nutrition Focus* 3, no. 5:1–5.

Spears, Marian C., and Allene G. Vaden. 1985. *Foodservice organizations: A managerial and systems approach:* New York: Macmillan Publishing Co.

Stokes, Judy Ford. 1979. *Cost effective foodservice: An institutional guide.* Germantown, Md.: Aspen Systems Corp.

Wessels, Janette. 1981. *Dietary policy and procedure guideline handbook.*

5

Work Relationships

"No man is an island" is particularly true of consulting dietitians. In order to do the best job possible, the consultant must have the support and cooperation of other members of the health care team, most notably the dietary manager, the administrator, and the director of nursing.

To achieve a good working relationship, the consultant must make an effort to understand the goals and objectives of each of these individuals and to help each of them, in turn, understand his or hers. In the beginning, the consultant dietitian must establish sound credentials and earn a place on the health care team of each facility.

WORKING WITH THE ADMINISTRATOR

The consultant dietitian is ultimately responsible to the administrator of the facility. It is therefore important to establish several things at the start of the consultant's employment:

1. What are the administrator's goals for the dietary department? The goals of the consultant must coincide with those of the administrator. It is unlikely that the dietitian will be able to accomplish anything that the administrator does not support.
2. What does the administrator want from the consultant dietitian? Some administrators expect a written report following each visit, while others may be content with a monthly summary. Does the administrator want the consultant to concentrate on clinical activities, food production activities, or both? The consultant may be expected to provide seasonal menus and input into food cost control. It is important to clarify exactly what is expected and at the same time to let the administrator know what can be done by an effective dietary consultant. Take this opportunity to market yourself and your skills.
3. What is the line of authority? Must any change be approved by the administrator in advance, or is the dietary manager authorized to make changes within specified boundaries? Some administrators will want to approve any change, particularly those with a cost factor such as a new set of menus and activities requiring additional consulting time. When dealing with administrators it is important to project yourself as a viable part of the facility health care team and to establish yourself as a resource person for all areas of the dietary department. Treat each account as if it were your most important

because while you are there, it is! Many dietary consultants make the mistake of "distancing" themselves from the facility staff since they are employed on a consultant rather than full-time basis. Successful consultants work to become an accepted member of each facility's team and are able to work much more effectively as an "insider."

With the administrator as well as the dietary manager, be honest. Try to hold an exit conference at least once a month to talk over the dietary department's progress as well as problems. Take care to project professionalism, concern for excellence, and a willingness to work within the established framework of the facility. Administrators generally do not like to receive written reports detailing numerous problems of which they were unaware. It is best to address these areas verbally first and to agree on a plan of resolution that can also be included in the report, making it much more positive in tone.

Learn to think over suggestions carefully, weighing any fiscal impact. Be prepared to justify your position. Once you have earned the confidence and trust of the administrator, you may be able to accomplish much more.

WORKING WITH THE DIETARY MANAGER

In many instances it could be said that the consultant is only as good as the dietary manager with whom he or she works. Most consultants would agree that a good dietary manager is priceless, and it is certainly true that neither the manager nor the consultant can function effectively without cooperation from the other.

In order to establish an effective working relationship with the dietary manager, the consultant must cultivate the following traits:

Integrity: A consulting dietitian must have sufficient job knowledge based on education and experience in order to assist the dietary manager effectively.

Flexibility: The consultant must be receptive to new methods and ideas and be able to set priorities. Input from the manager should be encouraged and incorporated into the consultant's plan. Each facility and manager is different and will require a different approach.

Objectivity: The consultant must have the ability to put aside personal feelings and to look at each situation objectively. Like or dislike of the dietary manager should not influence assessment of the manager's abilities or of the needs of the department.

Ability to communicate: The dietary consultant must be articulate, able to speak convincingly and communicate effectively both verbally and in writing. In the consulting process the dietitian must communicate with many people from diverse backgrounds.

Approachability: A good consultant is not intimidating or excessively demanding. The manager must feel able to come to the consultant with problems and suggestions and know that his or her input will be appreciated and useful.

Honesty: Above all the consultant must be honest and willing to admit a mistake and willing also to inform the manager directly of problems noted rather than communicating with the administrator behind his or her back. Honesty is necessary for trust to be built in the relationship. Without trust the consultant dietitian and the manager will not function effectively as a team.

Above all else, the role of the consultant dietitian with the dietary manager is that of teacher. The consultant has the skills to help the dietary manager increase his or her knowledge base and to function more effectively. It is often easier for the consultant to step in and make the needed changes than to motivate the dietary manager to do so. Changes initiated by the consultant, however, are not as long lasting or satisfactory as changes made by the dietary manager. Ultimately, any decisions made by the consultant dietitian to manage the department or enforce certain actions undermine the authority and responsibility of the dietary manager. It may be hard to sit back and wait for decisions or changes to be made and motivate others instead of doing the work yourself. You must bear in mind that the consultant does not have any direct line of authority in the facility. The role of the consultant is that of advisor, motivator, communicator, and sometimes mediator rather than supervisor. The consultant's goals must be accomplished through influencing other staff members. It takes great skill in communicating, for the consultant's success is measured in terms of the ability to get people to perform the desired tasks rather than his or her own ability to do them.

Discovering the specific strengths and weaknesses of each dietary manager that you work with and developing the strengths is one of the greatest challenges of the dietitian's job. It is unnecessary and fruitless to attempt to change a person's character; you should rather seek to use it for the greatest efficiency and to gain the highest degree of cooperation.

WORKING WITH THE DIRECTOR OF NURSING

In addition to starting off on the right foot with the administrator and the dietary manager, establishing a good working relationship with the director of nursing (DON) is essential. As with the administrator, it is important for the DON to perceive the consultant dietitian as a fellow professional and a member of the health care team. In addition, the consultant should strive to become a resource person to whom information and questions concerning nutrition will be referred.

When beginning consultation for a new account, the best course of action may be to approach the DON, introduce yourself, and request a meeting. It is vital to remember that both nursing and dietary share responsibility for the nutritional well-being of the patient and must work closely to achieve the desired results. At the meeting several points should be clarified:

1. To whom should the dietitian direct nursing-related suggestions or requests for information? For example, the consultant may suggest a three-day calorie

count for a patient with a poor appetite. To get this information, a detailed account of exact patient intake by nursing is necessary. The DON may prefer to handle these requests personally or may prefer them directed to a charge nurse or staff nurse. If the requests are directed to others, the DON may request a record of the requests.

2. When making a request of the physician such as a change of diet order, does the DON prefer that the dietitian make the request personally, or through one of the nursing staff? Which method would the physician be likely to prefer?
3. How should the consulting dietitian deal with care plans? If a nutritional problem has been identified can the dietitian write it on the plan, or should it be referred to the care plan committee to address?
4. How is information from the nutritional assessment transmitted to nursing or to the physician?
5. How will the consulting dietitian be notified of any patients requiring attention?
6. What has been the relationship between dietary and nursing in the past? What changes could or should be made?
7. What is the dietitian's role in inservicing the nursing staff on topics such as feeding techniques, therapeutic diets, and recording intake?

In general, the consulting dietitian should learn what the consultant's relationship to nursing has been in the past and what it could be in the future. Take the opportunity to express willingness to be part of the team and to help the director of nursing provide the best nutrition support measures possible with an alliance between nursing and dietary. Maintain frequent contact with the director of nursing at each consulting visit, if possible, to discuss recommendations and problems and goals. Once again, become a resource!

COMMITTEES AND STUDIES

Many nursing homes have a number of standing committees that may offer opportunities for the consulting dietitian. The most common committees are Utilization Review, Infection Control, Pharmacy, and Safety.

Utilization Review

The utilization review (UR) committee reviews records of patients who utilize Medicare funds. The committee approves initial access of these funds and reviews each patient for continued coverage throughout his or her stay in the facility.

The committee generally consists of several physicians, the administrator, the director of nursing, and any other staff members designated by the facility. Meetings are held every 30 days to meet Medicare guidelines.

The UR committee is also responsible for medical care evaluation studies to identify and analyze factors relating to patient care in the facility that might benefit the patients, staff facility, or the community. It is in this area that the consulting dietitian may contribute valuable expertise. Nutrition, as an important aspect of quality care, offers many areas of study that may prove beneficial to any or all of the groups. Examples of areas of study include, but are certainly not limited to

1. *Tube-fed patients:* Is there a common diagnosis for tube-fed patients? Is one specific formula more cost efficient for general use? Would an enteral feeding formula benefit the facility? Do all formulas used appear to be equally well tolerated by the patients? Do tube-fed patients receiving the formula by pump appear to have a better nutrition status than those fed by bolus or gravity drip?
2. *Weight loss:* Do an unusually large number of patients admitted to the facility show weight loss during the first year after admission? Is weight loss more significant in patients who must be fed? For patients on pureed diets?
3. *Diagnosis and modified diets:* Are patients admitted to the facility receiving the appropriate diet according to diagnosis?
4. *Pressure sores:* Is there a correlation between development of pressure sores and nutrition status?

The list above notes a few examples of possible nutrition topics that might prove interesting and beneficial for study. Such studies provide an excellent opportunity for the consulting dietitian to market his or her expertise to the medical staff and the facility while gathering data that may have an impact on the welfare of others.

Since the nursing department often has the primary responsibility for these studies, the director of nursing is often eager to have another department involved and assuming a share of the responsibility for studies.

Other benefits may include increased cooperation between departments through realization of a common goal and recognition of the consulting dietitian as a contributing member of the health care team. Summaries of two such studies developed by the Department of Health, Education, and Welfare follow (Benedict 1975).

DIAGNOSIS AND MODIFIED DIETS

Purpose: To determine if the diet that the patient is receiving is consistent with his diagnosis or condition
Personnel Initiating Study: Administrator, Director of Nursing, Consultant Dietitian
Time Period: February 1990
Population (choose one):
    A. All patients on modified diets
    B. 10 percent of all patients in facility regardless of diet (Population used for this study)

C. Review by diagnosis(es)

Criteria:

1. Diagnoses, particularly diabetes and circulatory problems
2. The type of diet ordered
3. The date the diet was ordered
4. How often is the diet reviewed or changed?
5. Who suggested a modified diet (M.D., family, patient, dietitian, etc.)?
6. Should the patient's diet be changed?
7. Should the modified diet have been instituted earlier?

Findings:

1. Most of the patients had a diagnosis of cerebrovascular accident or fracture of the hip.
2. A general diet was most often ordered regardless of the diagnosis.
3. Most diets were ordered at the time of admission.
4. The diets were never reviewed and rarely changed. They were changed only if there was a complaint from the patient or family.
5. Modified diets were generally suggested by the physician. Some were suggested by the patient's family.
6. Approximately 40 percent of the patients reviewed required some kind of diet change. All the changes should have been instituted earlier. For example, there were several patients receiving modifications for congestive heart failure who were not salt restricted, and there were two patients receiving insulin who were not on a diabetic diet.

Recommendations of the Utilization Review Committee:

1. All patients should be reviewed by the dietitian at the time of admission for the necessity of a modified diet. The dietitian should notify the physician if she believes that an appropriate modified diet has been omitted.
2. The nurses on each wing should notify the physician if the patient appears to be either dissatisfied or having problems with his or her meals.
3. Diets should be reviewed monthly by the dietitian for appropriateness. Dietary problems should be communicated to the physician, with suggestions for modification.

MODIFIED DIETS ORDERED BUT NOT RECEIVED

Purpose: To determine if patients for whom modified diets have been ordered are receiving these diets.

Personnel Initiating Study: Administrator, Director of Nursing, Medical Director, Consultant Dietitian

Time Period: October–November 1990

Population: All patients for whom a modified diet has been ordered

Criteria:

1. Was the ordered modified diet actually being received?
2. When was the modified diet ordered?
3. Was the modified diet ordered at the facility or sent with the patient?

4. What was the date the dietary department received the modified diet order?
5. Was the order verbal or in writing?
    a. Ordered by the physician
    b. Received by the dietary department
6. Is there a policy and a procedure for ordering a modified diet?

Findings:
1. 30 percent of the modified diets ordered were not being received.
2. Most modified diets were ordered at the time of admission. Some patients had diet orders sent with them from the hospital.
3. There was often a lapse of 2 or 3 days before the order was relayed to the dietary department.
4. The order was usually written on the chart by the physician but relayed to the dietary department verbally.
5. There is no standard procedure within the facility for ordering modified diets.

Recommendations of the Utilization Review Committee:
1. A written procedure for ordering modified diets should be developed.
2. A list of all patients on modified diets should be kept and checked weekly by the Nutritionist and the Director of Nursing.
3. The dietary department should be notified within eight (8) hours of the time the diet order is written by the physician.
4. All dietary orders or changes should be sent to the dietary department in writing.

Infection Control

Proposed Federal Regulation 483.65 Infection Control requires that both intermediate and skilled care nursing facilities conduct an active program for the prevention, control, and investigation of infections and communicable diseases. Skilled nursing facilities have been required to have an infection control committee for some time, but this has not been a requirement for intermediate care. With the merging of these levels under the new regulations, an infection control program is now a requirement.

The responsibilities of the committee, as stated above, make it quite broad in scope and involve many different disciplines within the facility. The committee may be composed of members from housekeeping, nursing, pharmacy, maintenance, and administration as well as dietary. Meetings are held quarterly. Since infection control is vitally important to the dietary department of any hospital or long-term care facility, it is imperative that the department be well represented. In these days of acquired immune deficiency syndrome (AIDS) and methicillin-resistant Staphylococcus aureus (MRSA) there is much to discuss and good infection control requires teamwork.

If time constraints placed on the consulting dietitian prevent involvement with this committee, the consultant should make sure the dietary manager attends the meetings. It may also be helpful to review minutes of the meetings occasionally to keep abreast of new policies or current issues discussed at the meetings. It is also necessary to check and become familiar with the infection control policies of each facility. The dietary department may be expected to culture particular areas at specified intervals or to report to the committee occasionally on the infection control policies implemented within the dietary department. A sample infection control checklist for the dietary department is shown below.

1. Refrigerator and freezer temperatures are checked and recorded twice daily, as soon as the kitchen is opened and right before closing.
2. Refrigerator temperatures do not exceed 40° F; freezer temperatures do not exceed 32° F.
3. Hot foods are maintained at 145° F or above.
4. Cold foods are held at 45° F or below.
5. Fresh fruits and vegetables are washed thoroughly before use.
6. Dry foods are stored off the floor.
7. Dry storage areas are 69–72° F.
8. Separation of clean and dirty functions is maintained in food preparation and dishwashing areas.
9. Dishwashing temperatures are 140° F or above for washing; 180° F or above for drying.
10. Equipment is cleaned and sanitized between uses.
11. Employees with respiratory illnesses, boils, diarrhea, or other contagious diseases are not allowed to work.
12. Trays and plate covers and bases are cleaned thoroughly between uses.
13. Tray cards and holders are cleaned regularly.
14. All ingredients for mixed salads and sandwich fillings are prepared from refrigerated ingredients.
15. Range top and drip pans are cleaned daily.
16. Ovens are wiped out daily and cleaned thoroughly weekly.
17. The steamtable is cleaned with de-scaler two times per week.
18. Coffee pots are cleaned weekly.
19. Sinks are cleaned daily.
20. Dishroom floors are swept and mopped daily, cleaned with special cleaner two times per week.
21. The dishroom is washed monthly.
22. The range hood, filters, drains, and vents are cleaned monthly.
23. Tray carts are cleaned weekly.
24. Disposable gloves are worn when handling food.
25. Hairnets or restraints are worn by all employees.
26. Dining room tables are sanitized after each meal.
27. All leftovers are placed in the cooler, covered, labeled, and dated; discarded if not used within three days.
28. Patients' water pitchers are washed weekly.
29. Frozen foods are thawed in refrigerator.

30. Patient water glasses are washed daily.
31. Trash containers are emptied each shift or as needed.

Pharmacy

The purpose of the pharmacy committee is to advise the facility on policies regarding evaluation, selection, procurement, distribution, use, safety practices, and other matters pertaining to drugs in the facility. This committee also recommends and assists in the formation of programs designed to educate the professional staff on matters related to drugs and drug practices.

The committee generally consists of the facility pharmacist, the director of nursing, the administrator, and a physician. Dietary may or may not be represented, although it obviously should be. With the current focus on food/drug interactions, the dietitian has a real opportunity to establish a place on the committee. These meetings also offer a chance to build a good working relationship with the consulting or in-house pharmacist. Such contacts are often beneficial for both parties.

Here again, time (cost) constraints may be a problem. Discuss the benefits of your potential input with the administrator when negotiating more time in the facility. Opportunities such as this demonstrate yet another reason why dietary consultants should sometimes concentrate on increasing time in existing accounts rather than seeking additional facilities.

Safety

Some facilities organize safety committees to develop programs and establish protocol for compliance with state and federal regulations pertaining to employee safety. The safety committee is instrumental in identifying possible occupational hazards and instituting corrective action to control accidents and minimize employee injuries.

Representatives of all departments within the facility should sit on the committee since there are potential risks associated with jobs in each department.

Although protocols may vary, committee members may be asked to survey their respective departments prior to the meeting and to report results of the survey to the committee. A sample checklist devised for this purpose is shown below.

1. Personnel
    a. Supportive, closed toe and heel, nonslip sole shoes worn by all employees
    b. No loose sleeves worn by employees working with grinders and mixers
    c. Only approved jewelry worn
    d. Hairnets worn

2. Kitchen
   a. Heavier and bulkier items stored on lower shelves
   b. Food containers covered unless in use
   c. Clear, easy access to all fire equipment
   d. No items protruding into aisles or shelves
   e. Light bulbs guarded
   f. No stock items stacked too high or improperly
   g. Stockrooms properly ventilated
   h. Proper lifting procedures demonstrated and in use
   i. Floors free from spills, grease, and clutter
   j. Adequate lighting in all areas
3. Dishroom
   a. Floors dry and free of clutter
   b. Dishes properly stored
   c. Proper techniques utilized with disposal and dishmachine
   d. Chemicals properly labeled and stored
4. Food preparation operations
   a. Only dry potholders or mitts used when handling hot utensils
   b. Minimum amounts of water used in cooking to avoid spills and boiling over
   c. Range tops and ventilation hoods free of grease
   d. Handles of cooking utensils turned away from edge of range
   e. Oven doors closed when not in use
   f. Oven clean and free of food particles
5. Equipment usage
   a. Machinery not operated with wet hands
   b. Proper use and cleaning of equipment in evidence
   c. Knives used and stored properly
   d. Dishes and glassware properly stored, not stacked too high
   e. Chipped or cracked utensils discarded immediately
   f. Carts and racks not overloaded
   g. Carts and racks pushed, not pulled
   h. Equipment in good repair

Any problems identified by the survey should be discussed and corrective action implemented. Problems noted may also pinpoint areas in need of further inservice efforts by the department head. The consulting dietitian should review the minutes of this meeting or discuss the meeting with the dietary manager to develop continuing education programs appropriate to the needs of the department. Examples of possible areas in need of review include proper lifting techniques, handling of knives, and the importance of learning the correct methods to use to operate and clean equipment in the department.

In summary, the consulting dietitian should become aware of the various committees within the facility that require representation by the dietary department. Each committee offers unique opportunities to develop effective programs and protocols necessary to the safe, efficient operation of the dietary department as well as the opportunity to enhance the image of the professional consulting dietitian.

COMMUNICATING WITH RESIDENTS

Although the entire health care institution revolves around care of the patient, it is sometimes the patient himself with whom there is the least direct contact once the initial assessment is completed. Care must be taken to maintain a personal relationship with as many of the patients as possible. To do this, the consultant must consider what opportunities are available and plan to create new opportunities as time allows.

If the consultant is involved with care plans it is good policy to visit patients individually as they come up for review. This is usually quarterly but may be sooner if a patient's condition indicates the need for more frequent revision of the plan. During this visit the consultant can talk with the patient about any problems experienced with the diet and can also observe any physical changes such as weight loss that may have become evident since the previous visit. Personal contact helps establish a rapport with the patient and puts the consultant in tune with the patient's perceptions of his or her nutritional care.

Another opportunity for one-to-one contact comes during routine meal observation, which should occur no less frequently than once a month. Although the consultant will be able to evaluate the appearance of the meal, the correctness of the diet, and so forth, it is still necessary to know the patient's perception to have the complete picture. Here again, personal contact gives the consultant an opportunity to establish a rapport with the patients and to build an atmosphere of caring and concern.

The yearly assessment offers a third occasion to visit each resident and to evaluate acceptance or tolerance of the diet and impressions of the meal service as a whole. Much can change from year to year. It is easy to overlook long-term residents who may be unwilling to talk about the meal service or diet unless asked directly.

If the facility has a residents' council, council meetings provide an avenue to meet with several of the patients at once and to obtain suggestions for meal planning and menu changes. Menus are often better accepted when patients have direct input in their development. Resident council meetings also offer a chance to explain principles of therapeutic diets, to update the patients' knowledge of nutrition, or to discuss current advances in the field.

Finally, the consultant dietitian may increase patient contact by providing one-to-one patient diet counseling as needed or by offering a weekly or monthly class for patients interested in updating their nutrition knowledge. Providing these classes and opening them to the public would make this opportunity an excellent marketing tool for both the consulting dietitian and the health care institution.

These suggestions are just a few ways to increase direct patient contact. Opportunities abound! Be original and never lose sight of the fact that the patients are what the health care business is about.

REFERENCES

Benedict, Sharon. 1975. *Medicare care evaluation studies.* Pennsylvania: U.S. Department of Health, Education, and Welfare.

Medicare and Medicaid: Conditions of participation for long term care facilities. 1987. *Federal Register* 52:200.

6

Purchasing and
Cost Control

MENU DEVELOPMENT

Menu development is often an important aspect of the dietary consultant's job in health care. As most consultants know, it is a far more complicated job than meets the eye. A successful menu cycle may have a big impact on administrative or resident satisfaction with consultant services.

In some settings, it may be traditional for the dietary manager to write the menu cycle and for the dietary consultant to extend the cycle for therapeutic diets. Or, if the dietary manager is particularly capable, the manager may write and extend the cycle and have the consultant review and approve the finished product.

Regardless of who writes the menu, the consultant should assure that the following areas are addressed:

Clientele

The menu planner must define the market to be served. In the case of long-term care facilities, the market is primarily geriatric patients. For hospitals the market may be much broader or may be very specialized as in a hospital for children. Whatever the situation, the market must be clearly defined before the menu can be written.

Once the market has been established, certain questions must be answered. What are the nutritional needs and preferences of the market? Skilled care residents, who are very ill, require different menu considerations than those who are ambulatory and active. Menus designed for children and growing adults will be different from those planned for geriatric patients because eating habits have changed significantly over the last 30 years.

Additional factors relating to clientele include regional food preferences and regional menu patterns.

Regional food preferences refer to foods common to and popular within a certain geographic area. These are foods or food combinations around which many residents have planned their own meals, foods they feel comfortable with and enjoy. It is important to identify these foods and include them in the cycle.

Regional menu patterns refer to when the clientele are traditionally served the heaviest meal and how meals are timed. Do residents prefer the heaviest meal at noon or in the evening? Are they used to a "full breakfast" at sunrise or a continental breakfast at 9 A.M.? Are special menus expected on Sundays? These questions must be considered and answered before menus can be developed.

There are other questions to be considered:

1. Do residents retire early? If so, they may prefer a light evening meal.
2. Are residents active well into the evening, perhaps receiving visitors or participating in an activity? If so, a heavier evening meal or a substantial snack at bedtime may be needed.
3. Does lunch follow soon after breakfast (3 to 4 hours)? If so, residents may not be hungry for a large lunch and lighter fare may be preferable.

The Number Served, Including Those on Therapeutic Diets

Two others factors to be considered by the menu planner are the number of people to be served and the number of therapeutic diets in the facility.

The number to be served will influence the types of foods on the menu. For example, it may be possible to prepare 25 fried eggs but not 200. Volume may have an impact on the degree of variety possible in the cycle.

By the same token, if a facility has a large number of residents on therapeutic diets, the menu should contain simpler meals consisting of foods easily adapted for a variety of diets. In this way regular menus can be easily modified to meet a variety of patient needs without placing undue strain on the dietary department. This is especially important when staffing or equipment is limited.

Budget

The budgetary goals of the administration must be your goals as well. It would be foolish to begin a menu cycle without consideration of these goals and a plan to stay within financial boundaries.

Know how much you have to spend. A daily log of food expenditures is an invaluable tool. Weekly totals allow the manager to see what has been spent and to calculate how much is still available.

Before beginning a new menu, take time to review food invoices and note any items that have become too expensive. Since market prices for food can fluctuate from month to month, this review must be ongoing. Regular price review with appropriate menu adjustments keeps menus cost effective.

The menu planner must also be knowledgeable about price per serving. This figure may be much higher than it appears for some items. Chicken is a good example. At $0.80/lb. chicken appears to be an inexpensive entrée, but what does it actually cost to serve a piece of chicken? If an average chicken weighs 2.5 lb. the cost of each chicken is $2.00. Each chicken serves four people for an average portion cost of $0.50. Compare this to a portion cost of $0.26 for five 3-oz. servings of ground beef at $1.30/lb. Cost per serving cannot always be based entirely on cost per pound. Some meats, like chicken, have a high percentage of waste. Learn to think in terms of yield.

By the same token, a serving of fruit for dessert may cost double that of a serving of cake with icing. If the fruit is not necessary to meet the recommended daily allowance on a given day, cake is more cost effective. Less expensive desserts can be used to balance out more expensive entrées for some menus and to add variety to menus.

All of these factors will have an impact on food cost and are an integral part of the menu planning process.

Equipment

Before beginning a menu cycle it is imperative to consider the equipment available. The planner must keep a mental image of the equipment when planning each meal or the consequences could be disastrous.

Care must be taken to utilize all equipment and not to overload any one piece. If the menu includes four items that require oven space and the facility only has one or two ovens, several things can happen. The menu may be modified by the cook, or several of the items will be prepared too early and will not be at peak quality when served.

The available equipment will also affect the variety of preparation that can be planned. Planning batter-dipped fish or French fries when the facility has no deep fat fryer can cause a hardship on the staff if they try to improvise. It can also result in poor quality products prepared inappropriately. In the examples considered here, when no deep fat fryer is available, the menu planner should specify "oven-baked batter-dipped fish" or "oven ready French fries." There are versions of these products developed for oven preparation and the consultant should first confirm their availability before including them in the cycle.

Staffing

Consideration must also be given to dietary staffing. First, evaluate the staffing pattern. If staffing is heavier for the morning shift, plan the heavier meals during this shift and have a lighter evening meal when staffing is reduced. If staffing on both shifts is equal, the choice can be made according to resident preference.

If resident preference is contrary to the present staffing pattern, consider altering the pattern. Try not to get into the habit of doing things only because "we've always done it that way." Be receptive to new procedures and ideas that may increase the effectiveness of the department.

Consider staffing when choosing specific menu items as well. If only one cook is scheduled for breakfast, preparing fried eggs for each resident may prove extremely difficult. This in turn may result in a poorly prepared meal or in the cook's ignoring the menu altogether and preparing something simpler.

Meeting with the dietary staff prior to menu planning may make it possible to avoid past mistakes and may yield valuable information. The end result can be greater menu compliance and fewer substitutions.

Dietary staff members will also be able to point out items from the present cycle that are not well accepted or are difficult to prepare, thus allowing the menu planner to avoid these items on the new cycle.

Distribution of Work

When writing menus always consider the impact of each day on the next. Although one day's menu may appear appropriate for staffing and equipment available, pre-preparation required for the following day may cause an overload on staff or equipment.

Season

Good, cost-effective menus are in sync with the current season, making use of foods that are plentiful. Season also affects resident acceptance. Heavy meals may not be well accepted in summer months when lighter fare is more desirable. Menus should be changed or revised at least twice a year to incorporate seasonal food changes.

Recipes

It would be foolish to plan meals the cook does not know how to prepare. The menu planner must either plan menus based on the file of existing recipes or furnish recipes for new items on the cycle.

When reviewing recipes the consultant should determine whether the available recipes yield amounts appropriate for the facility in which they are used.

If amounts are not appropriate, the cook may not be capable of adjusting the recipe satisfactorily and may prepare too much or too little food. In an attempt to modify the recipe amount, mistakes may be made leading to a poor quality product.

Standardized recipes are essential in a well-run food service. In addition to insuring quality control, they also contribute to cost containment. Using standardized recipes, a manager knows exactly what to order for each recipe. With specific instructions for each item on the menu, the cook can prepare unfamiliar foods and still obtain a quality product. This becomes especially important when training a new cook who is not familiar with the menu. With standardized recipes the quality of the food will be the same no matter who is cooking, and leftovers will be minimized.

Any recipe can be standardized. If a particularly talented cook claims to have a better recipe than the one being used, test the recipe the next time it comes up on the menu and, if it is better, standardize it. Some of the best recipes are obtained in this manner.

Portion Control

Menus should be specific about what is to be cooked for each diet to prevent varying and sometimes inaccurate interpretation. Portion sizes for each menu item should be stated in terms that correspond with the serving utensil to be used. For example:

1 egg—#16 dipper
Vegetable—#8 dipper (or 4-oz. spoodle)
Cooked cereal—6-oz. ladle

The serving size for meats should be listed in ounces. In cases where meats must be sliced, a commercial meat slicer should always be used. Before the entire piece of meat is sliced, several representative slices should be taken, weighed, and the slicer adjusted to the correct thickness for the portion size desired. For instance, if a 4-oz. serving of ham is specified, there are three alternatives for slicing: one 4-oz. slice, two 2-oz. slices, or four 1-oz. slices. In general, several thinner slices are more attractive and easier to chew (if this is a consideration). Several slices allow better plate coverage.

Aesthetic Factors

When all is said and done, the simple truth of menu writing is that the meal must look good to be good. Residents must be persuaded to try new menus and it is here that aesthetic factors become important.

Color

Many different aspects of the appearance of the meal combine to make it look good or bad. First, contrast in color is necessary to prevent the meal from looking too bland. One food may determine the success or failure of the look. For example, consider the following menu:

Roast pork with gravy
Cornbread dressing
Cabbage

This meal, although tasty, is colorless and bland. Cabbage is a poor choice for the vegetable because it provides no contrast in color. Peas would be a better alternative, particularly frozen peas that have been carefully prepared to preserve color and texture. With this menu change, the whole appearance of the meal is altered.

In some instances, when the menu writer is trying to plan for traditional combinations of foods, this is a difficult rule to follow. A boiled dinner of corned beef, cabbage and potatoes is traditional but colorless. In this situation a garnish may provide a contrast in color while preserving the traditional food combination. Two spiced apple rings or a sprig of fresh parsley would add color to the plate. A wide variety of garnishes is not necessary. A few carefully selected items will compliment many meals. Examples of versatile garnishes include parsley, tomato slices or wedges, lemon, spiced apple rings, and leaf lettuce. Using a limited number of items reduces both storage problems and waste.

Consistency and Texture

Consistency and texture must also be considered. If cream of potato soup is served as an entrée, applesauce and ice cream would be poor accompaniments. All are of a similar consistency and texture and the menu lacks eye appeal and interest. Changes in the fruit and dessert are necessary to provide variety in consistency and texture.

A revised menu might be:

> *Cream of potato soup*
> *Tomatoes vinaigrette on leaf lettuce*
> *Chocolate brownie with icing*

The varying textures and consistencies add the variety needed.

Shape

Variety in the shape of foods on the plate is also necessary to maximize eye appeal. Consider this menu:

> *Fried chicken planks*
> *French green beans*
> *Julienne beets in orange sauce*

All the foods are cut into strips resulting in a less than pleasing combination. All that is needed are a few changes in the shape of the foods to make the menu acceptable. Consider the following changes:

> *Fried chicken*
> *French green beans*
> *Sliced beets in orange sauce*

Taste

Certain flavor combinations compliment one another and have become traditional in menu writing: Corned beef and cabbage, sausage and fried apples, hot dogs and baked beans are a few examples. When these foods are served together, each enhances the flavor of the other.

It is important to be aware of and to utilize these special combinations when planning a menu cycle. Each region of the country uses certain flavor combinations that are unique to the area.

It is also important to consider what combinations of foods do not work. Avoid using too many foods of similar taste in the same menu. Balance out strong flavored foods with bland foods. Use rich foods sparingly in combination with lighter, fresh tasting foods.

Make your staff aware of the importance of aesthetic factors of food. Here are several suggestions for increasing staff involvement in this area:

1. Encourage the cook and dietary staff to taste food during preparation and make suggestions.
2. Develop a quality assurance program that has dietary staff members rating meals at periodic intervals.
3. Plan an inservice on aesthetic factors using examples from food magazines —"A picture is worth a thousand words!"

Additions to the Menu

A wise menu planner leaves nothing to chance. Good menus are complete and include all foods to be prepared by the department on any given day. This includes garnishes and nourishments.

Garnishes

Garnishes should be carefully planned to assure that they are both appropriate and cost effective. Including them on the menu will accomplish the following:

1. Assure that the garnish compliments the meal. You might be surprised to find that the cook may not choose appropriate garnishes when these are not specified.
2. Make ordering easier since it is clear what garnishes are needed for each meal.
3. Make certain that garnishes will actually be used since they are written as part of the menu.

Nourishments

Nourishments can be a tremendous drain on dietary finances if not carefully planned. Planning them into the menu is necessary to assure that the needs of the resident are being met in an appropriate manner. It assures that the nourishments will be ordered in a timely manner and be available when needed. It also enables the menu planner to avoid repetition in this area.

Before planning nourishments, take time to consider what the per serving cost will be. Remember that they must fit into the total budget for the day. It is also important to maintain good communication lines to determine if snacks are being accepted and to observe if they are being distributed appropriately.

Selecting a Cycle

A cycle menu is one that repeats at definite intervals. It may be as short as one week or as long as eight weeks. Length may be determined by precedent or may be negotiable. Hospitals function without difficulty on shorter cycles since most patients generally stay only a few days. Long-term care facilities require longer cycles since residents of these facilities generally stay for long periods of time, making variety more of a concern.

A cycle may be selective or nonselective. Selective cycles contain two or more foods in each category, allowing the resident a choice. This type of menu is generally well accepted and contributes to better resident satisfaction with the food service. A selective menu, however, is more expensive to offer since it requires more labor to prepare as well as skill in forecasting choices. Purchasing is also more difficult when items must be ordered and exact amounts are not known.

Nonselective cycles are set menus rotated at intervals. No choices are available although it is possible to incorporate a limited number of choices into the cycle, such as a choice of entrées or a choice of desserts.

Preplanned menus have several advantages. They are cost effective since forecasting is not a problem. They are "labor friendly" in that employees become familiar with menus and recipes and can standardize routines. They require less of the manager's time for purchasing. They can, however, become monotonous if not reviewed and revised frequently. It is good practice to run a new cycle twice, make revisions based on resident acceptance, and review the cycle again at set intervals. This increases resident satisfaction since unpopular menus and recipes are removed or revised in a timely manner.

Writing the Menu

After the menu planner has reviewed all contributing factors for menu writing and chosen a cycle length, the actual writing must begin. The following routine will make the process easier.

1. Choose a quiet place away from distractions.
2. Develop a list of recipes to be included in the cycle, making sure to incorporate a few new recipes in each cycle.
3. Have all necessary materials on hand. It is helpful to use a menu planning sheet, particularly one that displays the entire cycle. An example of a four-week cycle planner is shown in Appendix B.
4. First, plan all entrées in the cycle, making sure that food types are varied on consecutive days. For example, do not plan meatloaf one day and spaghetti with meat balls the next. Be specific about the method of preparation.
5. Next, plan all vegetables, pasta, and other side dishes. If this planning is done in one sitting, it is easier to avoid repeating foods at too frequent

intervals. The planner can make better use of traditional food combinations and it allows appropriate spacing of food types such as poultry and potatoes.
6. Plan breads and desserts, making fruit a dessert whenever necessary to meet standards for recommended daily allowances (RDA).
7. Plan nourishments and snacks.
8. Choose garnishes that compliment the meals.

The completed menu should then be reviewed for mistakes or revisions and recopied onto daily menu sheets. Be sure to specify the exact methods of preparation as well as portion sizes for each item on the menu. The menus are now ready to extend for therapeutic diets.

The consultant may have access to a computer. A computer can be programmed to extend and print the menus, thus saving much of the consultant's time. Menu changes are also easily made when menus are computerized.

DIETARY BUDGET

The dietary department budget represents the second largest area of expenditures in any health care facility. As consultant dietitians, we have a responsibility in assisting the dietary manager and health care administrator in establishing a realistic but cost-effective budget for dietary services. The amount of involvement will vary depending on the ownership of the facility. If a consultant dietitian is working with an independently owned facility, more input in the actual budget preparation can be realized than if one is working in a multi-chain operated facility. Regardless of the degree of involvement, it is important for the dietitian to be aware of industry standards for dietary costs as well as the current pricing trends in the food distribution industry.

Establishing dietary budgets that will allow high quality meal production and meet the therapeutic needs of the residents, while complying with management needs for cost-effective budgets, is difficult and challenging. A response of "it cannot be done" is not acceptable when dealing with these groundrules. Health care facilities look to the dietitian for viable solutions in meeting all the parameters.

The dietary service budget includes raw food cost, expenditures for paper and chemical supplies, nourishment (supplement) cost, labor, and expenditures for equipment. Preparation of an annual budget including these costs is shown in Figure 6-1 (except equipment expenditures). Equipment costs are usually considered a capital expenditure and would not be calculated in the dietary annual operating budget.

To establish an annual raw food cost budget, eight items need to be considered:

1. Historical data—average food cost per patient day (ppd) per month from previous year or years
2. Current industry standards for per patient day food cost

ANNUAL BUDGET

The following sample budget is based on a 150-bed long-term care facility.

1. Total Meals: *54,750 patient days × 3.0 meals/day = 164,250 (94%) of total meals served annually
   10,680 employee meals × 1.00 = 10,680 (6%) of total meals served annually
   174,930

   (Average, 29 meals/day × 365 days)

   * Patient days = 150 bed (100% census × 365 days/year)

2. Projected nonpatient cash receipts From employees and guests
   $2.25 meal value × 1.125 increase × 10,680 meals = $27,033.75
   (Based on projected 12.5% increase of employee/guest meals for budget year)

3. Preparation of an Annual Budget

   a. Calculate current cost of each dietary category (food, supply, labor, supplements).
   b. Multiply current cost of each category by estimated percent of increase based on projected inflation factors provided by the health care industry or associated company or owner.
   c. Multiply projected costs by total meals served to patients and employees (as calculated in #1).
   d. Totals represent operating expenses of each dietary category as well as projected operating expenses for dietary department.
   e. % of costs is the estimated distribution cost of the total dietary operating expenses, based on each category. "Breakdown" of each dietary cost category shows what percentage of the budget represents a specific category.
   f. Cash receipts is the total revenue estimated (see #2) from employee/guest meals for the budgeted year.
   g. Net operating expenses–operating expenses (percent of each category cost × cash receipts). Net operating expenses includes the projected nonpatient revenue anticipated.

Description	Current Cost		Estimated Increase %		Estimated Cost		Total Meals		Operating Expenses		% of Costs[a]	Cash Receipts	Net Operating Expenses
Food	$ 0.95/meal	×	6	=	$ 1.01	×	174,930	=	$ 176,679	less	32	$ 27,034	$ 168,028
Labor	3.15/day	×	8	=	3.40	×	174,930	×	594,762	less	58	27,034	579,082
Supply (paper, chemical)	0.25/day	×	5	=	0.26	×	174,930	=	45,482	less	7	27,034	43,590
Other costs (supplement)	0.10/day	×	2	=	0.102	×	174,930	=	17,843	less	2	27,034	17,302
Total									$ 834,766				$ 808,002

[a] *Distribution* based on historical usage by category. Percentages are examples showing a "breakdown" of dietary costs; 58% of total dietary costs is labor.

Figure 6-1. Sample figures for an annual budget.

3. Inflation factor of food costs for budgeted year
4. Type of menu served (selective, nonselective)
5. Type of purchasing program available to facility
6. Caliber of menu selections offered (steak versus ground beef)
7. Budgeted resident census
8. Projected revenue generating projects

Each of these factors plays a significant role in establishing a realistic, workable budget. A facility cannot budget $2.35 ppd food cost without realizing the limitations it will place on the variety of menu items available for its resident population, especially if the facility is not involved in an aggressive purchasing program with a food distributor or health care purchasing group.

In order to forecast price increases of paper, chemical, and equipment supplies, dietary personnel need to survey vendors, purchasing agents, or other foodservice administrators to obtain recommended or predicted percentages of increases.

Services that can be used to estimate anticipated wage increases for dietary staff include:

1. Federal and state government guidelines for wage increases
2. Current labor union predictions or demands in the area, if applicable
3. Health care facility guidelines for cost-of-living and merit raises
4. Economic conditions in the region or state

Once each of these areas has been researched, the dietary service personnel (including the consultant dietitian) and administrator can prepare a workable budget. One way to establish the most workable budget for the facility and its needs is to evaluate levels of activity based on specific budget levels (Rose 1984):

Minimum: This level, below the current budget amount, is the point at which activity could not be reduced without ceasing to exist entirely: for example, 75 percent of the current budget amount.
Current: This level indicates the current budgeted level of activity.
Adjusted current: This level is the budget required to perform the current level of activity adjusted for inflation.
Highest (maximum): This level of activity represents a budget for new programs or activities to be performed. Administration usually will establish a limit, such as 125 percent of the current budgeted amount.

By evaluating dietary services and meal quality obtainable at each level of budget, assumed expectations by administration as well as dietary personnel are eliminated. When a dietary manager, dietary staff, and a consultant dietitian are able to participate in the budgeting process, greater commitment by each health care team member is exhibited.

Once the budget is established, especially for raw food cost, controlling food cost becomes the next concern. There are basically five areas in the cost control system in which concentration is needed: purchasing, receiving, record keeping, production, and inventory control.

Purchasing is a specialized, essential component of the dietary service department. Responsibility for this task is assumed by the foodservice manager with input by the facility's administration and the consultant dietitian. The manager must constantly reevaluate decisions to assure that they remain appropriate and meet the purchasing goals of a health care facility. The main goals are (1) meeting the nutritional needs of the residents and (2) meeting the financial requirements of the facility.

The nutritional needs of the residents are mandated by the residents' diet orders, minimum dietary requirements as established by state and federal licensure and regulation agencies, and the planned menu that incorporates the nutrient requirements. The menu cycle will provide the dietary manager with essential information to make wise purchasing decisions. Information obtainable from the menus includes

- Foods needed to be purchased daily for each meal
- Amounts of specific items needed
- Forms in which food items are required (fresh, frozen, whole, canned)
- Quality of product needed to meet federal specifications as well as the facility's need

The financial requirements should be well known by the dietary manager, especially if he or she is involved in the budget process. In addition to knowing the monthly food cost budget, a dietary manager should also know the percentage of budget allocated to each major food group category. Within a food cost budget, meat and other protein items (including supplements) usually account for 35 percent of food costs; frozen and grocery items, 40 percent; dairy products, 13 percent; bakery, 4 percent, and produce, 8 percent. By using these spending guidelines, a dietary manager can avoid potential purchasing problems.

Before purchasing can begin, a vendor must be chosen. Vendors can be selected by using a bid procedure or by weekly shopping. The bid procedure is the best way to obtain formal price quotes of food and supplies based on product categories and acceptable quality. This procedure also establishes expected vendor services, delivery schedules, and payment arrangements. Use of this procedure assures the manager that vendors are quoting items of equal quality. To ensure equality of bids, the following information needs to be forwarded to each vendor:

1. Products required—specifying grade of product, pack size, and manufacturer's brand name
2. Guaranteed pricing for products—weekly or monthly

3. Anticipated dollar volume of business on a weekly, monthly, or annual basis; or projected patient census on monthly, annual basis
4. Delivery requirements—number of deliveries needed weekly, monthly; hours acceptable for deliveries
5. Payment terms and discount for early payment
6. Assurance of program compliance by facility
7. Request for pricing structure (Establish the type of price structure on which the bid is made. A cost-plus structure includes the vendor cost of the product, plus freight, plus a percentage to cover the vendor's cost of doing business, and profit. A quote can also be based on the foregoing, plus the percentage markup for delivery and profit.)
8. Effective dates of the contract (Rose 1984)
9. Method of placing orders—via marketing associate or telephone

Shopping is price comparison by line item based on weekly, monthly, or quarterly quotes. Using this system, the dietary manager can establish product requirements and receive price quotes by telephone, personal visit, or written proposal. Awards can be made by line item, product category, or the entire order. This is a less formal system, but does allow the manager flexibility to take advantage of vendors' specials. This method requires more of the manager's time because of the need for constant evaluation of bids and placing of orders. When evaluating the most effective bid system, a manager needs to weigh the costs versus the benefits. Will the savings realized by the shopping method outweigh the additional time (labor hours) required by management to use this procedure? Will the acceptance of a formal bid allow a vendor slowly to increase prices without notice by management? Price comparison still needs to be part of the purchasing system even with a formal purchasing program. Current monthly prices need to be compared with the previous month's to ensure that pricing is consistent and not out of line with bid guidelines and market trends.

Once bids are received, especially using a formal bid system, a primary vendor is usually selected. A primary vendor is one who meets all the bid criteria and can supply a full line of food, supplies, and equipment to a facility. To qualify for services and pricing offered by the vendor to a facility, the dietary manager must purchase at least 80 percent of total volume from the selected vendor. Using a prime vendor allows facility "price breaks" on items due to volume of purchases; increases the likelihood of obtaining new products or carrying a specific product line because of guaranteed business, and allows the facility to utilize special services such as menu analysis or costing at a nominal fee. It also reduces the amount of time spent by a dietary manager ordering and receiving purchases.

By using the shopping method and utilizing several vendors, a manager can take advantage of the competition between food distributors to obtain lower pricing. Also, deliveries may be more conveniently spaced and price "creeping" prevented.

In addition to the two direct purchasing programs discussed, a third option is for health care facilities to participate in an indirect group purchasing program. By participating in a group purchasing program, facilities can increase their purchasing clout, and are able to obtain lower prices. This type of program is especially beneficial to the individually owned facility that would have little bargaining power standing alone. In a group purchasing program, the formal bid procedure is handled by the organization. Decisions on vendor selection and some product lines are no longer made by the individual facility. Group purchasing has become popular in recent years, increasing the opportunity for any facility to participate regardless of location. Information on group purchasing programs can be obtained through state associations of health care facilities, homes for the aging, or hospital associations.

Once a vendor and purchasing program have been chosen, the dietary manager must establish good purchasing techniques. The consultant dietitian should assist the manager in developing an efficient, organized system. Key points to remember when organizing a purchasing system include the following:

1. Organize purchases. An up-to-date inventory of stock available plus a completed purchase guide (a complete list of items needed to meet the menu guidelines) are essential sources of information needed to make wise purchasing decisions.
2. Use a purchase order form (or purchase guide) to record orders. This form can also serve as a checklist when orders are received to assure that food items delivered match the order placed.
3. Always use specific product code numbers for items to be purchased or specific quality desired. A sales representative should not become part of the decision-making process when placing an order. Recommendations from a sales representative may be helpful but the final decision is the responsibility of the dietary manager.
4. Know approximate yields of various can sizes. This knowledge is important when evaluating case prices versus cost per serving. For example, whole canned tomatoes are less expensive per case than stewed tomatoes. However, the cost per serving of the whole tomatoes is greater than the stewed tomatoes due to poor yield.
5. Use standardized buying guides to assist in purchasing food items, especially meat. These guides provide helpful information regarding the quantity of specific foods to buy based on the patient census. Included in this chapter are four buying guides that have proven to be beneficial.
   A. *Protein Evaluation of Meat and Meat Alternatives:* A guide provided by the Indiana State Board of Health. It indicates ounces of ready-to-eat protein per pound of meat type. See Table 6-1.
   B. *Meat Purchasing Guide for 2-Ounce Yield:* A summary of the information provided in the Indiana State Board of Health protein evaluation guide. Total poundage of meat needed per patient census level is also provided in Table 6-2.
   C. *Food Buying Guide:* A summary of serving yields per unit purchased for

Table 6-1. Protein Evaluation of Meat and Meat Alternatives

Fresh, Frozen, or Processed Meats Poultry, Fish	Purchase Unit	Ready-To-Eat Protein (oz.)
Beef		
Dried, chipped	lb.	20
Ground beef	lb.	12
Liver	lb.	12
Roasts: brisket, chuck, rump w/bone	lb.	9
boneless	lb.	12
Round - w/bone	lb.	11
boneless	lb.	12
Short ribs	lb.	4
Steak, cubed	lb.	10
Stew meat	lb.	10
Pork		
Bacon	lb.	5
Chops—w/bone	lb.	9
Cured ham—w/bone	lb.	11
boneless	lb.	12
Sausage	lb.	8
Spareribs	lb.	4
Tenderloin roasts—fresh ham	lb.	12
Boston butt, picnic—w/bone	lb.	9
boneless	lb.	11
Lamb		
Chops, shoulder	lb.	9
Ground	lb.	11
Leg or shoulder roast—w/bone	lb.	9
boneless	lb.	12
Veal		
Chops	lb.	10
Cutlets	lb.	12
Roast—w/bone	lb.	7
boneless	lb.	11
Steak, chopped or cubed	lb.	10
Chicken		
Fryers	lb.	5
Chicken parts		
Breast halves	lb.	8
Legs	lb.	7
Thighs	lb.	8
Backs	lb.	3
Wings	lb.	5
Stewing, ready to cook	lb.	7
Turkey		
Whole, ready to cook	lb.	6
Breasts or thighs	lb.	8
Legs	lb.	6

Table 6-1. *(Continued)*

Fresh, Frozen, or Processed Meats Poultry, Fish	Purchase Unit	Ready-To-Eat Protein (oz.)
Cooked, diced	lb.	15
Roast or roll		
Ready to cook	lb.	11
Cooked	lb.	15
Fish		
Fillets	lb.	10
Breaded fish portions	lb.	8
Miscellaneous meats		
Frankfurters (all meat)	lb.	16
Luncheon meats (all meat)	lb.	16

Meat, Poultry, Fish Products (Canned-Frozen)

Barbecued beef, lamb, pork	lb.	7
Beef hash	lb.	5
Beef stew	lb.	2
Beef w/gravy	lb.	8
Beef, natural juices	lb.	11
Chicken or turkey, boned	lb.	14
Chicken salad	lb.	3
Chicken w/gravy	lb.	5
Creamed chicken	lb.	2
Chili con carne w/beans	lb.	5
Corned beef	lb.	16
Ham salad	lb.	4
Salmon	16-oz. can	13
Tuna	60–66 1/2-oz. can	58
Tuna	6–7-oz. can	6

Meat Alternatives

Cheese		
American, cheddar, Swiss	lb.	16
Cheese food or spread	lb.	8
Cottage	lb.	16
Eggs		
Fresh	doz.	12
Frozen	lb.	9
Peanut butter, beans, peas:		
Peanut butter	lb.	14
Beans, dried	lb.	12
Beans, canned	no. 10 can	24
Bean soup (reconstituted)	54-oz. can	11
	10-oz. can	2
Peas, dried	lb.	12
Pea soup (reconstituted)	50-oz. can	5

Table 6-2. Meat Purchasing Guide for 2-Ounce Yield

	Amount To Purchase To Serve										
	50	70	100	110	120	140	150	160	170	180	200
Beef											
Ground beef (12 oz./lb. ready-to-eat protein)	8.5	12	17	18.5	20	23	25	27	28.5	30	33.5
Liver	8.5	12	17	18.5	20	23	25	27	28.5	30	33.5
Beef (for roasting)	8.5	12	17	18.5	20	23	25	27	28.5	30	33.5
Gooseneck (boneless)	8.5	12	17	18.5	20	23	25	27	28.5	30	33.5
Cubed steak (10 oz./lb. ready-to-eat protein)	10	14	20	22	24	28	30	32	34	36	40
Fresh stew meat	10	14	20	22	24	28	30	32	34	36	40
Dried chipped beef (20 oz./lb. ready to eat)	5	7	10	11	12	14	15	16	17	18	20
Beef, canned (natural juices) (11 oz./lb. ready-to-eat protein)	9	13	18.5	20	22	25.5	27.5	29.5	31	33	36.5
Pork											
Pork roasts (11 oz./lb. ready-to-eat protein)	9	13	18.5	20	22	25.5	27.5	29.5	31	33	36.5
Cured ham (boneless)	8.5	12	17	18.5	20	23	25	27	28.5	30	33.5
Pork loin or tenderloin (12 oz./lb ready-to-eat protein)	8.5	12	17	18.5	20	23	25	27	28.5	30	33.5
Sausage (8 oz./lb. ready-to-eat protein)	12.5	17.5	25	27.5	30	35	37.5	40	42.5	45	50
Luncheon meats (all meats) (16 oz./lb. ready-to-eat protein)	6.5	8.5	12.5	14	15	17.5	19	20	21.5	22.5	25
Frankfurters (all meat)	6.5	8.5	12.5	14	15	17.5	19	20	21.5	22.5	25
Poultry											
Chicken fryers (16 to a chicken) (5 oz./lb. ready-to-eat protein)	20	28	40	44	48	56	60	64	68	72	80
Turkey (whole ready to cook) (6 oz./lb. ready-to-eat protein)	17	23.5	33.5	37	40	47	50	53.5	57	60	67
Turkey roll (pre-cooked) (15 oz./lb. ready-to-eat protein)	7	9.5	13.5	15	16	19	20	21.5	23	24	27
Boned chicken (canned)/ turkey (14 oz./lb. ready-to-eat protein)	7.5	10	14.5	16	17.5	20	21.5	23	24.5	26	29
Fish and other seafoods											
Fish fillets (10 oz./lb. ready-to-eat protein)	10	14	20	22	24	28	30	32	34	36	40
Fish portions (breaded) (8 oz./lb. ready-to-eat protein)	12.5	17.5	25	27.5	30	35	37.5	40	42.5	45	50
Salmon (16 oz. can) (13 oz./ can ready-to-eat protein)	8	11	15.5	17	18.5	21.5	23.5	25	26.5	28	31
Tuna (60–66.5 oz. can) (58 oz./can ready-to-eat protein)	8	11	15.5	17	18.5	21.5	23.5	25	26.5	28	31

foods other than meat. Recommended amounts to purchase per patient census levels are listed in Table 6-3.

D. *Purchasing Fresh Fruits and Vegetables:* A summary of percent yields, weights, and amounts to purchase for a 100-patient census is shown in Table 6-4.

6. Do not develop personal friendships with sales representatives. Friendships with these individuals tend to carry an obligation to buy "at least something." The buyer must remain objective at all times, buying only those items best for the facility.

7. Be aware of marketing trends and buy accordingly. Even though another person may be responsible for pricing menu items, the manager is responsible for the information and should review it monthly. Cost of frequently used items such as milk, bread, and produce should be known at all times since these prices fluctuate weekly.

8. Be aware that responsibility for purchasing should be limited to the dietary manager and his or her assistant. Anyone assuming the responsibility even temporarily should be trained not to deviate from established procedures.

9. Purchase food items according to appropriate use. Lower grade fruits and vegetables are as wholesome as higher grades, but have some cosmetic imperfections. Lower grade fruits and vegetables are better buys for casseroles, salads, and Jello molds, where imperfections in size or shape are not discernible.

10. Consider placing orders by phone. This can reduce the amount of time necessary to place orders, eliminate "visiting" with the sales representative, and serve as a bargaining point on overall pricing since the vendor cost is reduced.

RECEIVING

Accurate receiving techniques are as important as a good purchasing system. Without receiving controls in place, considerable money can be lost weekly. Since receiving of deliveries should be handled by the manager or a key employee, it is important to specify a delivery time that can fit into the manager's daily schedule.

When a delivery arrives, every item received must be checked against the invoice and purchase guide. The quality, quantity, and price of the item ordered should exactly match the item received. Vendors should not be allowed to substitute for items not in stock unless the terms of exchange have been agreed upon previously. Terms of right to exchange may include the following (Breeding, Foster 1989):

1. The vendor will only substitute an item of equal or higher quality at the same price as the item being replaced.

2. The vendor will call the manager prior to delivery for notification of a shortage and receive authorization for a substitute.

Table 6-3. Food Buying Guide

Food	Size of Standard Serving	Servings per Unit Purchased	Amount To Purchase To Serve					
			15	25	50	100	150	200
Bread								
White/whole wheat	1 slice	20 per 1 1/4 lb. loaf	3/4 loaf	1 1/4 loaves	2 1/2 loaves	5 loaves	7 1/2 loaves	10 loaves
		16 per 1 lb. loaf	1 loaf	2 loaves	4 loaves	8 loaves	12 loaves	16 loaves
		28 per 2 lb. loaf	1 loaf	1 loaf	2 loaves			
Rolls, Buns,	1	12 per doz.	1 1/4 doz.	2 1/4 doz.	4 1/4 doz.			
Hamburger	1–3 1/4"	24 per package	2/3 pkg.	1 1/4 pkg.	2 1/8 pkg.	4 1/4 pkg.	6 1/2 pkg.	8 1/2 pkg.
Hot dog	1–6"	30 per package	1/2 pkg.	1 pkg.	1 2/3 pkg.	3 1/3 pkg.	5 pkg.	6 2/3 pkg.
Cereals								
Dry	1/2 cup	18 per lb.	1 lb.	1 1/2 lb.	3 1/8 pkg.	6 1/4 lb.	9 lb.	11 1/4 lb.
		41 per 2 lb. 4 1/2 oz.		2/3 pkg.	1 1/4 pkg.	2 1/2 pkg.	3 3/4 pkg.	5 pkg.
		45 per 2 lb. 8 oz.		2/3 pkg.	1 1/8 pkg.	2 1/4 pkg.	3 3/8 pkg.	4 1/2 pkg.
Cooked	1/2 cup cooked	20 per 1 lb. cooked	1 lb.	1 1/4 lb.	2 1/2 lb.	5 lb.	7 1/2 lb.	10 lb.
		42 per 42 oz. box		2/3 box	1 1/4 box	2 1/2 box	3 3/4 box	5 box
Rice, macaroni, Noodles	1/2 cup cooked	17 per lb. cooked	1 lb.	1 1/2 lb.	3 lb.	6 lb.	9 lb.	12 lb.
Spaghetti	1/2 cup cooked	19 per lb. cooked	3/4 lb.	1 1/4 lb.	2 1/2 lb.	5 lb.	7 1/2 lb.	10 lb.
Dairy Products								
Milk	1/2 cup	16 per 1/2 gal.	1/2 gal.	1 1/2 (1/2 gal.)	3 1/2 (1/2 gal.)	7 (1/2 gal.)	10 (1/2 gal.)	13 (1/2 gal.)
		32 per gal.	1/2 gal.	3/4 gal.	1 3/4 gal.	3 1/2 gal.	5 gal.	6 1/2 gal.
	1 cup	16 per gal.	1 gal.	1 1/2 gal.	3 1/2 gal.	7 gal.	10 gal.	13 gal.
Cottage cheese	1/4 cup	8 per lb.	2 lb.	3 1/8 lb.	6 1/4 lb.	12 1/2 lb.	18 3/4 lb.	25 lb.
		40 per #5 cont.	1/3 cont.	2/3 cont.	1 1/4 cont.	2 1/2 cont.	3 3/4 cont.	5 cont.
	1/4 cup	4 per lb.	4 lb.	6 2/3 lb.	12 1/2 lb.	25 lb.	37 1/2 lb.	50 lb.
		20 per #5 cont.	2/3 cont.	1 1/3 cont.	2 1/2 cont.	5 cont.	7 1/2 cont.	10 cont.
Ice cream	1/2 cup	12 per doz.	1 1/4 doz.	2 1/16 doz.	4 1/8 doz.	8 1/4 doz.	12 3/8 doz.	16 2/3 doz.
	1/2 cup	25 per 1 lb.	2 qt.	1 gal.	2 gal.	4 gal.	6 gal.	8 lb.
Margarine	1 tsp.	96 per lb.	1/4 lb.	1/4 lb.	1/2 lb.	1 lb.	1 1/2 lb.	2 lb.

Quantities to purchase (amounts increase left to right across the six quantity columns)

Item	Serving size	Amount per container						
Groceries								
Canned fruit and vegetables	1/2 cup	7 per #2 1/2 can	2 can	3 1/2 can	4 can	5 can	6 can	7 can
		25 per #10 can	1/2 can	1 can	2 can			
Frozen vegetables	1/2 cup	10 per 2 lb pkg.	1 1/2 pkg.	2 1/2 pkg.	5 pkg.	8 pkg.	12 pkg.	16 pkg.
Broccoli, cauliflower, spinach, lima beans	1/2 cup	13 per 2 1/2 lb.	1 pkg.	2 pkg.	4 pkg.	10 pkg.	15 pkg.	20 pkg.
peas, corn, carrots	1/2 cup	5–6 per lb.	2–2 1/2 lb.	4–5 lb.	8–10 lb.	16–20 lb.	24–30 lb.	32–40 lb.
Miscellaneous								
French fries	8	20 per 4 lb. pkg.	3/4 pkg.	1 1/4 pkg.	2 1/2 pkg.	5 pkg.	7 1/2 pkg.	10 pkg.
Orange juice	1/2 cup	32 per 32 oz. can	1/2 can	1 can	1 2/3 cans	3 1/8 cans	4 2/3 cans	6 1/4 cans
Soup, tomato, mushroom	6 oz.	17 per #3 can	1 can	2 cans	3 cans	6 cans	9 cans	12 cans
Canned juice	1/2 cup	11 1/2 per #3 can	1 1/4 cans	2 1/4 cans	4 1/4 cans	8 1/2 cans	12 3/4 cans	17 cans
Potatoes, dehydrated sliced	1/2 cup	50 per 2 1/2 lb. pkg.	1/4 pkg.	1/2 pkg.	1 pkg.	2 pkg.	3 pkg.	4 pkg.
Miscellaneous								
Cake mixes, corn bread	1 piece (2 × 2 in.)	86 per 5 lb. box	1 lb.	1 1/2 lb.	3 lb.	1 1/8 boxes	1 3/4 boxes	2 1/3 boxes
Brownies, biscuits, muffins	1 square (2 × 2 in.)	100 per 5 lb. box	3/4 lb.	1 1/4 lb.	1/2 box	1 box	1 1/2 boxes	2 boxes
Pudding, regular	1/2 cup	81 per 4 1/2 lb. pkg.	1 lb.	1 1/2 lb.	3 lb.	1 1/4 pkg.	2 pkg.	2 1/2 pkg.
Pudding, instant	1/2 cup	40 per 2 lb. pkg.	1/4 pkg.	1/2 pkg.	1 1/2 pkg.	2 1/2 pkg.	3 3/4 pkg.	5 pkg.
Gelatin	1/2 cup	36 per 2 lb. pkg.	2/3 pkg.	1 pkg.	2 pkg.	4 pkg.	6 pkg.	8 pkg.
Eggnog mix	8 oz.	26 per 2 lb. pkg.	15 pkg.	25 pkg.				
Carnation Instant Breakfast	8 oz.	72 pkg. per case			3/4 case	1 1/2 cases	2 cases	2 3/4 cases
Milkshakes	8 oz.	36 per 1 1/2 lb. pkg.	2/3 lb.	1 lb.	1 1/2 pkg.	2 3/4 pkg.	4 1/2 pkg.	5 1/2 pkg.

Table 6-4. Purchasing Fresh Fruits and Vegetables

Vegetable/Fruit	% Waste	Measure	Approximate Measure	Amount to Purchase/100
Apples, A.P.	20	1 lb.	3–4 medium	30 lb. (1@)
Apples, A.P.		1.5 lb.	1 qt. sliced	20 lb.
Apples, diced 1.5" cubed, peeled		1 lb.	4 1/2 cups	14 lb.
Applesauce		1 lb.	2 cups	
Apricots, fresh		1 lb.	8 apricots	25 lb. (2@)
Asparagus, fresh		1 lb.	16–20 stalks	38 lb.
Bananas, A.P.	42	1 lb.	3 medium	17 lb. (1/2@)
Bananas, diced		1 lb.	2–2 1/2 cups	28 lb.
Beets, medium		1 lb.	3–4 beets	26 lb. topped
Beets, sliced, cooked		1 lb.	2 1/2 cups	20 lb.
Broccoli	38	1 lb.		35 lb.
Cabbage, A.P. shredded, cooked	20	1 lb.	1 1/2 cups	25 lb.
Cabbage, E.P. shredded		1 lb.	1 qt. lightly pck	
Cantaloupe	50	18 oz.	1 melon, 4.5" dia.	51 lb. (34 melons)
Carrots	20	1 lb.	4–5 medium	26 lb. topped
Carrots, diced		1 lb.	3–3 1/4 cups	
Carrots, ground raw, E.P.		1 lb.	3 cups	
Carrots, diced cooked		1 lb.	3 cups	
Cauliflower, head	69	12 oz.	1 small	50–60 lb.
Celery, diced E.P.	25	1 lb.	1 qt.	27 lb.
Cucumbers, diced E.P.	30	1 lb.	3 cups	
Eggplant	22	1 lb.	8 slices	26 lb.
Lemons (165#)		1 lb.	4–5	
Lettuce, head	31	9 oz.	1	

102

Item		Amount	Yield	Total
Lettuce, shredded		1 lb.	6–8 cups	17 lb.
Lettuce, leaf		1 lb.	25–30 garnish	9 lb.
Onions, A.P.	10	1 lb.	4–5 medium	25 lb.
Onions, chopped		1 lb.	2–3 cups	2 #10 cans dehyd.
Onions, dehydrated, chopped		1 lb.	7 1/2 cups	50 lb. raw
Oranges	43	1 lb.	2	43 lb. (1@)
Parsnips		1 lb.	4	24 lb.
Peaches, A.P.		1 lb.	4	
Peas, A.P. in pods		1 lb.	1 cup shelled	53 lb.
Peas, dried split		1 lb.	2 1/3 cups	5 lb.
Green peppers	20	1 lb.	7–9 medium	25 lb. (2 halves)
Green peppers, chopped		1 lb.	3 cups	8 lb.
Pineapple, fresh		2 lb.	1 pineapple, 2–3 cups	60 lb. (1/2 cup@)
				30 lb. (1 slice@)
Potatoes, A.P.	16	1 lb.	3	39 lb.
Potatoes, 2 lb. A.P. after cooking			1 quart	
Sweet potato	20	1 lb.	3 medium	35 lb.
Pumpkin, cooked		1 lb.	2 1/2 cups	
Spinach, raw	64	13 oz.	5 qts., light pack	31 lb.
Spinach, 1 lb. E.P. after cooking			2 3/4 cups	
Summer squash, A.P.	34	2 lb.	1 qt., 5" diam.	24 lb.
Hubbard squash	41	1 lb.	2 cups	46 lb.
Zucchini	2			25 lb.
Tomatoes, fresh	12	1 lb.	3–4 medium	23 lb.
Tomatoes, diced		1 lb.	2 1/4 cups	
Turnips, A.P.	20	1 lb.	2–3	25 lb.
Watermelon	54	1 lb.	1" slice, 6" diam.	100 lb. (3 melons)

3. The manager has the right to refuse any substitute and subtract the charge from the invoice.

Other techniques that should be practiced by the manager or designee when receiving stock are listed below.

1. See that meats and produce are weighed upon receipt. This is an area often ignored by managers, who may not realize the amount of money that can be lost by neglect. Meat scales (25 pound) can be purchased for less than $100. The cost of these scales can easily be recouped if a meat poundage shortage is discovered. For example: A 40 lb. roast beef is ordered at $2.75 per pound, but actual weight received is 37 lbs—a discrepancy of $8.25 for one item! Considering that roast beef is served one time per week, a continuing discrepancy could result in overpayment of several hundred dollars for one item in a 12-month period.
2. Do not allow the delivery person to stock the shelves.
3. Take time to review the order thoroughly for accuracy, no matter how impatient the delivery person becomes. Remember that once the invoice is signed, the order becomes the property of the facility. Consider the cost incurred by a facility when a 40-lb. box of roast beef "fails to appear" after the invoice is signed and the delivery person is gone. If the roast costs $2.75/lb., $110.00 is lost.
4. Make sure that credits are received prior to the delivery person's departure for all missing items as well as food items not meeting weight specifications or quality standards.
5. See that deliveries are recorded immediately in the inventory record book.

STORAGE

The cost of deliveries can continue to rise if food items are not properly stored. Boxes of frozen food are often left on the kitchen floor for long periods before an employee decides to place them in the freezer. In order to protect valuable purchases, it may be helpful to schedule an additional employee on delivery days to alleviate handling problems.

When stock is stored, the date of delivery should be marked on each item to help prevent using new stock first. Stock should be placed on the shelves and old stock rotated to the front. The storeroom should be organized by food category, and counts should correspond with the inventory record forms. A well-kept storeroom allows for easy utilization of stock and makes ordering and inventory faster and more accurate.

INVENTORY CONTROLS

Since a typical inventory may be worth several thousand dollars, depending on the size of the facility, a good inventory control system is vital! There are two types of inventory systems—physical and perpetual. At least one type of system should be used in every facility. An inventory system helps a dietary manager control against theft, calculate food costs, and purchase food items in an organized manner.

A physical inventory involves the actual count of product in stock on a monthly basis. The advantages of this system are simplicity, ease of implementation, and the minimal amount of time required to perform the task. Disadvantages include lack of information on the quantity of products that *should* be in stock versus the actual count of products available; the need for frequent counts prior to purchasing; and lack of daily control over inventory to prevent possible theft.

A physical inventory is advantageous for a small facility, but a simplified perpetual inventory may be necessary along with it for weekly purchases such as meats and produce.

The main advantage of a perpetual inventory is that it maintains a "running balance" of products in stock and automically alerts the manager to the need to reorder specific items. Other advantages include the possibility of holding every employee accountable for deliveries to or withdrawals from inventory; the elimination of physical counts before placing an order; and greater control of product in stock against pilferage. If a perpetual inventory system is not accurately kept, however, greater errors can result in purchasing and time requirements for inventory control will increase. It is important that the dietary manager complete a daily random review of items removed from inventory compared to actual items used. Inventory withdrawals should match production sheet requirements. Employees need to understand the role of the perpetual inventory as it relates to purchasing. If they realize that keeping accurate records helps to control cost, they may be more motivated to complete the records accurately. Even with the implementation of an accurate perpetual inventory system, it is recommended to complete a monthly physical inventory for verification and calculation of actual dollars in inventory.

Food inventory levels must be in compliance with state and federal requirements (to maintain a 3-day supply), but an excessive level of inventory can be costly to the facility. At its lowest point, the inventory should be no less than 25–30 percent of budget. In larger facilities (100 or more beds) a good minimum inventory level is 40–45 percent of total budget. This level may be difficult to achieve in small facilities because of less frequent usage of some products. A maximum of 50 percent of the budget in inventory is feasible for any size facility. If a facility spends approximately $10,000 per month for food, the inventory should run about $5,000 for the month. Occasionally, the inventory percentage may be elevated due to an additional delivery received in a month. For example, if a facility receives deliveries every Tuesday, there will be several months with five Tuesdays rather than four. This additional expenditure should not increase a month's food cost because it is primarily stock for next month rather than actual used items (Breeding, Foster 1989). An inventory in excess of 50 percent inflates food cost and ties up available cash.

COST CONTROL

Controlling costs of dietary expenditures can be achieved by maintaining an accurate record-keeping system. It is difficult to track spending if purchases are not recorded throughout the month. Health care facilities that are owned and operated by chain operations usually have excellent dietary cost control procedures in place. Amazingly some independently owned facilities have no control systems or forms in place and do not understand why costs, especially food, are not within budget. When these situations occur, the consultant dietitian must work with the facility and dietary manager to implement effective cost control measures.

One of the most important forms to maintain is a monthly report that provides a daily log of actual & budgeted expenditures for food and supplies (Fig. 6-2), which should be viewed as the dietary manager's checkbook. At the beginning of each month, the amount of money allocated to food and supplies is logged. If the spending percentages for each food category have originally been determined during the purchasing process, the monthly cost of each category needs to be recorded also. For example, if the monthly food cost budget is $10,000 and it has been established that 35 percent of the budget should be meat and meat product cost, $3,500 should be noted initially as the monthly budget for meat items. As deliveries are received, the delivery date, vendor, invoice number, and the amount of the invoice are recorded (by category and total amount) on the daily log. Invoices should be posted the actual day of delivery. Once recorded, the amount of the invoice can be subtracted from the previous totals. The total of this calculation is the amount of budget remaining for the month (total expenditures as well as by categories). It is important when recording daily purchases to separate supplies and minor equipment (such as portion scoops and serving spoons) from actual food cost. If the daily log of purchases has been kept up to date and accurate throughout the month, the dietary manager or consultant dietitian will not be surprised by the bottom line.

A "Monthly Cost Report Analysis" (Fig. 6-3) should be completed at the end of each month. A typical monthly cost report requests the beginning inventory value of food and supplies, making it necessary to take a physical inventory of food items in stock. An ending inventory needs to be taken on the last day of the month to establish the amount of the food budget presently in stock. Of course, this value becomes the beginning inventory of the following month and only one physical inventory is required per month. The actual cost of food used during the month is derived from the value of the beginning inventory plus the cost of food purchases within the specific month, subtracting the ending inventory value. In order to translate the total food cost into cost per meal, a meal census form should be kept daily (Fig. 6-4), documenting the number of patient/resident and employee meals served.

Most of the time, food cost budgets are expressed in terms of cost per patient day (ppd). Patient day censuses for the specific month need to be obtained from the bookkeeping department.

The monthly cost report analysis may also include information pertaining to supply cost, nourishment cost, and/or activity and marketing cost. Each of these cost areas should be expressed in total dollars as well as cost per patient day in order to evaluate actual cost versus budgeted cost. By comparing total dollars spent and per patient day cost, one can determine if costs have been adjusted to reflect the in-house census, especially when the census is lower than the budgeted amount.

Regardless of the purchasing and food cost reporting system in place, cost containment problems can occur when attention to detail is lacking. The following are key control areas that can save a facility hundreds of dollars yearly.

1. *Awareness of market trends and pricing.* As mentioned earlier in this chapter, the dietary manager should be aware of marketing trends and buy accordingly. The price of frequently purchased items like bread, milk, and produce should be known at all times. Clerical tasks such as recording pricing or inventory may be delegated to a key employee, but it is still the responsibility of the dietary manager to know pricing and be accountable for all purchasing functions.

2. *Random costing of like items to obtain cost per serving* (rather than total cost). Total cost of an item is deceiving because it does not indicate yield. An example of this is bone-in meats in which the edible portion makes up only half the total weight (thus doubling actual price per pound).

3. *Production sheets.* Production sheets need to be used to control the quantity of food produced daily based on the patient census and employee meals (see Fig. 6-5). The production sheet should be completed by the dietary manager or designee with information on what food to prepare (including therapeutic variations), cooking times, and preparation needs for the following day's menu. If used effectively, production sheets can reduce leftovers and waste and contribute to food cost control.

4. *Purchase of appropriate items.* Lower grade fruits and vegetables are as wholesome as higher grades, but have some cosmetic imperfections. The lower grade items are "better buys" for casseroles, salads and Jello molds, in which imperfections in size or shape are not discernible.

5. *Use of standardized recipes and ingredient measuring.* The dietary manager must enforce the use of standardized recipes even by the most experienced cook, to assure that production and quality of food items are consistent with the daily meal census.

6. *Portion control.* Portion control of menu items must be emphasized and enforced by the dietary manager and/or the consultant dietitian. In order to enforce portion control, sufficient tools must be available and the correct portion size for each food item must be indicated on the production sheet and diet menus. Each employee should be trained in determining portion utensil size and using the correct utensil during meal service. The dietary manager should check the serving area prior to meal service time to assure that proper portion control utensils have been selected for each menu item.

MONTHLY BUDGET AND COST REPORT

MONTH _____ YEAR _____
FACILITY _____

Date	Day	Meat Fish, Fowl 30%	Fruits & Vegetables 30%	Dairy 16%	Cereal & Breads 10%	Fats & Oils 2%	Misc. 12%	TOTAL FOOD
		Budget						
1		Invoice						
		Balance						
2		Invoice						
		Balance						
3		Invoice						
		Balance						
4		Invoice						

	Balance		
5	Invoice		
	Balance		

30	Balance		
	Invoice		
31	Balance		
	Invoice		
	Balance		

FOOD COST COMPUTATION

Total Food Cost/Patient Day = _____ $ Amount in Inventory = _____

_____ _____

FOOD SERVICE SUPERVISOR   ADMINISTRATOR

Figure 6-2. Daily log of food and supply costs.

```
┌─────────────────────────────────────────────────────────────────────────┐
│                    MONTHLY COST REPORT ANALYSIS                           │
│                                                                           │
│  Facility name              _____                      │
│  Monthly patient days       _____                      │
│  Food expenditures          $_____                      │
│  Food cost ppd              _____                      │
│  Total nourishment cost     _____                      │
│  Nourishment cost ppd       _____                      │
│  Total marketing cost       _____                      │
│  Marketing cost ppd         _____                      │
│  Total activities cost      _____                      │
│  Activities cost ppd        _____                      │
│  Food inventory             _____                      │
│  Percent of budget in inventory  _____                      │
│  Meal revenue               _____                      │
│  Number of guest/employee meals served _____ │
│  Reasons for exceeding food cost ppd _____ │
│  _____ │
│  _____ │
│  _____ │
│  _____ │
│  Number of grocery orders received this month _____ │
│  Date last order called into CFS/distributor _____ │
│  Date last order received from CFS/distributor _____ │
└─────────────────────────────────────────────────────────────────────────┘
```

Figure 6-3. Analysis of monthly expenditures.

7. *Meal substitutions.* Substitutions must be carefully planned so that they can be used as a regular diet substitute as well as an alternative for residents on modified diets. This eliminates overproduction and controls cost.

8. *Monitoring the purchase of special diet products.* Special diet products such as diet gelatin and low sodium soups can be costly, especially if they are not acceptable to the targeted clientele. Menu items substituted for modified diets should be applicable to a variety of dietary needs (diet pudding, for example, that is low in both calories and sodium). The more menu items introduced, the higher the cost involved in labor, purchasing, inventory as well as the incidence of error.

9. *Nourishment and snack costs.* Food cost can escalate if control of nourishment and snack costs are not in line. To control nourishment costs, a dietary manager or consultant dietitian must review the list each month to assess continued need for the product. Standardize products as much as possible on the nourishment list. Use fortified milk-based products in place of commercial supplements for oral supplementation. Supervise nourishment distribution at the nursing stations. Maintain accurate records of nourishment expenditures. Know the cost of an 8-oz. serving of instant breakfast as compared to an 8-oz. serving of a commercial supplement.

MEAL CENSUS
FOR MONTH OF _____

WORK SHEET FOR _____ 19 _____

DATE	PATIENTS				EMPLOYEE				GUEST				TUBE FED	TOTAL	COMMENTS
	B	N	E		B	N	E		B	N	E				
TOTALS															

Figure 6-4. Daily record of meals served.

DAILY DIETARY PRODUCTION SHEET

DATE _____ DAY_____

RECIPE NO.	BREAKFAST	SIZE SERV	AMT TO PREPARE	RECIPE NO.	NOON	SIZE SERV	AMT TO PREPARE	RECIPE NO.	EVENING	SIZE SERV	AMT TO PREPARE
	Cereal - Hot				Entree				Entree		
	Cold				Ground				Ground		
	LS				Puree				Puree		
	Egg				LS				LS		
	LS				Other				Other		
	Meat				Vegetable/Soup				Vegetable/Soup		
	Bread				Puree				Puree		
	Juice				LS				LS		
					Other				Other		
					Salad/Fruit				Salad/Fruit		

	PULL FROM FREEZER	PRODUCTION FOR FOLLOWING DAY:	AMOUNT LEFT OVER	PLANNED USAGE
Puree			Puree	
DB			DB	
Bread		Bread	Bread	
Dessert		Dessert	Dessert	
Puree		Puree	Puree	
DB		DB	DB	
Other		Other	Other	
ENTREE SUB		ENTREE SUB	ENTREE SUB	
VEGETABLE SUB		VEGETABLE SUB	VEGETABLE SUB	

LS - Low Sodium Restriction Variation
DB - Diabetic Variations

Figure 6-5. Production sheet used to control the quantity of food produced.

Under the federal survey regulations, snacks are required to be given at least at bedtime to all residents. In some states, snacks must be given three times daily as diet allows. Unless medically indicated, between meal snacks should be light, consisting of fluids only (juice) with a more substantial snack in the evening. To control snack costs, specific food choices should be listed on the daily menu and the amount of snacks delivered to the nursing stations must be monitored.

10. *Security control of all storage areas.* All storage areas—storerooms, freezers, and refrigerators—should be locked and accessible only to authorized employees. Food storage areas should be locked throughout the day, with withdrawals made only once per shift. Access to keys should be limited. Keys should be issued only by the dietary manager—never hung in a public area.

Suggestions for controlling costs of specific types of food are listed below.

Meats

1. Purchase quantities as indicated by meat protein guidelines and recipes.
2. Consider purchasing ground meat items for puree preparation. Ground chicken is considerably less expensive to puree than baked chicken breasts.
3. Specify amounts of meat to thaw and amounts to use on production sheets. If a partial piece of meat is to be used, specify usage of the remaining quantity (e.g., cook or slice). Specify when leftover meats are to be thawed and used on the product sheet.
4. Check cooking methods to avoid excess shrinkage. Utilize the meat thermometer.
5. Take five meat samples to check for accuracy of portion size.

Groceries

1. Avoid unplanned menu substitutions. Substituting canned fruit because the cook did not make the baked dessert will raise cost.
2. Again, utilize production sheets to avoid overproduction of vegetables, salads, and desserts.
3. Cooks must use recipes and must measure and weigh ingredients. They must prepare food according to instructions. For example, whipping mashed potatoes in the mixer increases yield.
4. Watch portion control. Use correct scoops, ladles, and spoodles when serving. Are cakes cut in 2 × 2 in. squares?
5. Check quantities of leftovers and utilize them appropriately. Employees should check with the dietary manager before throwing any food down the garbage disposal.

    Collect "appropriate" leftover vetetables in a stock pot in the freezer for the next time vegetable soup is on the menu. Use leftover fruit by mixing together and adding bananas for fruit cup or as fruited gelatin.

6. Bulk cereal rather than individual boxes should be used for significantly increased savings.

Eggs

1. In many facilities, there is a standing order for eggs or eggs are left in the cooler at the discretion of the delivery person and deliveries are often made at times the dietary manager is not present, such as early morning. Check to be sure you are receiving the amount of eggs indicated on the invoice.
2. Recalculate the amount of eggs necessary to feed residents. Allow one egg per person, then count the number of tray cards that call for two eggs. Also, record how many eggs to crack on the production sheet.
3. Check how scrambled eggs are mixed to be certain the proportion of eggs to milk is correct. Beat scrambled eggs in the mixer to increase yield.
4. Check portion size. One egg is a #20 scoop. This dipper should be used, but instruct cooks to spread the eggs out a little with the scoop so they are not in the shape of a "ball." Of course, additional eggs may be served to residents who request them or to those who need extra protein at the direction of the physician.
5. Remember to watch for those residents who dislike eggs and never consume them. Add this to their tray card and add the equivalent protein to their diet in some other form.
6. Evaluate the best price of eggs. Medium sized eggs are the better buy if there is more than a 7-cent difference between these and large. However, large eggs should only be used in scrambled eggs to increase yield. Also, evaluate the cost of frozen pasteurized eggs versus fresh. At times, frozen eggs can be more cost effective than fresh.

Milk

1. Use powdered milk for all cooking. Since employees may not want to take the time to mix it during food preparation, check to make sure it is always prepared and available. Assign one cook the job of checking the "cooking milk" supply daily. Keep a large container made up in the cooler. If the supply is low or more than 48 hours old, this cook is responsible for making more. The container must be labeled and dated. Follow package directions for reconstitution of powdered milk.
2. Now that you have reduced the amount of milk used for cooking, go back and recalculate how much other milk you will need for the residents to drink. Allow at least 16 oz. per person, then count the number of tray cards calling for additional milk.

EXAMPLE

16 oz. × 100 residents = 1,600 oz.
Plus ten 8-oz. portions =   80 oz.
                              1,680 oz.

Quantity needed per day:

No. of gallons	=	1680 ÷ 128	=	13 1/8
No. of half-gallons	=	1680 ÷ 64	=	26 1/4
No. of 5-gallon bags	=	1680 ÷ 640	=	2 2/3
No. of 8 oz. cartons	=	1680 ÷ 8	=	210

Add to this the amount of milk needed daily for nourishments such as Carnation Instant Breakfast, eggnog, or milkshakes.

3. Check your milk usage regularly to be certain of an adequate but not excessive supply.

Margarine

1. Check the amount of bulk margarine used for toast at breakfast. What happens to the leftover melted margarine for the toast? Use of a butter wheel rather than a pastry brush for toast will cut down on the amount of margarine used.
2. Consider "buttering" the bread in the kitchen using bulk margarine rather than serving margarine pats. Bulk margarine can be whipped to increase yield and lower cost. Calorie-controlled diets should continue to be served pats.

Bakery

1. Save all stale bread, leftover toast, and bread heels. These leftovers, kept in an airtight container in the freezer, can be the bread supply for bread pudding and dressing. No fresh bread need be used for such items.
2. Leave a written order for the bread man. Do not let him decide what to leave. The best way to do this is to post what you need each delivery day in an area where he will see it. Remember, if you have items such as buns, dinner rolls, or cornbread, you will need fewer loaves of bread. If sandwiches are on the menu, you will need more bread.

Coffee

1. Compare coffee prices on your buying guide. Packs with the most bulk coffee are substantially cheaper per pound.
2. Evaluate coffee brewing procedures. Do employees measure how much coffee they are using per urn or pot full? If so, is this amount appropriate?
3. Write beverage preferences on tray cards to avoid serving excessive amounts of coffee.
4. Check leftover coffee that is returned from the nursing unit after meals (if sent in bulk for nursing to pour). Cut down on the amount sent if too much is left over but be sure nursing is not running out before all residents are served.

The dietary department represents a significant percentage of the facility's total operating budget, requiring attention be paid to cost control.

Controlling dietary costs, especially food costs, is a difficult task.

A dietary manager must work with the facility's administrator and the consultant dietitian to develop an effective and efficient system by which dietary costs can be controlled within the budgetary guidelines.

REFERENCES

Breeding, Carolyn, and Donna Foster. 1989. *Cost effective recipes for 10-100*. New York: Van Nostrand Reinhold.

Cabot, Elaine, and Ellsworth Cabot. 1973. *Handbook for menu makers*. Chicago: McGraw-Hill.

Molt, Mary, Grace Shugart, and Maxine Wilson. 1985. *Food for fifty*. New York: John Wiley & Sons.

Ninemeier, Jack D. 1985. *Managing foodservice operations*. West Lafayette, Ind.: Purdue Research Foundation.

Rose, James, 1984. *Handbook for health care food service management*. Rockville, Md.: Aspen Systems Corp.

Unicare Health Facilities. 1985. *Food purchasing and cost control*. Milwaukee: Unicare Health Facilities.

7

Sanitation and Safety

SANITATION WITHIN THE DIETARY DEPARTMENT

It is the goal of every foodservice department to provide clean, wholesome food. Because certain diseases can be transmitted through food, specific practices are recommended to control the growth of foodborne organisms (AHA 1972). In order to protect the patient's health, there must be a continuous program of education in sanitation designed so that every worker will understand his or her role in preventing the spread of infection. Staff education at regular intervals using a variety of teaching aids and techniques will help break bad work and personal habits and stimulate an interest in helping create a clean, healthy, and safe work environment.

One of the keys to sanitary foodservice is healthy employees who are well trained in safe food handling and practice good personal hygiene by keeping themselves clean. The worker with clean clothing is apt to perform his work in a similarly "clean" manner. It can be difficult to impress upon people the dangers involved in bad work habits. Because bacteria cannot be seen, it is easy when rushed to become careless about handwashing, handling food, or monitoring food temperatures. Many cases of food poisoning can be traced directly to the foodservice worker.

The consultant dietitian can assist facilities in developing a successful sanitation program—one that functions on a day-to-day basis, not just for state inspection or the day of the consultant's visit. The heart of a good program is self-evaluation and prompt corrective action. It involves looking at equipment, facilities, and food, as well as close observation of personnel, their appearance, clothing, and food-handling practices. The dietitian can help develop a comprehensive self-evaluation tool to be used by dietary managers and other dietary employees to increase individual awareness of the advantages of maintaining a sanitary operation.

The second part of such a program is employee education. Providing stimulating inservice programs that inspire the employee to do a good job is a challenge to the dietitian. Involving employees in the training program and focusing on the contribution of each staff member to the sanitation program help employees perform to their maximum capabilities.

An important tool for education and self-evaluation is the sanitation checklist. The checklist should be based on the state foodservice code. Although federal regulations for sanitation exist, each state has developed an individual code based on the federal code. A copy of the state code is usually available from the local health department free of charge.

Any checklist developed should be applicable to the facility and company policies, practices, and procedures and be compatible with local foodservice sanitation regulations. It should be organized by areas to permit inspection of specific functional units of the department. The general areas of sanitation are (1) personal hygiene, (2) food-handling practices, (3) equipment and facilities, and (4) patient concerns.

The sanitation survey that follows is included as a guide to developing a sanitation program.

Personnel
1. Do any food handlers have infected cuts or boils? Are they free from colds or other communicable diseases?
2. Are employees clean, neat, and well groomed with clean uniforms and aprons?
3. Are food handlers wearing effective hair restraints?
4. Are food handlers' hands clean and good handwashing techniques used frequently throughout the day?
5. Do employees eat or smoke only in designated areas?
6. Are disposable gloves used by food handlers?
7. Are fingernails short, clean, and unpolished?
8. Do employees wear a minimal amount of jewelry?

Food-handling practices
1. Is all food stored off the floor?
2. Are potentially hazardous foods held at room temperature?
3. Are fruits and vegetables thoroughly washed prior to preparation and serving?
4. Are food warmers or steamtables used to reheat prepared foods?
5. Are frozen foods properly thawed under refrigeration or under cold running water?
6. Are raw and cooked or ready-to-serve foods prepared on the same cutting board without washing and sanitizing the board between use?
7. Are hands used to pick rolls, butter, bread, ice or other foods to be served?
8. Are food servers touching food contact surfaces of plates, glasses, cups, and silverware?

Receiving
1. Is food inspected on receipt for spoilage or infestation?
2. Is perishable food stored promptly under refrigeration?
3. Are nonfood supplies inspected for infestation?
4. Is the receiving area clean and free of food debris, boxes, cans, and other refuse?

Dry storage
1. Is food stored at least 6 in. off the floor to permit floor cleaning?

2. Are walls, floors, and shelves clean?
3. Is the storage area dry and well ventilated, and is temperature maintained lower than 70° F?
4. Are nonfood supplies and chemicals stored separately from food stock?
5. Have empty cartons and trash been removed?
6. Are food supplies stored in a manner to insure "first in, first out" use?
7. Are bulk foods (such as sugar and flour) if no longer stored in original package, now stored in a covered container with an identifying name?
8. Is there evidence of insects or rodents?

Refrigerator storage

1. Are refrigerators equipped with properly functioning thermometers?
2. Are temperatures maintained 45° F or lower in refrigerators and 0 degrees or lower in freezers?
3. Is all food stored off the floor?
4. Is cooked food stored above raw food?
5. Are all foods properly wrapped or covered to prevent contamination?
6. Are walls, floors, and shelves clean and free of debris and objectionable disorder?
7. Are any spoiled foods present?
8. Are foods arranged to permit good air circulation?
9. Are cooked foods or other products removed from original containers in clean, sanitized, covered containers and identified?

Food preparation

1. Is the food preparation area clean and free from accumulated debris?
2. Are the floors of the kitchen and other foodservice areas clean and dry?
3. Are food preparation equipment and utensils not in use clean, sanitized, and stored in a manner that will protect them from contamination?
4. Is preparation equipment such as slicers, grinders, and mixers cleaned and sanitized after each use?
5. Are cleaning supplies and pesticides present in the food preparation area?
6. Is the cook's sink being used for employee handwashing or dumping mop water?
7. Are ventilation hoods free from grease and dust?
8. Are soiled cloths stored in a covered container?
9. Are can openers clean and sanitized?
10. Are there an adequate number of trash receptacles conveniently placed and frequently emptied and kept clean?
11. Is holding equipment maintaining food at or above 140° F or at 45° F or lower?

Dining room

1. Are dining room floor, tables, and chairs clean and dry?
2. Is tableware clean and sanitized and stored in a manner to prevent contamination?

   3. Are single service items disposed of after single use?
   4. Are the cloths used to wipe dining room tables clean and sanitary and stored in sanitizing solution between uses?

Warewashing
   1. Is the rinse temperature of 170° F being maintained?
   2. Are tableware and utensils scraped and flushed before washing?
   3. Do personnel wash or sanitize hands between handling soiled tableware and sanitized tableware?
   4. Do automatic detergent and sanitizer dispensers operate properly?
   5. Are tableware and utensils air-dried after sanitizing?
   6. Are dishwashers and sinks thoroughly cleaned after use?

Restroom facilities
   1. Are employee facilities clean, dry, and odor free?
   2. Are adequate soap and towels available for employee needs?
   3. Is sanitary equipment operational and clean?
   4. Are adequate waste receptacles available and clean?

Equipment

Sanitary features should be a major consideration in the selection and purchase of equipment. Equipment that is easily disassembled for cleaning and installed in a manner that allows accessibility for easy removal of soil, food, and other debris is recommended. Some older institutions, without the advantage of new equipment, need to exercise particular vigilance regarding comprehensive training and supervision in order to keep the facility looking its best (AHA 1954). Cleaning should be regularly scheduled using a specific cleaning schedule that designates who cleans what, when, and how often in order to prevent the accumulation of dirt. Food contamination can be prevented through effective cleaning practices. Clean surroundings are the first step in good sanitary practices.

TEMPERATURE CONTROL

Several million cases of bacterial food poisoning occur every year, and the number of cases increases each year. Salmonellosis, one type of food poisoning, has more than doubled in the past 10 years. Why is this happening? One reason is the increase in our elderly population, who are more susceptible to food poisoning. In addition, the rapid expansion of the foodservice industry, including food technology and processing, and the shortage of qualified staff has contributed greatly to the increase of foodborne illness. Although great progress has been made by various regulatory agencies in formulating adequate legal safeguards, foodborne illness will never be eliminated by government inspection of meat and poultry. Food contamination can be prevented, however, through careful handling and storage as well as special attention to time and temperature.

One study done by the Centers for Disease Control lists the most common factors leading to food poisoning (Bailey 1985):

1. Inadequate cooling
2. The lapse of a day or more between preparing and serving food
3. Food handling by infected persons
4. Inadequate time or temperature, or both, during heat processing
5. Insufficiently high temperatures during storage of hot food on the steamtable

Of these, inadequate control of food temperature is the most common factor contributing to outbreaks of foodborne disease. The temperatures for food commonly called the "danger zone" are between 45° and 140°F. The temperature most favorable to bacterial growth is body temperature, or about 98°F; temperatures below 45°F markedly inhibit bacterial growth and the high food temperatures of 165° to 212°F reached in boiling, baking, frying, or roasting kill most food poisoning bacteria.

The consultant dietitian plays a key role in educating dietary workers in the area of temperature control. Routine visits to facilities should always include an infection control check of equipment and food being served to patients (see the infection control checklist in chapter 5). At least annually a mandatory inservice program on time and temperature control should be planned in order to impress on employees the importance of temperature checks and holding food at safe temperatures. Figures 7-1 and 7-2 show procedures for daily recording of equipment and food temperatures.

There are two terms that are important when considering food safety. One is *potentially hazardous food,* which is defined by Kentucky's State Food Service Code as

> any food which consists in whole or in part of milk and milk products, eggs or egg products, meat or meat products, poultry or poultry products, fish or fish products, shell fish (oysters, clams, mussels and edible crustacea) or shell fish products, cooked rice, or other ingredients including synthetic ingredients, in a form capable of supporting rapid and progressive growth of infectious or toxigenic microorganisms. This term does not include clean, whole, uncracked, odor-free shell eggs or food which have a pH level of 4.6 or below or a water activity (wa) value of 0.85 or less, nor does it include hard-boiled, peeled eggs, commercially prepared, packaged and properly labeled.

The other is *safe temperature,* which means, "when considering potentially hazardous food, food temperature of forty-five (45) degrees Fahrenheit or below and one hundred forty (140) degrees Fahrenheit or above, except for frozen food, which should be stored at zero (0) degrees Fahrenheit or less." Food may safely remain between 45° and 140° for up to four hours; however, food should not be in the 60°–100°F range for longer than two hours.

During preparation much of the food is handled at room temperature or

Dietary Temperature Control Chart   Month of _____

All refrigerators and freezers are to be checked twice each day to insure they are in proper working order.
Dishwasher, pots and pans temperature are to be checked and recorded AM & PM daily.
T = Temperature I=Initials

Date	Time	Freezer 1		Freezer 2		Freezer Walk-in		Refrig. 1		Refrig. 2		Refrig. Walk-in		Dishw. Wash		Dishw. Rinse		Pot & Pan		Milk Mach.	
		T	I	T	I	T	I	T	I	T	I	T	I	T	I	T	I	T	I	T	I
1																					
2																					
3																					
4																					
5																					
29																					
30																					
31																					

Figure 7-1. Form for recording equipment temperatures.

123

Steamtable Temperatures

Temp	Foods	Mon Reg	Mon Pur	Tue Reg	Tue Pur	Wed Reg	Wed Pur	Thurs Reg	Thurs Pur	Fri Reg	Fri Pur	Sat Reg	Sat Pur	Sun Reg	Sun Pur	Comments
	BREAKFAST															
180	Hot cereal															
160	Eggs															
190	Coffee, tea															
	LUNCH															
170	Meat, fish															
160	Potatoes															
180	Vegetables															

170	Casseroles														
180	Soup, gravy														
165	Cream soup														
190	Coffee, tea														
	SUPPER														
170	Meat, fish														
160	Potatoes														
180	Vegetables														
170	Casseroles														
180	Soup, gravy														
165	Cream soup														
190	Coffee, Tea														

Reg = regular; Pur = pureed.

Figure 7-2. Form for recording hot food temperatures.

above, which is ideal for bacterial growth. Workers must be impressed with their responsibility to keep foods refrigerated except during preparation. Meat and poultry especially need to be cooked thoroughly without interruption and should not be partially cooked, refrigerated, and recooked at a later date. Cooks should be taught to take the temperature of food before it leaves the oven to ensure that the interior temperature is within the safe range. If not served immediately, hot food should be transferred from deep containers into shallow ones and placed at once in the refrigerator or freezer to chill. As the American Dietetic Association points out, "Refrigerating foods in large, deep pots that cool too slowly is one of the riskiest food handling mistakes" (ADA 1989). Because food can take up to 12 hours or longer to chill in a deep container, bacteria will multiply in the warm center of the food, increasing the risk of food poisoning. Current recommendations specify that "for hot food to be cooled quickly it should be no more than 2 inches deep in shallow containers, and the center of the food mass should reach 45 degrees F within 4 hours" (Spears, Vaden 1985).

The National Institute for the Foodservice Industry (NIFI) has developed 10 key practices that can be used as a reference when instructing and/or training foodservice personnel (Spears, Vaden 1985).

- When refrigerating potentially hazardous foods, make certain an internal product temperature of 40°F or less is maintained.
- Use extreme care in storing and handling food prepared in advance of service.
- Cook or heat-process food to recommended temperatures.
- Relieve infected employees of food-handling duties and require strict personal hygiene on the part of all employees.
- Make certain that hot-holding devices maintain food at temperatures of 140°F or higher.
- Give special attention to inspection and cleaning of raw ingredients that will be used in foods that require little or no cooking.
- Heat leftovers quickly to an internal temperature of 165°F
- Avoid carrying contamination from raw to cooked and ready-to-serve foods via hands, equipment, and utensils.
- Clean and sanitize food-contact surfaces of equipment after every use.
- Obtain foods from approved sources.

Encouraging employees to be knowledgeable in these areas will help prevent outbreaks of foodborne illness. The old adage "Keep hot foods hot and cold foods cold" is still the best rule to follow. An equally important guideline is "When in doubt, throw it out."

SAFETY IN THE DIETARY DEPARTMENT

Dietary employees are at particular risk of accident because of hazards that are inherent in a foodservice operation. There are few occupations that confront an employee with such a multitude of hazardous equipment and working conditions. Daily, the foodservice worker is involved in the use of knives; cutting, chopping, grinding, mixing, and slicing equipment; high-pressure steam; hot ovens and grills; hot cooking fats and other hot liquids; open gas flame; slippery floors as the result of spillage of liquids or grease; and other hazards resulting from working with several people to meet meal service deadlines.

As well as emphasizing good sanitation practices, the consultant dietitian must be concerned about developing safety techniques to prevent accidents within the department. Preventive measures are too often put into effect only after an accident has occurred. Employee safety training programs are a priority, and a careful inspection of safe working habits is the key to prevention. Comprehensive safety training begins with orientation and is kept ongoing through inservices, posters, and safety reminders that keep employees alert to safety hazards.

The Federal Occupational and Safety Health Act (OSHA) places a legal obligation on employers to provide a safe environment. OSHA places legal responsibility on employers to meet certain conditions in operating a business, including provision of adequate work space; proper lighting and ventilation; an adequate number of exits; flooring that is clean, dry, and free from hazards; suitable storage for food and other materials; and safe equipment that is cor-

Safety Checklist			
Evaluation Query	If Yes, list problem and location	Follow Up	Completion Date
Is any electrical cord frayed?	Y N _____	_____	_____
Is any grounding device missing or not in use?	Y N _____	_____	_____
Is any electrical cord on portable equipment resting on the floor?	Y N _____	_____	_____
Is any electrical outlet broken or damaged?	Y N _____	_____	_____
Is a drop cord routinely used for any specific connection?	Y N _____	_____	_____
Is any drop cord noncompliant with policy?	Y N _____	_____	_____
Is any electrical panel physically obstructed?	Y N _____	_____	_____
Is any personal appliance noncompliant with policy?	Y N _____	_____	_____
Is any electrical connection in danger of splash, by chemicals, water, or other liquids?	Y N _____	_____	_____

Continued

Figure 7-3. Sample safety checklist (reprinted by permission from *Hospital Food & Nutrition Focus*, Vol., 2, No. 7, pp. 4–5, Aspen Publishers, Inc., March 1986).

Safety Checklist

Evaluation Query		If Yes, list problem and location	Follow Up	Completion Date
Is any electrical appliance in need of repair?	Y N			
Is any temperature gauge inoperable?	Y N			
Is any emergency light missing or inoperable?	Y N			
Is any lightbulb broken, missing?	Y N			
Is any lightbulb cover missing?	Y N			
Is any compressor fan or fan guard obstructed, missing, or lint-filled?	Y N			
Is any gearworks or similar exposed?	Y N			
Is any equipment cleaned while the power is on?	Y N			
Does any faucet leak?	Y N			
Is there a steam leak?	Y N			
Is there a water tank leak?	Y N			
Is any drain cover too high? Too low?	Y N			
Is any drain clogged?	Y N			
Is any drain slow to drain?	Y N			
Is there any standing water?	Y N			
Is the hot water temperature ok in handsinks?	Y N			
Is any steam pipe not properly insulated?	Y N			
Is any gasket missing or needing repair?	Y N			
Is any pressure valve in disrepair?	Y N			
Is any drain set-up non-gapped?	Y N			
Is any disposal not fitted with a guard?	Y N			
Does any floor drain look as if it needs flushing?	Y N			
Is any hose cracked or leaking?	Y N			
Is any cut-off valve missing or in disrepair?	Y N			
Is any dishmachine temperature incorrect?	Y N			
Is any pipe sweating?	Y N			
Is any fire extinguisher missing or in disrepair?	Y N			
Is any fire safety signage missing?	Y N			
Is any employee using incorrect lifting techniques?	Y N			

Figure 7-3. (*Continued*)

Safety Checklist

Evaluation Query		If Yes, list problem and location	Follow Up	Completion Date
Is any long-haired employee without a hair covering?	Y N	_____	_____	_____
Is any employee wearing dangling jewelry?	Y N	_____	_____	_____
Is any employee operating equipment while wearing rings?	Y N	_____	_____	_____
Does any employee have unsafe shoes?	Y N	_____	_____	_____
Does any employee near hot equipment have on a plastic apron?	Y N	_____	_____	_____
Does any employee handling hot equipment have on plastic gloves?	Y N	_____	_____	_____
Does any employee not understand the fire procedures?	Y N	_____	_____	_____
Is any employee handling a knife incorrectly?	Y N	_____	_____	_____
Is any storage unit unsafe?	Y N	_____	_____	_____
Is any toxic item stored with food or supplies?	Y N	_____	_____	_____
Is any heavier item stored higher on shelving than lighter items?	Y N	_____	_____	_____
Is any broken tile a hazard?	Y N	_____	_____	_____
Is there any hazardous projection (walls, floors, etc.)?	Y Y	_____	_____	_____
Is any ladder unsafe?	Y N	_____	_____	_____
Can you be trapped in a refrigerator or freezer?	Y N	_____	_____	_____
Can you be trapped in any other appliance?	Y N	_____	_____	_____
Can you be trapped in any work area?	Y N	_____	_____	_____
Is any cart in disrepair?	Y N	_____	_____	_____
Is any dish in use that is cracked or chipped?	Y N	_____	_____	_____
Is any service tray in use that is cracked or chipped?	Y N	_____	_____	_____
Is any knife stored incorrectly?	Y N	_____	_____	_____
Is any knife in disrepair?	Y N	_____	_____	_____
Is any lid on an opened can not removed entirely?	Y N	_____	_____	_____
Is any broken dish or glass in the area?	Y N	_____	_____	_____
Is any broken dish or glass in open garbage cans?	Y N	_____	_____	_____

Continued

Safety Checklist			
Evaluation Query	*If Yes,* *list problem* *and location*	*Follow* *Up*	*Completion* *Date*
Is any grease filter clogged with grease?	Y N _____	_____	_____
Does any food thermometer contain toxic substances?	Y N _____	_____	_____
Is any safety guard missing from slicers?	Y N _____	_____	_____
Is any safety guard missing from a dishmachine?	Y N _____	_____	_____
Is any serving utensil or small equipment in disrepair?	Y N _____	_____	_____
Is any blade on slicers or other such equipment chipped or missing?	Y N _____	_____	_____
Is mopping occurring without wet floor signs being used?	Y N _____	_____	_____
Is any ladder stored incorrectly?	Y N _____	_____	_____
Is any mop or broom stored incorrectly?	Y N _____	_____	_____
Is any spill not cleaned up immediately?	Y N _____	_____	_____
Is any aisle blocked?	Y N _____	_____	_____
Is any cleaning compound mixed incorrectly?	Y N _____	_____	_____
Are any two or more chemicals being mixed together?	Y N _____	_____	_____
Is any chemical being poured into hot water?	Y N _____	_____	_____

Figure 7-3. (*Continued*)

rectly installed. In addition to the OSHA requirements, the operator has an obligation to protect both workers and customers from careless accidents.

A safety inspection conducted monthly, or more often if indicated, is a means to detect problem areas that should be addressed in the consultant dietitian's report and corrected immediately. A safety program enables the dietitian to promote cost effectiveness, by preventing costly workman's compensation claims to the facility and loss of employee time and services. The dietitian needs to be involved in the development of programs assuring that employees are properly instructed in safe work practices.

A comprehensive safety inspection checklist can be designed to include the following major areas of concern:

- Fire prevention
- Burns and cuts
- Falls
- Back strain or injury
- Injury from mechanical equipment
- Physical plant

A foodservice operation should develop its own safety inspection checklist that is pertinent to company policy and procedure and is compatible with federal, state, and local safety regulations. A good example of a safety checklist is provided in Figure 7-3.

REFERENCES

American Dietetic Association (ADA). 1989. Of interest to you. *Journal of The American Dietetic Association 89*, no. 11:1635.

American Hospital Association (AHA). 1954. *Hospital food service manual*. Chicago: AHA.

———. 1972. *Food service manual for health care institutions*. Chicago: AHA.

Bailey, Janet. 1985. *Keeping Food Fresh*. New York: The Dial Press, Doubleday & Co.

Harger, Virginia F., Bessie B. West, and Levelle Wood. 1966. *Food service in institutions*. New York: John Wiley & Sons.

National Restaurant Association (NRA). 1979. *Sanitation operations manual*. Chicago: NRA.

Spears, Marian C., and Allene G. Vaden. 1985. *Foodservice organizations*. New York: Macmillan Publishing Co.

Tufts University. 1989. Cooling food the safe way. *Diet and Nutrition Letter 7*, no. 9:2.

8

Equipment and Layout

The role of the dietary consultant in relation to dietary equipment and kitchen design will vary depending on the condition of the department and the plan of the facility. If the building is old, the consultant may be requested to evaluate existing conditions and equipment and formulate suggestions for changes to achieve increased efficiency and productivity. On the other hand, the consultant may be influential in implementing a plan for updating and/or replacing existing equipment or a complete renovation of kitchen facilities. Larger renovation or construction projects may require work with an architect, kitchen planner, equipment vendor, and administrator.

In any facility, the consultant should be actively involved in developing and maintaining an effective equipment management program. Information about the facility and equipment is vital in making appropriate recommendations for the facility. Equipment programs include procedures for cleaning, maintenance, and replacement.

THE IMPORTANCE OF EQUIPMENT TO THE FOODSERVICE OPERATION

Every dietary consultant knows the impact of equipment on dietary operations. The type and design of available equipment affect all areas of foodservice systems.

Menu

The menu must be planned according to the type and availability of equipment. It is unwise to plan pancakes for 50 when a griddle is not available, or fried catfish and hushpuppies when the department does not have a deep fat fryer. By the same token, it would be a mistake to plan a menu that includes three oven-prepared items when only one oven is available.

Productivity

Some pieces of equipment increase employee productivity. A food processor or a vertical cutter may allow an employee to prepare coleslaw, grate cheese, or

This chapter was contributed by Deborah H. Sutherlin.

prepare bread crumbs more quickly than these tasks can be done by hand. Dough can be kneaded by machine with the proper attachments. Convection ovens and steamers allow faster preparation of food items. Adequate refrigeration space makes it possible to complete some steps in pre-preparation of items ahead of time, allowing more efficient use of "down times."

Safety

Proper equipment increases safety within the dietary department. The use of the appropriate equipment in good working order reduces the likelihood of accidents in the foodservice department.

Quality of Food

The quality of the food will be affected by the type and availability of the equipment to be used during food preparation and holding. Fast food establishments are capable of holding fried items such as French fries without loss of quality because of specialized holding equipment. If health care establishments attempt to hold the same item on a steamtable, loss of quality will result. With adequate equipment, batch cooking can be done so food can be prepared in smaller amounts and will not require long periods in holding equipment that may be unsuitable for the product.

Energy Efficiency

Equipment manufactured in recent years is generally more energy efficient and may cost considerably less to operate than older comparable pieces of equipment.

INITIAL REVIEW OF PLANT AND EQUIPMENT

The physical characteristics of an existing kitchen affect many areas of food service production. A consultant may be involved in menu planning, recipe development, and training of employees in new procedures. In making these plans for departmental operation, it is helpful to have available information pertaining to the existing equipment and its function.

Upon contracting with a new account, it would be advisable to conduct a review of existing plant and equipment. Information needed includes a list of equipment, its current condition, date of purchase, and maintenance history. This will aid the consultant in making recommendations for its continued use or replacement and for planning foodservice operations. The following areas and types of equipment should be considered in conducting an initial review:

Receiving
  Scales
  Hand trucks
  Weather protection
Dry storage
  Shelving
  Lighting
  Ventilation
Refrigerated storage
  Walk-in refrigerator
  Walk-in freezer
Chemical storage (Location)
Other storage (specify)
Production
  Range
  Ovens (type)
  Steam equipment
  Deep fat fryer
  Tilting skillet
  Mixer
  Other
Small equipment
  Blender
  Food processor

Toaster
Other
Tray assembly
  Starter station
  Steam table
  Conveyor
  Refrigerator
  Carts
  Tray system
  Other
Work areas
  Salad/veg
  Beverage
  Other
Dishwashing
  Dishmachine (type)
  Disposal
  Other
General
  Floors
  Walls
Other
  Galvanized shelving
  Hoods and ventilation systems[1]

Additional comments could relate to how well the equipment functions and whether capacity is acceptable or if replacement is desirable.

THE EQUIPMENT MANAGEMENT PROGRAM

Every facility should have a system for the maintenance and use of equipment in the foodservice department. Whether for a new facility with new equipment or for an existing facility, department policies should detail the procedures for purchase, operation, and review of equipment.

The planning of a successful equipment program begins with purchase and continues as a result of the policies determined by the facility. A successful program would address the following areas:

Purchase and installation
Training

1. These pieces of equipment have been improved in recent years so that they are much more energy efficient than in the past. The decision to replace this type of equipment might be made on the basis of energy efficiency, even though existing equipment may still be useful and in good operating condition.

Equipment operation and equipment records
Routine maintenance and inspection
Equipment replacement

Purchase and Installation

Equipment purchase should be a planned program of the facility. The department should determine the requirements of the purchasing system regarding bids, equipment selection, specifications, and vendor requirements. The facility should make decisions concerning the responsibility of installation of the equipment since this may be an added cost or may be included in the quoted price.

Characteristics of Good Equipment

Equipment should be functional, durable, and compatible with the needs of the facility. The National Sanitation Foundation maintains standards of acceptance for equipment. NSF approval indicates that the equipment meets certain sanitation and safety standards.

Manufactured equipment is usually the first source to explore. If appropriate equipment is not available, the facility should investigate the option of designing fabricated equipment to meet its needs.

Developing a Cost Estimate

A cost estimate for foodservice equipment should include (1) the cost of the equipment; (2) the model number, unless fabricated; and (3) a price estimate for each piece of equipment not installed, delivered to site, uncrated and set in place. The estimate generally represents an amount more than the dealer's cost of equipment but less than list price. Equipment dealers generally discount equipment 30 to 50 percent of list price (Birchfield, 1988).

Developing Specifications

Equipment specifications should contain detailed, clearly written information about the requirements of specific pieces of equipment. The goal is to obtain the lowest possible price for equipment that matches the specifications.

To submit the lowest price, the dealer may attempt to substitute inferior equipment. It is the responsibility of the facility and design consultant to inspect the dealer's bid and specification of equipment priced (Birchfield 1988). Limiting acceptance of equipment to the model number on the specification prevents inappropriate substitutions.

The following specification checklist was developed by John C. Birchfield and published in *Design & Layout of Foodservice Facilities* (1988).

- Item number: The number used on the drawing, in the specifications, and on the equipment schedule

- Name: The generic name of the equipment (work table, range, etc.)
- Number: The quantity to be purchased
- Model and manufacturer: The model number, name, and location of the manufacturer. This is the first choice of the client.
- Measurement (size): Height, width, depth
- Description: Specification of the quality and standards, and a description of the standard parts normally furnished with the equipment
- Utility requirements: Listing of the electrical, plumbing, steam, and ventilation requirements for the equipment
- Accessories: The optional finishes, features, and parts that have a substantial impact on the price
- Approvals: Underwriters Laboratories (UL), National Sanitation Foundation (NSF), American Society of Mechanical Engineers (ASME), and American Gas Association (AGA)
- Other notes: Special installation notes or instructions that will assist the bidder and/or contractor in understanding the desires of the client; special local codes or regulation for this particular piece of equipment

The consultant should maintain an active role in the bid system and approval of equipment as it is being delivered and/or fabricated.

Training

The purchase of new equipment creates a need for training of employees who will operate and maintain the equipment. Equipment vendors will provide the facility with operating and maintenance manuals pertaining to the specific equipment purchased. Vendor or manufacturer representatives should be scheduled to conduct training programs on the initial purchase of a piece of equipment. This training should include equipment operation, specific features, cleaning, and maintenance. The manuals should be used to prepare written procedures for employees using the equipment. It is helpful to provide written and graphic operation and cleaning information near the equipment. Laminating these materials can protect them from soiling in the production and cleaning areas.

Equipment Operation and Equipment Records

Employees are a valuable asset in identifying equipment operating needs. Employees should be trained in routine care of equipment and in recognizing improper operation.

Maintenance of adequate equipment records is essential to the foodservice operation. Many health care facilities do not maintain these records and therefore cannot properly evaluate equipment performance or status. The dietary consultant should establish a system to monitor equipment if one is not being used.

Complete information should be available on each piece of equipment in the dietary department. This information can be recorded on an index card, in a notebook, or on a special form prepared for this purpose (see Fig. 8-1).

Important information to be recorded includes

1. Equipment manufacturer and model number
2. Purchase price
3. Date of purchase
4. Equipment vendor
5. Warranty information
6. Maintenance and repair record

Failure to record specific information about equipment can be costly to the facility. Keeping records of the date of purchase, for example, can protect the right to a repair or replacement under the warranty. The dietary consultant should assist the manager in establishing a system for recording information for major pieces of equipment like ranges, steamers, and ovens as well as small equipment such as toasters, slicers, and food processors.

Routine Maintenance and Inspection

The department should adopt a system for routinely inspecting each piece of equipment. Routine maintenance programs are cost effective, help prevent breakdowns and unsafe operation, and maintain the quality of service. Detailed

Figure 8-1. Form for recording information on maintenance and repair of equipment.

instructions should be prepared to allow thorough inspection of major equipment parts. Facility maintenance employees may be trained for routine inspection and minor repair of foodservice equipment. The facility equipment program should indicate the appropriate procedures to be followed for both emergencies and needed routine maintenance.

A number of factors influence decisions regarding equipment maintenance. Managers must evaluate the availability of in-house maintenance staff, procurement of parts, warranty and service requirements, and cost to the facility of nonfunctional equipment. For example, when comparing service options, the manager must decide if timely repair of a dishmachine would help maintain service quality and be less costly than utilization of disposable serviceware.

Large facilities may retain skilled employees who are qualified to evaluate and repair electrical, mechanical, or refrigeration equipment. Other options include service contracts with the equipment vendor or local businesses (Puckett and Miller 1988). Regardless of service procedures, the facility should be aware of the availability of parts in order to avoid costly delays in equipment repair. It is important to remember that the warranty covering new equipment requires that certain procedures be followed to insure the validity of the coverage.

Equipment Replacement

Replacement of foodservice equipment is a frequently overlooked function that should be included in the overall equipment management program. The equipment records described above can be a valuable tool in determining the need for replacement and should be reviewed periodically. This review is especially important when preparing budget recommendations. Timely replacement of equipment is cost effective and should be addressed by the consultant and the dietary manager on a regular basis.

A number of factors affect the decision to replace equipment. The age of the equipment is an important factor in deciding to repair or replace. All equipment has an expected useful life. Basic guidelines for the probable useful life of kitchen equipment can be found in Table 8-1. The actual life span of equipment may vary since this will depend on the degree of use and maintenance a particular piece of equipment has received.

Initial outlay for the equipment must also be considered. If repairs are minor and inexpensive whereas a new model is very costly, it may be wiser to continue to repair. The cost of the repair should also take into consideration the length of time the equipment is expected to continue to be functional in the operation.

The future plans of the facility should also be considered. If total renovation is planned within the next few years, it may be wiser to delay buying major pieces of equipment until plans for the renovation are complete. This may help avoid costly mistakes in purchasing new pieces that may not be appropriate in the new facility.

In general, the dietary consultant may want to recommend a new piece of equipment for any of the following reasons (Birchfield 1988):

- The equipment is part of a new food facility.
- Existing equipment needs to be replaced.
- Changes in the menu or volume of production require an addition to the facility.
- The equipment will reduce labor costs.
- The equipment will reduce maintenance costs.
- The equipment will produce energy savings.
- The equipment will improve food quality.

Unsafe equipment creates a liability for the facility and can have the potential for harm to employees. Poorly functioning equipment can affect food quality or safety. For example, an oven with a malfunctioning thermostat can result in an unacceptable product. A malfunctioning refrigerator may pose a threat to food safety and reduce the quality of the products held in the unit.

When preparing to recommend equipment replacement or purchase, it is

Table 8-1. Probable Useful Life of Kitchen Equipment

Item	Useful life (years)
Convection oven	7–10
Deck oven	10–15
Rotary oven	12–20
Mixers	15–25
Ranges	10–15
Steam-jacketed kettles	15–25
Food choppers	10–15
Vertical cutter mixer	12–15
Tilting fry pans	12–20
Grills	8–12
Fryers	8–12
Broilers	8–12
Steamers-high pressure	10–15
Steamers-low pressure	12–15
Steamers-no pressure	8–12
Refrigerator/freezer-walk-in	12–20
Refrigerator/freezer-reach-in	12–20
Carts and cabinets	8–12
Coffee urns	8–12
Dishwashing machines	10–15
Stainless steel tables, sinks, and counters with stainless steel legs	unlimited
Galvanized tables and sinks	8–12
Stainless steel shelving	unlimited

Source: John C. Birchfield. 1988. *Design and Layout of Foodservice Facilities.* New York: Van Nostrand Reinhold.

helpful to complete an equipment need analysis. Figure 8-2 details the areas that should receive evaluation. You may wish to use this form to develop one appropriate to your use.

Operating in a Less Than Perfect Kitchen

When working with an existing facility, the consultant often finds poorly designed kitchens that have inadequate or older equipment. Especially in older facilities, production equipment may only include a range and conventional

---

EQUIPMENT NEED ANALYSIS

Type of equipment: _____

Replacement or new? _____

If replacement, what is the condition of the existing equipment?

_____ Old and worn out

_____ Energy hog

_____ Capacity too small

_____ Cannot get replacement parts

_____ Produces an inferior product

_____ High repairs and maintenance costs

Costs to fix the existing piece of equipment: $ _____

Useful life if the equipment is repaired: _____

If equipment is new: _____

Capacity needed: _____

Features wanted: _____

Costs

1. List price: $ _____

   Budget price: $ _____

2. Cost to install: $ _____

3. Annual operating costs (energy): $ _____

4. Annual maintenance costs: $ _____

5. Labor costs

   A. Estimate of additional labor costs (if any) to operate equipment: $ _____

   B. Estimate of actual labor costs saved as a result of buying the equipment (subtract from A): $ _____

6. Annual interest expense on investment: $ _____

   Useful life of the equipment in years: _____

7. Divide purchase price and installation cost by the useful life to determine annual costs.

   Total annual cost (add items 3 through 7): $ _____

Figure 8-2. Evaluation form for purchase or replacement of equipment. *Source:* John C. Birchfield, *Design and Layout of Foodservice Facilities* (New York: Van Nostrand Reinhold, 1988).

ovens. Tray preparation may be hindered by lack of a steamtable and other support equipment. Planning and creative use of available equipment can improve foodservice operations.

The use of steam in food preparation is recommended for many items to help retain nutrients and the quality of the product. Facilities without steam equipment often prepare all items on the range with direct heat. Vegetables may be cooked in deep stock pots with water.

Using a combination of steamtable pans and the range, foodservice employees can create steam equipment. The use of a deep (6- or 8-in.) solid pan and a more shallow (2 1/2-in.) perforated pan will provide the employee a method of steaming vegetables. To use, place 2–3 in. of water in the deep pan and place the perforated pan on top. The use of a lid or other covering while cooking will help retain the steam produced and reduce cooking time. When using this method, employees should only place a shallow layer of food to steam so that the product will cook evenly. Steaming works especially well for fresh or frozen vegetables such as broccoli, cauliflower, and carrots.

To create a large "double-boiler" unit, place a 2 1/2-in. solid steamtable pan over the deeper pan of water. This method provides a larger cooking surface (depending on the sizes of pans used) and is quite suitable for cooking foods requiring medium heat such as eggs, sauces, and soups.

Tray assembly is another area that often was poorly planned in smaller or older facilities. Support equipment such as steamtables, starter stations, and even delivery carts are frequently absent or inappropriate for use by the dietary unit. Also, procedures for assembly may not make the best use of available equipment and labor. For example, trays may be prepared in numerous steps. Employees may stack trays containing silverware, desserts, and so on for use later—when the plate of hot foods is placed on the tray. This procedure wastes space, increases the number of times a tray must be handled, and increases total time required for tray preparation.

A workable solution for tray assembly in the absence of proper equipment requires evaluation of existing equipment, space, and number of employees available at each tray assembly time. The procedure for tray assembly should follow a logical sequence with all needed items organized in a local area.

The number and formation of trayline stations may vary depending on the needs of the system or the availability of employees. The following is an example of a centralized tray assembly system utilizing three employees in three stations. Also provided is a suggested list of equipment needed and items each station may place on the tray.

Trayline starter (employee #1): Stacked trays, identification cards, silverware, napkins, condiments

Hot foods station (employee #2): Plate, base (type depends on system), hot foods, plate garnish

Cold foods station (employee #3): Salads, beverages, bread, desserts, plate cover or dome

In the absence of appropriate equipment, a cart or table can be useful in organizing the trayline starter station. The range may be the only available equipment for holding hot foods. The technique described above for cooking can be used to create "steam" equipment for holding foods on the range. The use of deep steamtable pans and shallow pans to create steam heat can provide an improved holding system as compared to direct heat from the range. Arranging the tray system around the range may be a workable solution to tray preparation in this situation.

The final station can also utilize carts or table space. Mobile baker racks can be especially useful with limited space. Most items needed can be arranged on trays or baking sheets and moved to the tray assembly area when needed.

The above suggestions relate to only two of many problems in poorly equipped kitchens. Many other opportunities exist for the consultant to be effective in improving efficiency and quality. Depending on the facility, the creative use of existing equipment may provide some solutions to design inefficiencies.

DESIGN PREPARATION

The preparation of the foodservice design is an important step in planning a foodservice facility. The planning method selected by an institution often depends on the cost of the preparation. The following are descriptions of common approaches to design preparation.

- The facility may utilize the services of a construction firm to prepare the design and oversee the construction and selection of equipment. This method is usually the lowest in initial cost, but may result in poorly placed equipment or costly equipment that may not meet the needs of the facility (Birchfield 1988).
- The facility may utilize the services of an architect, without the assistance of a foodservice design consultant. The design may be prepared by the firm or with the assistance of an equipment vendor. This also can be disastrous for the facility in terms of cost and poor design (Birchfield 1988).
- The facility may utilize the services of a professional design consultant. This option seems to be the least commonly used, especially by smaller facilities. The use of a design consultant helps insure that the design will meet the needs of the facility and provide the most efficient use of space and equipment. Poor design results in losses related to labor and operational costs. These costs are difficult to measure but have a great impact on the foodservice operation. Even small errors in design and equipment selection can be quite costly (Birchfield 1988).

The design consultant usually charges fees on an hourly basis. The amount is generally based on 6 to 10 percent of the cost of the equipment (Birchfield 1988). For example, for a project in which $100,000 of equipment was purchased, design fees of $6,000 to $10,000 would be expected. The savings realized are noted in the following areas (Birchfield 1988):

Operational costs related to efficiency
Equipment costs related to proper selection
Construction costs related to space utilization
The purchase price of equipment related to specifications

Depending on the nature and scope of the project, the dietary consultant may be involved in the preparation of the design, selection of equipment, and other decisions related to the renovation or construction project. Even with the services of a design consultant, the consultant dietitian should maintain an active role in evaluating the design and selection of equipment throughout the project.

KITCHEN DESIGN AND LAYOUT

In planning foodservice facilities, it is necessary to consider many factors affecting the operation. The design must reflect a system that addresses the following items (Puckett and Miller 1988):

Goals and objectives of the facility and foodservice department
Number of beds and institution design
Additional services or programs supported by dietary
Labor policies and labor availability
Budget, including initial costs and operating costs

Once the above factors are considered, detailed information must be obtained about the operation of the foodservice department. Specific factors directly affecting the design include

Menu type (selective or nonselective)
Menu pattern and the length of the cycle
Desired production system (cook/chill, cook/freeze, prepare/serve)
Variety and numbers of modified diets
Energy availability (gas, electric, steam)

Design Principles

Although each facility will require individualized assessment to obtain the best design for the operation, certain basic principles must be considered in the preparation of any plan.

Locating the Kitchen

The kitchen should be located with easy access to receiving, storage, dining areas, and elevators. The transportation of trays to patient areas should be evaluated in respect to efficiency and the type of tray delivery system selected. Depending on the system, the actual distance to these areas may be less important because of advancements in tray delivery systems in maintaining food temperatures (Puckett and Miller 1988).

Work Flow: Materials and Personnel

The design should reflect the most efficient movement of food, supplies, and personnel. The flow begins with the receiving of materials and ends with service, waste disposal, and dishwashing. The design should eliminate as much cross-traffic and backtracking as possible. Figure 8-3 illustrates the main functional areas of a foodservice operation and relationships between them (Puckett and Miller 1988).

It would be helpful for the dietary consultant to evaluate the location of the functional areas to determine efficiency and traffic patterns of materials and equipment. This evaluation can be made using colored pencils or markers to indicate flow of materials and employees.

Sanitation

The design of the foodservice facility can reduce difficulties in cleaning and time required to complete this function. Finishes of walls and floors that are grease resistant and easily cleaned require less time and effort. Use of wall-mounted equipment eliminates legs, which create difficulty in cleaning. Garbage disposal should be convenient to production and dishwashing areas. The sanitation function requires significant time and should be given special consideration in the preparation of the layout of the facility.

Supervision

One key to supervision is visual access to foodservice production areas. Open floor plans increase supervisory effectiveness. The use of half-walls (4 ft. in height) between lines of equipment and between work departments can be useful in providing visually open spaces in production areas (Birchfield and Miller 1988).

DETERMINING SPACE REQUIREMENTS

In evaluating space needs of a foodservice department, the following areas should be considered:

- Receiving
- Storage: dry, paper, cleaning supplies, refrigerator, freezer, utensils, tray delivery carts
- Office
- Food preparation: Pre-preparation, hot food, salads, beverage, baking
- Tray assembly and distribution
- Dining areas
- Warewashing
- Employee locker areas and toilets

Total space needs for the department should be determined as a result of evaluation of specific functions and equipment needed. The following review of

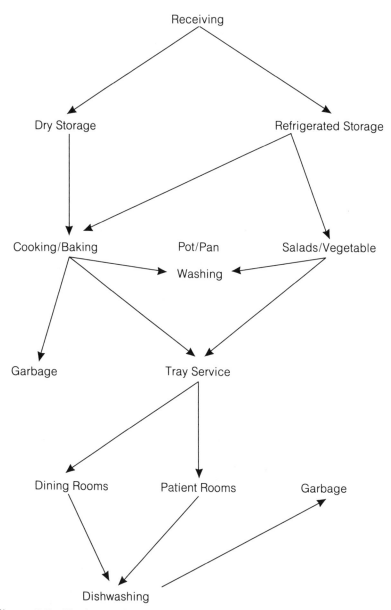

Figure 8-3. The layout of functional areas.

functional areas provides general guidelines for determining space requirements (Birchfield 1988).

Receiving

Small institution   80–100 sq. ft.
(300–1000 meals/day)   (7.44–9.30 m²)

Dry Storage

Small institution	200–300 sq. ft.
	(18.60–27.90 m^2)

The figures given for dry storage are based on twice weekly deliveries and the assumption that cleaning supplies and paper are stored separately.

Cleaning Supplies

Small institution	120–175 sq. ft.
	(11.16–16.28 m^2)

Walk-in Refrigeration

Small institution, two	180–240 sq. ft.
units	(16.7–22.3 m^2)

Walk-in Freezer

The size of the freezer should be based on the menu, number of meals served, and the frequency of deliveries. Frozen foods are usually packaged in cartons that can be stacked. The size of a freezer should be calculated based on the cubic feet of space needed. A sample menu may be used to calculate the frozen space needed. Keep in mind items kept on hand such as margarine and juices when evaluating the menu cycle.

Paper

No standard space requirement is possible because of the variability in the use of paper products by a particular facility. Planning for paper storage should be based on the specific practices of the facility.

Office

Small offices	60–80 sq ft.
	(5.58–7.44 m^2)

The size and number of offices is directly related to facility operations. If the office is to be used by managers, clerical staff and other support personnel, the facility may elect more offices or larger office space. Also, the use of equipment (i.e., computers) affects space needs.

Tray Assembly

Standard recommendations are not available. The amount of space needed can be determined using the following steps:

1. Evaluate the menu and the production/tray assembly system.
2. Compile a list of all equipment to be included in the facility.

3. Prepare a schematic drawing of the functional areas.
4. Prepare templates for equipment (common scale: 1/4 in. = 1 ft.).
5. Arrange equipment and measure the total space needed.

Dining Areas

Standard recommendations are not available. The amount of space needed can be determined using the following steps:

1. Determine the number of residents to be served in the dining area at any one time (consider policies on multiple use of the dining area during meal service).
2. Determine the type of service.
3. Compile a list of numbers and sizes of tables and chairs to be included in the dining area.
4. Prepare templates for equipment (common scale: 1/4 in. = 1 ft.).
5. Arrange tables and chairs and measure the total space needed.

Warewashing

Type of dish system	Size of space
Single-tank dishwasher	250 sq. ft. (23.25 m^2)
Single-tank conveyor	400 sq. ft. (37.20 m^2)
Two-tank conveyor	500 sq. ft. (46.50 m^2)
Flight type conveyor	700 sq. ft. (65.10 m^2)

The above data assumes the inclusion of a three-compartment pot sink with drainboards.

Employee Locker Area and Toilets (combined)

Number of employees	Size of space
5 or fewer employees	60 sq. ft. (5.58 m^2)
5–10 employees	100 sq. ft. (9.30 m^2)
10–20 employees	150 sq. ft. (13.95 m^2)
20–40 employees	225 sq. ft. (20.93 m^2)

PLANNING FUNCTIONAL AREAS

Each area in the foodservice facility should be planned to make the best use of materials and labor. The following discussion briefly addresses important facets of each area, including design features and typical equipment required.

Receiving

The receiving area should be designed to accommodate the needs of the particular foodservice facility—the intended use as well as institutional policies. If the area is a multiple purpose receiving area, all departments may receive deliveries at the same point. In that case, the location should be determined by institution design and the needs of other departments. If a receiving area is intended for foodservice use, it should be located adjacent to the department.

Design Features

CONTROL

Management staff will need visual access to monitor food and supplies as they are transported into and out from the kitchen (for example, from a manager's office or receiving office).

PROTECTION

Deliveries should be protected from the weather by roof overhangs or recessed docks.

DOORS

If the area is planned with two doors, a total width of 5 ft. is needed. If the area is planned with one door, a total width of 4 ft. is needed (Birchfield 1988).

Common Equipment

HAND TRUCKS

These should be heavy duty and have either two or four wheels (Puckett 1988).

SCALES

Scales should be used by all foodservice operations to verify actual weights of products purchased by weight. This step is often omitted since most will have been marked with the weight by the vendor when the product was packaged (Birchfield 1988). It should not be assumed that these weights are accurate at time of delivery. For most facilities, a scale with a maximum capacity of 250 pounds is adequate (Puckett and Miller 1988).

Storage

Storage areas should be planned to create the most efficient flow of material. Storage requirements are affected by a number of factors:

- The number of meals per day
- The variety of menu items
- The type of menu and the length of the menu cycle
- The frequency of deliveries
- Meal distribution procedures
- Policies regarding stock levels, inventory turnover, and so on

A number of recommendations are offered for calculating space needs for dry, refrigerated, and frozen foods. One factor that makes the estimation of storage requirements for institutional foodservice operations difficult is the routine revision of menus. Menus are customarily revised on a seasonal basis and the introduction of new food items is common. It would be advisable to conduct an analysis of typical menus to estimate the type and amounts of foods to be purchased and stored.

Cleaning supplies should be stored in a separate area. The type of cleaning system used will dictate the actual amount of storage needed. If equipment is also stored with supplies, this should be considered in the analysis. Frequency of deliveries will affect needs. Infrequent deliveries by chemical companies may require the facility to purchase larger amounts per delivery.

Adequate space should be planned for storage of tray delivery carts. The number and sizes of carts required can be evaluated for total space needs. The space should be adjacent to the cart washing area and the tray assembly area.

Storage areas that should be planned in the foodservice facility are:

DRY STORAGE

These areas should be planned considering floor, wall, and ceiling material; ventilation and temperature control; and security. Surfaces should be resistant to moisture, smooth, and easily cleaned. Floors should be level with adjacent areas to allow the use of mobile equipment (Puckett and Miller 1988).

FREEZER STORAGE

The requirements of freezer storage will depend on the type of production system. Standard freezers operate between $-10°F$ and $0°F$. The use of a cook/chill system will require equipment that can quickly chill and freeze foods (Puckett and Miller 1988).

REFRIGERATED STORAGE

Standard refrigerators operate between $32°F$ and $40°F$. Walk-in and reach-in units should be in convenient locations for delivery, production, and service.

Work Areas

Work areas should be planned to obtain the highest efficiency possible. Human engineering takes into consideration physical capabilities and the design of the facility and placement of equipment and supplies in the work environment. In planning work areas, the following basic areas should be provided (Birchfield 1988):

Work surface
Sink
Cutting surface
Utensil storage
Pot/pan storage
Adequate aisle space

Production

Design Features

EFFICIENCY

The arrangement of equipment should promote the best use of materials and labor. Equipment may be arranged in lines or islands, or in a U-shape, or an L-shape (Puckett and Miller 1988). The arrangement should provide a direct route from ingredient storage to service areas. The number of employees is an important factor in this design element.

SAFETY

Equipment should be placed to reduce the potential for accidents. Adequate work surfaces should be provided to give the employee space to place hot utensils and pans. For example, a work table beside ovens and deep fat fryers reduces the amount of time and distance the employee needs to transport hot containers.

Common Equipment

OVEN

Ovens cook with heat from either convection, radiation, or microwave. The most common use of the microwave is for small quantities of individual items (Puckett and Miller 1988).

The convection oven cooks with the use of a heat source and a motor-driven fan that circulates air inside the oven. This provides more even cooking and uses less energy than conventional ovens. Further, oven temperature settings can be reduced from 25 to 75 percent (Scriven and Stevens 1989). Some models offer a feature that allows the fan to be turned off, allowing operation as a conventional oven. The capacity of the oven is related to the size of the interior space, the number of racks it holds, and the distance between rack supports. Controls usually indicate both temperature and load, since the amount of food that can be cooked varies with the item and production requirements. Space efficiency can be obtained by purchasing two units that can stack for use (Puckett and Miller 1988).

Conventional ovens cook with radiant heat. The most common and least expensive is referred to as a standard oven and is purchased in combination with a range, grill, or broiler. These are generally not recommended because they are difficult to use, energy inefficient, and difficult to clean (Puckett and Miller 1988). Other oven models should be evaluated for inclusion in the production area.

Deck ovens can handle a variety of baking and roasting needs. The heat is produced from top and bottom units, providing a more even heat source as compared to the conventional oven (Puckett and Miller 1988). These can be stacked in double or triple units. The small facility may not desire this selection since it requires more floor space.

GRILL

Grills can be purchased as freestanding, part of a range top, table model, or a modular unit to be mounted on an equipment stand. Grills are available in widths of 2, 3, 4, 5, or 6 ft. and are generally 21 to 34 in. deep. Large grills have multiple controls that allow varying temperatures in 12-in. sections of the grill. A grooved grill is also available. An alternative to the broiler, it allows improved control during cooking and uses less energy (Scriven and Stevens 1989).

TILTING SKILLET OR BRAISING PAN

The tilting braising pan is a versatile piece of equipment: It can be used to fry, stew, simmer, grill, or boil a wide variety of foods. It is available in 10- to 40-gal. capacities (Puckett and Miller 1988) and may be purchased as a table model, a wall-mounted unit, or free-standing unit on legs. The ability of the pan to tilt allows for easy removal of foods. For ease in cleaning, a floor drain should be placed at the front of the skillet (Scriven and Stevens 1989).

RANGE

In many facilities, the bulk of food production is completed on the range, requiring the use of a variety of pots and pans. For many foods this method of cooking is the least desirable, and it increases the time required for pot and pan washing. With the variety of cooking equipment available, the need for large or multiple range units is limited.

Electric ranges have solid tops or round individual units. Solid surfaces should have multiple controls so that the entire unit is not operating when only a small area is needed. Individual units have separate controls for each unit. Gas ranges have solid tops and open individual burners. As with the electric, the solid tops should have separate controls. Individual open burners direct gas flame to the surface of the cooking container and can be operated individually (Puckett and Miller 1988).

STEAM EQUIPMENT

Steam equipment has been found to be useful in reducing energy usage in the foodservice facility. Common steam equipment includes high-pressure, low-pressure, or no-pressure steamers and steam-jacketed kettles. The source of steam for these pieces may be a central steam line, separate boilers with each piece, or a combination of steamer and steam-jacketed kettle operated from a shared boiler. Steam equipment is more energy efficient than open or closed surface range units since the energy used for cooking is contained inside the cooking compartment.

High-pressure steamers operate at approximately 15 lb. per sq. in. The cooking process is faster than low- and no-pressure steamers since the cooking temperature is higher (Birchfield 1988). The higher temperature allows foods to be prepared in small amounts during the meal service, reducing holding time and helping to improve the quality and nutrient value of foods. Food cooked in steamtable pans and used directly in meal service reduces the number of pans to wash.

Low- and no-pressure steamers allow cooking of large quantities of food. Low-pressure steamers operate at approximately 5 lb. per sq. in. They may be purchased with one, two, or three compartments. These steamers are especially suited to cooking starch products, vegetables, and eggs (Birchfield 1988).

Steam-jacketed kettles operate with steam heat contained within a double-walled jacket. Foods are cooked as a result of heat conducted through the walls of the kettle. Stationary kettles have a valve at the base of the kettle through which food is removed. Tilting kettles are manually operated or may have a powered tilting mechanism. The capacity of kettles ranges from 2 1/2 to 120 gal. (Puckett and Miller 1988). The size and type of kettle selected should reflect intended usage by the facility.

DEEP FAT FRYERS

Fryers come in many capacities with a wide range of features. They may be free-standing or built in with capacities ranging from 15 to 30 lb. Features to consider are accurate thermostats, an easily accessible drain, timers, and basket lifters (Puckett and Miller 1988). The facility should evaluate the menu for intended use and capacity needed.

SLICER

Slicers are useful in producing uniform slices of meat and other foods. The most common in small facilities is the gravity-fed machine with a slanted carriage.

Manual or automatic slicers are available. The thickness of the food is adjusted with a dial. The machine should be easy to operate and clean and provide safety protection from the blade while in operation (Puckett and Miller 1988).

MIXER

Mixers are available in bench or floor models. Bench models range from 5 to 20 qt. while floor models may be as large as 140 qt. (Puckett and Miller 1988). The facility should evaluate intended use of the mixer to select capacity and accessories. Most mixers come equipped with a bowl, a wire whip, and a flat beater.

BLENDER

Blenders are a common piece of equipment in institutional foodservice. The need for texture modification for many long-term care residents requires the use of pureed foods. Common container sizes of blenders include 24, 44, 64, and 128 oz. (1 gallon). The container may be glass, Lexan, or stainless steel. Motors may be 115 or 220 v. The size of the motor and blades varies (Scriven and Stevens 1989). Smaller facilities may be accustomed to the use of home type blenders that are less powerful and are not designed for the heavy use required by many institutions. Institutional type blenders are recommended because of their longer life and greater production capacity.

OTHER EQUIPMENT

A variety of small pieces of equipment is needed in foodservice production. The facility will need to purchase an assortment of pots and pans for cooking and baking; scales; toasters; measuring equipment; portioning equipment; knives; and mixing bowls. The complete line of small equipment needed will depend on the production system and menu.

The above list is typical of equipment in institutional foodservice. Additional items may be needed depending on the facility. For example, if the facility plans to prepare yeast products, the addition of proofing equipment may be indicated. In addition, holding equipment for hot foods may be needed by the foodservice facility.

Tray Service

Design Features

TYPE

The type of tray assembly equipment needed depends on the tray system components.

CONFIGURATION

Equipment arrangement around a straight line conveyor is most common. Other options include the use of a circular or oval conveyor with support equipment arranged around the conveyor or conveyors with one or more turns (Puckett and Miller 1988).

ASSEMBLY SYSTEM

Tray assembly in a central kitchen is the most utilized in institutional foodservice. It allows greater control of materials and labor as compared to multiple tray assembly areas.

DESIGN

The basic design of the tray assembly system involves the selection of the conveyor and arrangement of supporting equipment. The number of employees available at tray assembly times is the factor that dictates the number of stations planned.

Common Equipment

TRAY CONVEYOR

The conveyor should be selected to accommodate the width of the tray. The purpose of the conveyor is to transport the tray past assembly stations. This may be accomplished by the use of rollers, or motor-driven belts. The roller conveyor is manually operated with employees moving the tray past each station.

TRAY STARTER STATION

Tray starter stations are designed to organize the assembly of the tray. The station should contain trays, napkins, silverware, condiments, and tray cards. Depending on the temperature system used, this station may also contain insulated bases or heated pellets placed on the tray at this time. Specialized eating equipment may be used including spill-proof cups, plate guards, scoop plates, suction plates, and large-handled silverware.

STEAMTABLE

Steamtables may be either gas or electric and may contain dry or wet wells. The typical openings are rectangular and 12×20 in. in size. The number of wells available ranges from two to six. Steamtables can be purchased with separate controls on each well, allowing varying temperatures depending on the product being served.

REFRIGERATION

Refrigeration units at the trayline aid in efficiency since food can be stored at the next point of use immediately after being prepared. Upright reach-in units are commonly selected. Refrigerators equipped with air curtains maintain cooler interior temperatures while allowing easy access to foods. The facility may desire to place a separate milk cooler at the tray assembly area to reduce handling. Freezer equipment may also be positioned at the trayline to serve frozen items such as ice cream.

TRAY SERVICE

The type of tray service selected depends on the size of the facility and the time from tray preparation to service to the resident. Among other things, the system should also be evaluated for the appearance desired by the facility. The following are common selections in temperature maintenance systems.

Heated plate
Insulated bases and domes
Heated bases with domes
Compartmentalized insulated bases and domes
Insulated glasses, bowls, coffee cups
Dual trays for hot and cold foods, to be combined at the time of service

TRAY DELIVERY CARTS

The number and size of tray delivery carts will be determined by the meal system and the numbers of trays to be served in various locations in the facility. The carts should be easily moved and cleaned. The decision to select open or closed carts remains with the facility. It should be remembered that all items should be covered or wrapped if open carts are used. Carts that maintain hot and cold temperatures are also available and allow separation of foods on two trays to be combined at the time of service.

OTHER EQUIPMENT

Additional equipment that may be required for the tray assembly system includes beverage equipment; toasters; self-leveling dish dispensers; units for holding cups, saucers, glasses, and covers,; and heated plate dispensers.

Dishwashing

Design Features

LOCATION

This area should be located near the tray assembly, dining, and production areas. Centralized cleaning improves efficiency and control of materials and supplies.

LAYOUT

The layout of the area should promote efficiency, safety, and productivity (Puckett and Miller 1988). Evaluations must be based on procedures, the type of service, the number of meals, and meal service times. Adequate space must be planned for scraping, sorting, and racking dishes to be washed. Wall-mounted shelves are helpful in racking glasses and cups. Landing space for clean dishes needs to be adequate for air drying of dishes (Puckett and Miller 1988).

VENTILATION

Adequate ventilation is necessary in this area. Excessive heat and moisture create unpleasant working conditions. Hoods should be placed above the dish-machine to exhaust steam and heat. Adequate air conditioning should be provided (Puckett and Miller 1988).

Common Equipment

GARBAGE DISPOSAL

The size of the disposal is related to the number of meals served. A motor of 3/4 HP is recommended when serving up to 100 persons per meal, 1 HP when serving 100–150, and 1 1/4 HP when serving 150–175 (Scriven and Stevens 1989).

DISHMACHINE

A variety of dishmachine sizes and styles is available. The sanitizing system can use either hot water or chemicals; hot water sanitizing is the most common. Dishwashers are categorized as single-tank stationary, single-tank conveyor, or multiple-tank conveyor. A basic guide to the selection of the dishmachine is the number of meals per hour. For 50–250 meals per hour a single-tank stationary machine is recommended. For 250–400 meals per hour, a single-tank conveyor is recommended (Scriven and Stevens 1989).

Single-tank stationary machines utilize standard 20 × 20-in. racks. The washing action is done by wash arms above and below the racks. The dish-machine operator manually lifts the doors to place the rack in the machine.

Single-tank conveyors operate in much the same way as single-tank station-ary machines except that conveyors automatically transport the dish rack through the machine either by chain or pawl. The pawl mechanism uses a single rod to pull racks through (Scriven and Stevens 1989).

Other features available with the dishmachine are automatic detergent and rinse agent systems and booster heaters.

OTHER EQUIPMENT

A variety of other equipment is available for inclusion in the dishwashing area. If the facility chooses centralized sanitation, the design and selection of a three-pot sink should be planned in this area. Depending on the needs of the facility, specialized equipment such as sinks for soaking, silverware washing equipment, glass washers, and pot washers may be purchased.

CONCLUSION

The successful management of foodservice equipment in an existing facility requires continual involvement of the consultant dietitian in the operation. Monitoring of the department is a joint effort between the consultant, dietary manager, and administrator. Systems must be developed that address the needs of the facility and allow timely review.

In planning foodservice facilities, the consultant must make thorough evaluations of the needs, budget constraints, and departmental procedures. Foodservice facilities should be planned to make the best use of human and material resources. Equipment selection should be based on function, the need for the equipment, and levels of quality required. Proper design and equipment selection can be an asset to the dietary manager in maintaining department operations.

REFERENCES

Birchfield, John C. 1988. *Design and layout of foodservice facilities.* New York: Van Nostrand Reinhold.

Jernigan, Anna, and Lynne Ross. 1980. *Food service equipment.* Iowa: Iowa State University Press.

National Restaurant Association. 1979. *Sanitation operations manual.* Chicago: National Restaurant Association.

Puckett, Ruby, and Bonnie Miller. 1988. *Food service manual for health care institutions.* American Hospital Association.

Scriven, Carl, and James Stevens. 1989. *Food equipment facts.* New York: Van Nostrand Reinhold.

Spears, M. C., and A. Vaden. 1985. *Foodservice organization: A managerial and systems approach.* New York: John Wiley & Sons.

9

Nutritional Care

NUTRITION ASSESSMENT

Resident assessment is a key component of the new Omnibus Reconciliation Act of 1987 (OBRA) and the Interpretive Guidelines of the Long Term Care Requirements for Medicare and Medicaid. With the implementation of these requirements in 1990 comes an increased emphasis on accurately and thoroughly assessing the resident's status upon admission to a long-term care facility. Within the total resident assessment is an increased emphasis on the resident's nutritional status. This emphasis on nutrition opens the door of opportunity for consultant dietitians to provide dietary services required to comply with federal regulations.

What is a nutrition assessment? Nutrition assessment is a process of gathering information from a number of sources to evaluate an individual's nutritional status (Jernigan 1987). Assessing the geriatric resident is frequently difficult because of the unreliability of some nutritional measures, the lack of standards for nutritional sufficiency of individuals over age 55, and changes in nutritional requirements that occur with normal aging. The process of aging affects the nutritional status of the resident. The normal bodily changes that occur with the passage of time include changes in the body's different organs and tissues. Aging of specific organs proceeds at different rates for different people, however. Advanced age is associated with nonuniform changes in various body tissues. Some common changes in biological aging are the following (Kittelberger et al. 1984):

- Decreased acuity of senses—sight, smell, taste, and hearing
- Changes in gastrointestinal function
  Loss of teeth/ill-fitting dentures
  Decreased taste sensation
  Decreased secretion of digestive juices and enzymes
  Decreased mobility of GI tract
- Decrease in basal metabolic rate (BMR)
  The BMR decreases 20 percent between ages of 30 and 90 because of the reduction of the number of metabolically active cells
- Decrease in bone mass
  Average bone loss is approximately 25 percent in females by the age of 80
  Average bone loss is approximately 12 percent in males by the age of 80

- Changes in body composition, resulting in
  Decreased lean body mass
  Decreased total body water
  Increased body fat, up to 30 percent
- Decrease in cardiovascular function
  Declining cardiac output
  Reduced elasticity of blood vessels
- Decrease in respiratory system with 50 percent reduction in maximum breathing capacity
- Decreased capability of the kidneys to excrete metabolic end products
- Decreased immune function
- Decreased ability to maintain glucose levels
- Increased fragility of skin

The initial assessment is designed to pinpoint the presence of nutritonal problems. Once problems are identified, they are clearly defined and measurable approaches are formulated during the care-planning process.

Completing the resident assessment requires teamwork. All disciplines, including nursing, social services, activities, and auxiliary services such as physical therapy, must work together to identify and develop workable solutions of interdisciplinary problems involving the nutritional status of the resident. The initial assessment is cost effective for the facility since preventive nutritional measures may be less costly than measures required to restore the nutrition status of a malnourished resident/patient.

For example, 3 percent of our nation's annual health care budget or $60 million is spent treating pressure sores, only one of the many nutrition-related problems that may occur in the institutionalized aged population (Johnson 1989).

The assessment should be initiated within 24 hours of admission via the resident interview and completed within the specified time frame mandated by state and/or federal regulations. The OBRA requirements specify that the assessment must be done promptly upon admission but no later than 14 days after the date of admission.

Initial Interview

The initial interview is step 1 of the nutrition assessment process. Talking with someone about food preferences is a relatively simple task, but preplanning is necessary. Prior to interviewing a new resident, scan the medical chart for documented analysis of the resident's hearing, vision, and speech capabilities; mental status; prescribed diet; and admitting diagnosis. Good listening and observation skills are key factors in a meaningful interview. It is important to establish good communication with the resident initially and to be honest about which services and individual preferences can be met by the facility. Initial promises that cannot be kept will only create anxiety and distrust between the resident and the facility.

Specific physical handicaps may be noted during the chart scan. Some common handicaps and accepted approaches by the dietary consultant are reviewed below:

Speech disorders: Use closed-ended questions; provide paper and pencil or use food models or pictures as appropriate to the individual being interviewed.

Hearing loss: Look directly at the resident when speaking, speak slowly and clearly, use short sentences, and repeat words as needed; write information or questions on paper if necessary.

Vision loss: Introduce yourself and maintain one position in room with the resident; ask about feeding assistance and adaptive devices that may be needed.

Impaired mental status: If the resident is unable to answer questions coherently, a follow-up with family members or observation during mealtime might reveal food preferences and dislikes.

Clinical Examination

Clinical examination, step 2 of the assessment process, is also completed during the initial interview. By observing the physical status of an individual, one can look for clues to possible nutritional deficiencies. If a resident appears to be underweight, inquire about recent weight changes and historical weight. Check for physical signs that may be the result of protein or calorie malnutrition and/or vitamin and mineral deficiency. Table 9-1 gives examples of physical signs of malnutrition.

Once signs have been observed, document any abnormalities noted on the nutrition assessment. Discussion with other health care team members (nurses and physicians) is vital to verify the possible physical signs noticed before developing a plan of care. Much practice is needed in this particular area to develop a high percentage of accuracy.

During this step of the assessment process, one can also observe for possible signs of dysphagia. Dysphagia is defined as difficulty in swallowing, and refers to a wide range of impairments caused by many underlying conditions. Possible observable signs include drooling, poor lip closure, weakened facial muscles, pocketing of food and/or medications in the weakened facial area, and poor tongue control.

Anthropometric Assessment

Step 3 of the nutrition assessment is the anthropometric assessment, the measurement of body size, weight, and proportions (Chumlea et al. 1987). Obtaining and recording anthropometric measures as part of the nutritional assessment is essential. Currently used methods of nutritional anthropometric

Table 9-1. Physical Signs of Malnutrition

Body Area	Signs	Possible Cause
Hair	Dull, dry, thin, sparse; lack of natural shine; loss of curl; changed color; easily plucked; depigmentation	Protein-calorie deficiency; zinc deficiency; other nutrient deficiencies; manganese, copper deficiency
Eyes	Small, yellowish lumps around eyes; white rings around both eyes	Hyperlipidemia
	Pale eye membranes	Vit. B_{12}, folacin, and/or iron deficiency
	Night blindness, dry membranes, dull or soft cornea	Vit. A, zinc deficiencies
	Redness and fissures of eyelid corners	Niacin deficiency
	Angular inflammation of eyelids	Riboflavin deficiency
	Ring of fine blood vessels around cornea	Generally poor nutrition
Lips	Redness and swelling of mouth; angular fissures, scars at corner of mouth	Niacin, riboflavin, iron, and/or vit. B_6 deficiency
Gums	Sponginess, swelling, bleed easily, redness, gingivitis	Vit. A, C, niacin, riboflavin deficiencies
Mouth	Chelosis, angular scars	Riboflavin, folic acid deficiency
Tongue	Sores, swelling, scarlet and raw	Folacin, niacin deficiency
	Smooth with papillae Glossitis, purplish color	Riboflavin, vit. B^{12}, pyriodoxine, iron, or zinc deficiency
Taste	Sense of taste diminished	Zinc deficiency
Teeth	Gray-brown spots	Increased fluoride intake
	Missing or erupting abnormally	Generally poor nutrition
Face	Skin color loss, dark cheeks and eyes, enlarged parotid glands, scaling of skin around nostrils	Protein-calorie deficiency; niacin, riboflavin, pyridoxine deficiencies specifically
	Pallor	Iron, folacin, vit. B_{12}, C deficiencies
	Hyperpigmentation	Niacin deficiency

Continued

Table 9-1. Physical Signs of Malnutrition (*Continued*)

Body Area	Signs	Possible Cause
Neck	Thyroid enlargement, symptoms of hypothyroidism	Iodine deficiency
Nails	Fragility, banding	Protein deficiency
	Spoon-shaped	Iron deficiency
Skin	Slow wound healing	Zinc deficiency
	Psoriasis	Biotin deficiency
	Scaliness	Biotin deficiency
	Black and blue marks due to skin bleeding	Vit.. C and/or vit. K deficiency
	Dryness, mosaic, sandpaper feel, flakiness	Vit. A deficiency or excess
	Swollen and dark	Niacin deficiency
	Lack of fat under skin, bilateral edema	Protein-calorie deficiency
	Yellow-colored	Carotene deficiency/ excess
	Cutaneous flushing, pallor	Niacin, iron, folic acid deficiency
Gastrointestinal system	Anorexia, flatulence	Vit. B_{12} deficiency
Muscular system	Weakness	Phosphorus or potassium deficiency
	Wasted appearance	Protein-calorie deficiency
	Calf tenderness, absence of knee jerks	Thiamin deficiency
	Peripheral neuropathy	Folacin, pyridoxine, pantothenic acid, thiamin deficiencies
	Muscle twitching	Magnesium or pyridoxine excesses/deficiencies
	Muscle cramps	Chloride deficiency, sodium deficiency
	Muscle pain	Biotin deficiency
Skeletal system	Demineralization of bone	Calcium, phosphorus, vit. D deficiencies
	Epiphyseal enlargement of leg and knee	Vit. D deficiency
	Bowed legs	Vit. D deficiency
	Growth failure in children	Protein, vit. D deficiency
Nervous System	Listlessness	Protein-calorie deficiency
	Loss of position and vibratory sense; decrease and loss of ankle and knee reflexes	Thiamin and vit. B_{12} deficiencies

Continued

Table 9-1. Physical Signs of Malnutrition (*Continued*)

Body Area	Signs	Possible Cause
	Seizures, memory impairment and behavioral disturbances	Magnesium, zinc deficiencies
	Peripheral neuropathy, dementia	Pyridoxine deficiency

Source: Barness, Coble, MacDonald, and Christakis, *Nutrition in Medical Practice* (Westport, Conn.: AVI Publishing, 1981).

assessment are not always satisfactory for elderly persons, however, because of individual differences in the aging process. Measurements such as stature, tricep skinfold thickness, and mid-arm circumference can reflect a variety of physiological factors.

Of the anthropometric measurements, weight is the most commonly used. Each resident/patient should be weighed upon admission with follow-up in a timely manner based on facility policy. A majority of long-term care facilities weigh residents monthly unless physical/physiological conditions indicate the need for greater frequency. The usual methods of obtaining weight include the use of an upright balance beam, an electronic scale, a wheelchair scale and a bed scale. Regardless of what type of equipment is used, accuracy depends on the health care giver obtaining the weight. Because of the importance of accurate measurements, facilities should be encouraged to train specific care givers to obtain weights.

When a resident/patient is nonambulatory and appropriate scales are not available or a resident requires casting or traction due to bone fractures, weight can be estimated using recumbent measurements. Recumbent measures are made while a person is lying on a bed or on a flat surface that has adequate support for the arms and legs. Some recumbent measures require bending or lifting an arm or leg. All measurements should be made on the left side of the body. If the left side cannot be measured, the corresponding right side is used. The recumbent measurements used to determine an appropriate weight include calf circumference (calf C), knee height (knee H), mid-arm circumference (MAC) and subscaplar skinfold thickness (subsc SF). Each of these measurements is multiplied by a factor, adding the results and then subtracting a constant. All measurements are to be recorded in centimeters. The formulas used for weight determination (Chumlea et al. 1987) are

$$\text{Body weight for men} = (0.98 \times \text{calf C}) + (1.16 \times \text{knee H}) + (1.73 \times \text{MAC}) + (0.37 \times \text{subsc SF}) - 81.69$$
$$\text{Body weight for women} = (1.27 \times \text{calf C}) + (0.87 \times \text{knee H}) + (0.98 \times \text{MAC}) + (0.4 \times \text{subsc SF}) - 62.35$$

The process for obtaining recumbent measurements will be discussed later in this chapter.

Once the resident's weight is obtained, a comparison of the weight factor based on the resident's height and sometimes age, provides the basis for estimating whether an individual is over or under ideal body weight (IBW). Establishing an ideal body weight formula for elderly persons can be difficult. Tables used include the Metropolitan Life Insurance Weight-Height Tables, 1983; Gerontology Research Center Weight Range for Men and Women by Age; and the Calculation of Desirable Body Weight. The calculation of desirable body weight using height as the main index and allowing for a ±10 percent range for body frame is one of the most widely used indicators for ideal body weight, regardless of the resident's age. For men, calculate 106 lb. for 5 ft., adding 6 lb./in. above 5 ft. For women, calculate 100 lb. for 5 ft. adding 5 lb./in. above 5 ft. Calculating ideal body weight for the geriatric person (especially women) can be difficult because of the unavailability of a standardized formula. However, a chart for females under 5 ft. tall has been developed by a dietetic consulting firm on the basis of information from the Metropolitan Life Insurance Company (Table 9-2). This chart is to be used as a guideline only.

When estimating body weight for residents or patients with amputations, the commonly used formula is based on the following percentages of body weight per body part (Brunnstrom 1972): the upper body, 43.0 percent; the arm, 6.5 percent; the entire leg, 18.5 percent; and the leg below the knee, 9.0 percent.

The accuracy of initial weight measurement is as important as the accuracy of subsequent weights. Weight loss is evaluated not only in actual pounds, but in percentage of weight loss in a designated time period. In the new Interpretive Guidelines of the Federal Long Term Care Requirements for Medicare/Medicaid, the following weight loss formula has been designated as the guideline to use in evaluating weight status of residents:

$$\text{Percent weight loss} = \text{usual weight} - \text{current weight}$$
$$\div \text{current weight} \times 100$$

For example: $130 - 115 \div 115 \times 100 = 13\%$

Interval	Significant Loss %	Severe Loss %
1 Week	1.0–2.0%	>2.0
1 Month	5.0	>5.0
3 Months	7.5	>7.5
6 Months	10.0	>10.0

Source: Blackburn et al. 1977. Nutritional and metabolic assessment of the hospitalized patient. *Journal of Parenteral and Enteral Nutrition.* 1:11.

Table 9-2. Height-Weight of Short Stature People: Females under 5 Feet Tall

Height	Weight		
	Small Frame	Medium Frame	Large Frame
4'-11"	93–101	98–110	106–120
4'-10"	90–98	95–107	103–117
4'-9"	87–95	92–104	100–114
4'-8"	84–92	89–101	97–111
4'-7"	81–89	86–98	94–108
4'-6"	78–86	83–95	91–105
4'-5"	75–83	80–92	88–102

Source: C. L. Gerwick and Associates, Overland Park, KS.

Policies and procedures should be established by each facility detailing the nutrition intervention implemented based on percentage of weight loss. When significant weight loss is documented by nursing services, the physician, dietitian and/or dietary manager should be notified immediately. This information should be transmitted in written form, especially to physicians. The form letter in Figure 9-1 is an excellent example of a written communiqué for physicians regarding resident weight loss.

Another common anthropometric measure that is equally vital to establishing nutrition status parameters is height. For measurement of stature, an individual should be able to stand upright with assistance. Even when elderly persons are able to stand, inaccuracies may be recorded because of physical conditions related to aging such as osteoporosis. When stature cannot be measured, the use of recumbent measurements is a solution. One alternative measure in estimating stature is the measurement of total arm length. It is, that long-bone length does not decrease with age and total arm length measurement does correlate closely with height (Chernoff et al. 1987). No information currently exists documenting the correlation of the arm-length measurements, however. Another method involves measuring the length of the bedfast resident from the crown of the head to the bottom of the heel with the individual facing the ceiling (Jernigan 1987). Again, accuracy of results using this method is questionable.

The most reliable recumbent measurement for establishing stature is knee height. Knee height changes little with increasing age but correlates closely with stature (Chumlea, et al. 1987). To obtain knee height, a sliding broad-blade caliper is used. A device used specifically for this purpose is available from MediForm Printers & Publishers (5150 S.W. Griffith Drive, Beaverton, OR 97005) and Ross Laboratories (Columbus, OH 43216). The following technique is used for measuring knee height (Chumlea et al. 1987):

1. All measurements are obtained on the left side of the individual.
2. Left knee and ankle of the individual are bent at a 90° angle.

To: Dr. _____
From: _____
Date: _____
Reference: Weight Loss

   In reviewing the records of resident _____ , I feel I should notify you of the weight loss this patient is experiencing. Please review the following information and notify facility of any additional measures you would like us to take.

Comments from Nursing Staff:

Comments from Physician:

Please return to: _____   _____
                                                    Physician's Signature

Figure 9-1. Sample letter to the physician concerning patient weight loss.

3. One blade of the caliper is placed under the heel of the left foot while the other blade is placed over the anterior surface of the left thigh, above the condyles of the femur and just proximal to the patella. The shaft of the caliper is held parallel to the shaft of the tibia.
4. Pressure is applied to compress the tissue and measurements are recorded to the nearest 0.1 cm.
5. Two measurements are made in immediate succession and should agree within 0.5 cm.

Once the knee height is obtained, the stature of an individual can be computed. Two formulas are used, one for men and another for women. The formulas are

Stature for men: $(2.02 \times knee\ H) - (0.04 \times age) + 64.19$
Stature for women: $(1.83 \times knee\ H) - (0.24 \times age) + 84.88$

Knee height measurement is recorded in centimeters and age is rounded to the nearest whole year.

Other recumbent measurements that can be obtained include calf circumference, mid-arm circumference, tricep skinfold thickness, and subscapular skinfold thickness. All of these values must be obtained if a computed weight versus an actual weight is to be documented.

The calf circumference value is primarily used as part of the computed weight calculations and is obtained using an insertion measuring tape with the left knee bent at a 90° angle (Chumlea et al. 1987).

The mid-arm circumference and triceps skinfold thickness can be used together to estimate body mass by calculation of the mid-arm muscle area. Again, an insertion measuring tape is used, measuring the upper left arm at midpoint to obtain the mid-arm circumference. For accuracy of measurement, the left arm is extended alongside the body, with the palm facing upward. Measurements should always be recorded to the nearest 0.1 cm with successive measurements within 0.5 cm.

The triceps and subscapular skinfold thickness measurements provide an indirect estimate of body fat. Using a skinfold caliper, the triceps skinfold measurement is obtained on the back of the left arm over the triceps muscle (at midpoint), while the subscapular skinfold thickness is measured just posterior to the left scapula, or shoulder blade. When both measurements are made, the individual is lying on the right side with the right arm extending from the front of the body. The upper body is in a straight line while the legs are bent and slightly tucked. The left arm rests along the trunk, palm down. Both of these measurements are recorded to the nearest 2 mm with successive agreements within 4 mm.

Obtaining accuracy in these measurements requires practice. The accuracy of these recumbent measures, especially the triceps skinfold thickness, has been questioned in the case of elderly persons, however, because of changes in body composition. The body fat of an elderly person, for example, may increase to 30 percent of the total weight.

Assessment of Basal Energy Needs

Anthropometric measures are key factors in completing the resident's nutrition assessment and are needed to evaluate the basal energy, protein, and fluid needs of an individual resident. Establishing the basal needs of a resident is Step 4 in the assessment process.

The Harris-Benedict equation, with adjustment for sex, age, activity, and injury, is the most common formula used for estimating basal energy expenditure (BEE):

$$\text{Men: BEE} = 66 + (13.7 \times W) + (5 \times H) - (6.8 \times A) \times \text{activity factor} \times \text{injury factor}$$

$$\text{Women: BEE} = 655 + (9.6 \times W) + (1.7 \times H) - (4.7 \times A) \times \text{activity factor} \times \text{injury factor}$$

Key
W = Actual weight
  in kilograms
H = Height in
  centimeters
A = Age in years
Activity Factors
  Confined to bed = 1.2
  Ambulatory = 1.3
Injury factors
  Minor surgery = 1.1
  Major surgery = 1.2
  Mild infection = 1.2 (stage I
  and II pressure sores)

Injury factors
  Moderate infection =
  1.4 (stage III pressure sores)
  Severe infection =
  1.8 (stage IV pressure sores)
  Skeletal trauma = 1.35
  Head injury with
  steroids = 1.6
  Blunt trauma = 1.35
  40 percent body
  burn = 1.5
  100 percent body
  burn = 1.95

Establishing protein needs is based on the Recommended Dietary Allowance for adults of 0.8 grams of protein/1 kg body weight. For ease of calculation, it is rounded to 1 g/kg body weight. Protein needs increase as injury factors are identified. For residents with pressure sores, fractures, or infection, 1.2 to 1.8 g of protein/kg body weight may be needed for positive nitrogen balance. When calculating protein needs of residents significantly over or under ideal body weight, the ideal body weight is used as the weight factor rather than actual weight.

Calculating daily fluid needs is equally important especially for those residents with tube feeding and poor fluid intake. Thirty cc/kg body weight is often used as the standard for calculating fluid needs for elderly persons.

Establishing these basal requirements is essential in estimating appropriate nutrient needs for oral or enteral feeding levels.

Review of Laboratory Data

Step 5 of the nutrition assessment process is reviewing and evaluating laboratory data. Locating laboratory data for some residents may be a major challenge, although the availability of data has improved over the years. Increased emphasis on laboratory data is noted in the newly revised Interpretation Guidelines of Federal Long Term Care Requirements for nursing homes as well as in recent literature on nutrition assessment. It is essential that recent laboratory data be available upon admission of a resident. If a resident has been admitted to a long-term care facility from a hospital, laboratory data may be available but may not be transferred with admission histories. This problem can be resolved by having the facility's coordinator of admissions notify the hospital with instructions to include laboratory records in the admission history. If a resident is admitted from the home setting, however, laboratory data is usually absent. In these instances, the consultant dietitian may need to initiate the process by recommending laboratory data be obtained as soon after admission as possible. This request may be made by the dietitian or through the nursing department.

Laboratory data in a long-term care facility is not obtained as frequently as in acute care settings, but parameters should be established for obtaining data in a timely manner. Fasting blood sugar levels need to be obtained at least monthly for residents diagnosed as diabetic, while electrolyte levels, particularly potassium, are needed for residents receiving diuretic therapy without potassium supplementation. Residents with hematologic data or any other laboratory data noted as abnormal on the initial screening should be retested within three months or sooner, depending on the severity of the abnormality.

When evaluating nutritional status in the aged population, serum albumin is often considered to be a predictor of malnutrition. Serum albumin is minimally affected by aging, but related conditions can skew test results. Tests of serum albumin level may not be valid when liver disease and/or urinary and gastrointestinal protein losses are occurring. Also, recent literature has indicated that bed rest alone will significantly decrease serum albumin levels (Chernoff et al. 1987). Typically, serum albumin will reveal depleted body protein levels after approximately two weeks of starvation. Research indicates that serum transferrin is the most accurate indicator of protein calorie malnutrition, however. Serum transferrin will usually show protein depletion earlier than serum albumin—within a few days of the beginning of "starvation." Despite its accuracy, the serum transferrin test is seldom available due to cost. In reality, the consultant dietitian must work within the financial limitations of the facility and the resident when recommending additional laboratory data.

When evaluating a resident's nutritional status based on laboratory data, one must still use the parameters established as acceptable for persons 51 years of age or younger. In 1988, however, The American Journal of Nursing established a guide to changing lab values in elders, and it was published in Geriatric Nursing, May/June, 1989 (Table 9–2A). Research is continuously being conducted in this area to establish definite guidelines.

Drug/Nutrient Interactions

Step 6 of the initial assessment process is identification of possible drug/nutrient interactions, which can manifest themselves in two ways: (1) as the effect of a medication on nutrient metabolism or utilization, or (2) as an effect of ingested food on drug uptake or utilization. Often it is the responsibility of the consultant dietitian to identify and alert the health care team to the possibility of nutrient imbalances caused by medications or the effects food may have on the absorption of drugs. The food/medications interactions booklet (Powers and Moore 1988) is a valuable tool for dietitians to use in documenting possible drug/nutrient interactions. The drug/nutrient interactions listed in Table 9-3 are limited to those for which there are well-documented studies and/or case reports and which may occur at therapeutic doses.

The nutrion assessment process identifies those residents at risk of nutri-

Table 9-2A. Guide to Changing Lab Values in Elders*

Lab Test	Adult (20–40 yr)	Changes with Age	Why	Caution
Urinalysis				
Protein	0–5 mg/100 ml	Rises slightly.	May reflect changes in kidney basement membrane, renal pathology, or sub-clinical urinary tract infection.	Proteinuria is more common in elders than younger adults. A 1+ (30 mg/100 ml) may be of no clinical significance, but renal pathology or a urinary tract infection should be ruled out.
Glucose	0–15 mg/100 ml	Declines slightly.	Same as protein above.	Glycosuria may not occur until the plasma glucose exceeds 300 mg/100 ml. Urine glucose checks in diabetic elders are highly unreliable.
Specific gravity	1.032	Declines to 1.024 by age 80.	33%–50% decline in the number of nephrons impairs kidneys' ability to concentrate urine.	
Hematology				
Hemoglobin (HGB)	Man: 13–18 g/100 ml Woman: 12–16 g/100 ml	Men: Drops 1–2 g/100 ml (10–17 g/100 ml).	As bone marrow diminishes,	Just because hemoglobin declines with age, do

Component	Normal value	Age-related change	Cause	Nursing implications
		Women: No change documented.	hematopoiesis declines. Mens' drop in androgen activity lowers hemoglobin further.	not assume a low hemoglobin is normal in an elder. When hemoglobin and hematocrit are low, look for other signs of anemia: pale skin, pale conjunctiva. Protect elders from infections since they have fewer and weaker lymphocytes with which to fight invading organisms. Immune system changes diminish antibody–antigen response.
Hematocrit (HCT)	Men: 45–52% Women: 37–48%	Sight decline hypothesized, but specific changes not documented in studies to date.	Decreased hematopoeisis as above.	Encourage elders to have pneumococcal, tetanus, and influenza vaccines.
Leukocytes	4,300–10,800/cu mm	Total count drops to 3,100–9,000/cu mm. Decrease in proportion of lymphocytes, but exact decline not documented.	Decreased hematopoeisis as above.	
Lymphocytes	500–2,400/cu mm 50–200/cu mm	T lymphocytes fall. B lymphocytes fall.		
Platelets	150,000–350,000/cu mm	No change in number, but characteristics change: decreased	Unknown. Possibly related to diminished bone marrow.	No conclusive evidence that clotting increases, but some

Continued

Table 9-2A. Guide to Changing Lab Values in Elders* (*Continued*)

Lab Test	Adult (20–40 yr)	Changes with Age	Why	Caution
		granular constituents, increased platelet-release factors.		suggest fibrinogen levels increase with age.
Prothrombin time (PT)	11–15 s	No change in healthy elders.		
Partial thromboplastin time (PTT)	60–70 s			
Blood Chemistry Albumin	3.5–5.0 g/100 ml	Before 65, levels in men higher than women. After 65, values equalize and decline at the same rate, but what that rate is has not been documented.	Related to declines in liver size, blood flow, and enzyme production.	Low serum albumin produces edema. If there is no liver dysfunction, teach elder to increase protein intake by eating fish, meat, nuts, grains, peanut butter, vegetables, eggs, and milk products. Elders need more protein per kilogram body weight than does a younger person.
Prealbumin (Northwest Clinical Lab, 1990)	16–40 mg/dl (10– 16 mg/dl—moderate	Unknown	More reliable than albumin. To identify	

Test	Normal value	Age-related change		
	to mild Pro/Kc malnutrition. 10 mg/dl—severe Pro/Kc malnutrition).		malnutrition and a more effective monitor for outcome of nutrition intervention. With adequate nutrition support pre-albumin can increase 1 mg/dl/day.	Decreased total protein may signal malnutrition, infection, or liver disease.
β-Globin	2.3–3.5 g/100 ml	Increases slightly.	Increased β-globin balances decreased albumin.	
Total serum protein	6.0–8.4 g/100 ml	No change.		
Sodium	135–145 meq/L	Interval widens: 134–147 meq/L		
Potassium	3.5–5.5 meq/L	Increases slightly.		Avoid salt substitutes largely composed of potassium. Teach elders to check food labels for potassium and to learn signs of hyperkalemia.
Carbon dioxide	24–30 meq/L	No change.		
Chloride	100–106 meq/L	No change.		
Blood urea nitrogen (BUN)	Men: 10–25 mg/100 ml; Women: 8–20 mg/100 ml	Increases, sometimes as high as 69 mg/100 ml.	Declines in cardiac output, renal blood flow, and glomerular filtration rate	A slightly elevated BUN causes no problems unless such stressors as infection or

Continued

Table 9-2A. Guide to Changing Lab Values in Elders* (*Continued*)

Lab Test	Adult (20–40 yr)	Changes with Age	Why	Caution
			compromise renal function.	surgery are added.
Creatinine	0.6–1.5 mg/100 ml	Increases, sometimes as high as 1.9 ml/100 ml in men.	Endogenous creatine production falls as lean body mass shrinks.	Consider the creatinine and the creatinine clearance levels to prevent toxicity when giving drugs excreted via the urinary system.
Creatinine clearance	104–125 ml/min	Formula for calculating age-referenced interval in men; (140 − age × kg body wt) − 72 × serum creatinine. Women: 85% of this.	Glomerular filtration rate slows with age.	
Glucose tolerance	1 h: 160–170 mg/100 ml 2 h: 115–125 mg/100 ml 3 h: 70–110 mg/100 ml	Fasting plasma glucose rises more quickly in the first 2 h, then drops to baseline more slowly.	Pancreatic insulin supply declines and release is slower with age. With decline in lean body mass, less tissue is available for glucose uptake. Some cellular resistance to insulin develops with age.	Drugs such as alcohol, MAO inhibitors, and beta blockers can contribute to a rapid fall in glucose. A rise in glucose can quickly precipitate nonketotic hyperosmolar acidosis. A drop in glucose triggers

confusion as brain cells are deprived of glucose.

Determination	Normal Value	Change with Age	Cause	Comments
Triglycerides	40–150 mg/100 ml			
Cholesterol	120–220 mg/100 ml	Men: Increases to age 50, then decreases. Women: Lower than men to 50, then increases to 70 and decreases after 70.	Unknown Women have "postmenopausal shot" when the drop in estrogen triggers cholesterol rise.	After menopause, womens' risk of cardiovascular problems increases to the level of mens'. Diet high in fiber and in fish oils (e.g., from tuna, salmon, sardines, trout) can lower cholesterol. Weight loss and exercise can raise HDL.
HDL	80–310 mg/100 ml	Women consistently higher than men, then difference disappears in elders.		
Thyroxine (T₄)	4.5–13.5 mcg/100 ml	Decreases 25%.	Thyroid gland slows production.	
Tri-iodothyronine (T₃)	90–220 ng/100 ml	Decreases 25%.		
Thyroid-stimulating hormone (TSH)	0.5–5.0 mcg U/ml	Increases slightly.		
Alkaline phosphatase	13–39 IU/L	Increases 8–10 IU/L	May be due to decline in liver function, or to vitamin D	

Continued

Table 9-2A. Guide to Changing Lab Values in Elders* (*Continued*)

Lab Test	Adult (20–40 yr)	Changes with Age	Why	Caution
			malabsorption and subsequent bone demineralization.	
Acid phosphatase	Men: 0.13–0.63 U/ml Women: 0.01–0.56 U/ml	No change.		
Serum glutamic oxaloacetic transaminase (SGOT)	0–40 U/L	No change.		
Creatinine kinase (CK)	17–148 U/L	Increases slightly.	May be related to age loss of muscle mass and decline in liver function.	
Lactate dehydrogenase (LDH)	45–90 U/L	Increases slightly.		

* Aging, even without disease, changes physiology, which can alter laboratory test results. Thus, the data is summarized to assist you.
Copyright 1988, American Journal of Nurs. Co. Reprinted with permission from Geriatric Nursing, May/June, 1989. All rights reserved.

Table 9-3. Drug/Nutrient Interactions

Drug	Possible Interaction	Recommendation
Alcohol	Affects the action of more than one hundred different drugs	
Acetaminophen (Anacin-3, Tylenol) [analgesic]	Cruciferous vegetables speed up metabolism of drug, reducing its effect	Avoid excessive quantities of cabbage, brussel sprouts, cauliflower, broccoli
Aspirin [analgesic]	Long term use, vit. C and potassium loss; chronic use, empty stomach irritation	Take with food or milk if taking ASA regularly
Apresoline (hydralazine) [antihypertensive]	B_6 (pyridoxine) antagonist; B_6 decrease may cause peripheral neuropathy	May need vit. B_6 supplement
Calcium [supplement]	High-fiber diet may decrease calcium absorption by decreasing transit time, complexing	Give calcium away from fiber meals
Captopril (Capoten) [antihypertensive]	Food (fat) may decrease absorption 30–40%	Give one hour before meals
Carafate [antiulcer]	When given with or after food, decreases its ability to coat ulcers	Give 1 hour before meals and at bedtime
Correctol (phenophthalein) [laxative]	Routine use cuts down nutrient absorption by speeding the passage of food through the gut	Stimulant laxatives should not be used routinely
Cuprimine (penicillamine) [antiarthritic]	Absorbs iron from metals in food; decreases B_6 (pyridoxine)	Take 1 hour before or 2 hours after meals; give B_6 supplement
Chemotherapy: Cyclophasphamide Doxorubicin Vincristine Methotrexate	Taste sensation altered, nausea, vomiting, digestive disturbance Folate antagonist Fluorouracil thiamine depleting	Change food temperature, portions; give favorite foods, use antiemetics Good nutrition is vitally important for cancer patients; they feel better, show improved resistance to infection
Colchicine [antigout]	May cause lactose intolerance; may cause	Lactose-free diet; add lactate enzymes

Continued

Table 9-3. Drug/Nutrient Interactions (*Continued*)

Drug	Possible Interaction	Recommendation
	malabsorption of sodium, potassium, and vit. B_{12}	
Dulcolax Tabs [laxative]	Milk will dissolve enteric coating.	Give away from milk
Decongestants [pseudoephedrine, phenylpropanolamine]	Appetite depressants	Observe for change in appetite
Digoxin (Lanoxin) [cardiac glycoside]	High-fiber (bran) diet may decrease Digoxin absorption	Give Digoxin away from bran
Dilantin (phenytoin) [anticonvulsant]	Increases need for vit. D, causing malabsorption of calcium; tube feeding absorption interaction	May need to increase vit. D in diet or supplement
Desyrel (trazadone) [antidepressant]	Food may increase absorption, and decrease incidence of drowsiness or light headedness	Give with food
Estrogens (Premarin) [hormones]	Cause sodium and fluid retention	May need sodium-restricted diet
Ferrous sulfate [iron]	Vit. C may enhance absorption	
Furosemide (Lasix) [diuretic]	Potassium-wasting diuretic that also causes loss of magnesium	Increase intake of high-potassium foods (bananas, oranges, potatoes), high magnesium foods (nuts, legumes, seafood)
Griseofulvin [antifungal]	High-fat diet increases absorption and decreases risk of G.I. distress	High-fat foods (nuts, cream, fats, oils, butter, chocolates, cheese)
Inderal (propranolol) [antihypertensive]	Absorbed more efficiently if taken with food	Take with meals or a nutritional supplement
Hismanal (astemizole) [antihistamine]	Food decreases absorption; Hismanal decreases appetite	Take on empty stomach 2 hours after meal; do not eat for 1 hour
Isoniazid (INH) [tuberculostat]	May cause B_6 (pyroxine) deficiency	Increase foods rich in B_6 or supplement

Continued

Table 9-3. Drug/Nutrient Interactions (*Continued*)

Drug	Possible Interaction	Recommendation
Levodopa (Larodopa) [antiparkinsonian]	Drug effect is reversed by B_6	Avoid excessive quantities of B_6 foods (beans, milk, pork, tuna, avocados, enriched bread, cereals)
Lithium (major tranquilizer)	Sodium can reduce therapeutic response; with increased sodium lithium is decreased	Avoid excessive salt
Mandelaine [antibacterial]	Vit. C acidifies urine to allow mandelaine to convert to formaldehyde	Cranberry juice, critrus juice, vit. C supplement
Mineral oil (laxative)	Traps fat soluble vitamins (A, D, E, K); causes loss calcium and phosphorons	Use other laxative for chronic treatment
Nitrofurantoin (Macrodantin) [antibacterial]	Absorption enhanced and stomach protected with food	Take with food
Periactin (cyproheptadine) [antihistamine]	May stimulate appetite	Take for weight gain
Prednisone [glucocorticoid]	Increases sodium and fluid retention; causes loss of calcium and potassium and increases appetite	Sodium-restricted diet; monitor weight
Prolixin (tranquilizer)	Vit. C may cause return to manic behavior	Monitor for behavior changes
Prozac [antidepressant]	Decreases appetite	Monitor weight
Phenobarbital [sedative, anticonvulsant]	Increases turnover of vit. D and eventually calcium loss	Increase intake of vit. D foods or supplement
Questran (cholestyramine) [hypocholesterolemia]	Interferes with absorption of vit. A, D, K, B_{12}, folic acid	May need vitamin supplements
Quinidine gluconate	Excess intake of vit. C may increase blood drug levels	Decrease intake of citrus fruits and other high-vit. C foods (green peppers, tomatoes)
Sulfamethoxazole [Sulfonamide]	Inadequate fluid intake may result in crystaluria	Drink full glass of water with each dose

Continued

Table 9-3. Drug/Nutrient Interactions (*Continued*)

Drug	Possible Interaction	Recommendation
Tetracycline [antibiotic]	Calcium and iron bind drug so neither drug nor the Ca and Fe is absorbed	Take on empty stomach, avoid dairy products (eggs, milk, cheese); avoid taking with iron-rich foods
Theophylline [antiasthmatic]	High-protein diet and smoking decrease theophylline level, increase clearance of theophylline	Monitor theophylline levels
Warfarin (coumadin) [anticoagulant]	Blocks vit. K blood clotting factors; excessive amounts of vit. K-rich foods interfere with coumadin	Avoid excessive quantities of food rich in vit. K (turnip greens, broccoli, lettuce, cabbage)

Source: Printed by permission of Jeffery E. Arnold, 1989.

tional depletion. Optimal nutritional status is considered at risk in the following cases:

- Recent weight loss or gain of 10 percent or more of usual body weight
- Grossly overweight or underweight status
- Nothing By Mouth (NPO) status for more than 10 days on simple intravenous solutions
- Increased metabolic needs as related to disease states, injury, or stress
- Impairing drug/nutrient interactions
- Prolonged nutrient losses and therefore malabsorption, renal dialysis, or draining of wounds
- Other conditions, such as alcoholism that may affect nutritional status

Once the nutrition-related problems are identified, the consultant dietitian can develop goals for the care plan. These goals must be realistic, attainable, measurable, and congruent with the resident's perception of his or her needs, problems, and goals.

If the six steps of initiating the nutritional assessment are performed thoroughly, the plan of care will be developed easily. The consultant dietitian must ensure that the current status of the resident is reflected in the plan of care with changes being made as needed.

Documentation by the consultant dietitian and dietary manager is critical throughout the processes of assessment, planning, implementation, and evaluation. Documentation facilitates communication among the health care disciplines in resolving the multi-disciplinary nutrition-related problems.

Assessing the nutritional status of the elderly resident is challenging because of the lack of standards for nutritional sufficiency in persons over the age of 55 and physiological changes that occur normally with the aging process. However, the nutrition assessment process is vital in establishing baseline measurements for subsequent reassessment in monitoring a resident's nutritional status.

ENTERAL FEEDING OF ADULT PATIENTS BY TUBE (Beagle 1989)

Introduction

Quality assurance in patient care can be described as making certain that the right person receives the right therapy at the right time. How does one achieve this goal in dietetic services? Whether it is a tray of solid food, a feeding through a tube into the gastrointestinal tract, or an intravenous feeding, one must make these decisions correctly. The director or manager of dietetic services in the health care facility is responsible for assuring that decisions are made regarding what, why, when, and how each patient is fed. If the director is not a registered dietitian, then a clinical dietitian needs to be assigned to make these judgmental decisions. This individual needs to know (1) how to assess a patient's nutritional status, (2) how to select the optimal formula or diet, and (3) how to decide on the mode and method of feeding to use.

This section is devoted to methods of providing specific nutrients and calories to an individual via a tube in the gastrointestinal tract. Enteral formulas that are provided through a tube distal to the oral cavity are designed for patients who are physically or psychologically incapable of consuming food by mouth. These patients present a special challenge to the consulting dietitian.

Who Are These Patients?

Some cannot eat adequate amounts of food voluntarily because of weakness or nausea. Others have existing conditions of the mouth, throat, or esophagus such as sores, inflammation, or partial obstruction. Many individuals have increased nutritional requirements that cannot be met by oral intake because of disease states, including thermal injury, trauma, cancer, or major infections. Lastly, others are prevented from eating orally by physical conditions such as stroke, coma, neurological disorder, or surgery of the upper gastrointestinal tract.

When individuals are unable to take food by mouth but have a functional gastrointestinal tract that is safe to use, enteral feeding via tube should be used before a total parenteral nutrition solution is given by intravenous route. Enteral feeding is preferred for two major reasons:

1. The presence of food in the digestive tract helps maintain the integrity of the mucosa of the gastrointestinal tract.
2. Enteral feedings are safer and considerably less expensive than complete feedings by intravenous routes.

If the patient has optimal function of the tract but simply cannot take food by mouth, a complete formula with intact nutrients should be used. Only when the gastrointestinal tract has limited ability to digest and absorb nutrients should elemental feeding be used. Figure 9-2 illustrates how to select the mode and type of feeding.

Before determining the kind of formula needed and the mode of feeding, the patient must be evaluated to determine specific nutrient needs. Most complete formulas base their nutritional value on caloric and/or volume content. Therefore, a good assessment of the need for calories, protein (or nitrogen), and fluid will assist one in determining the patient's individual needs.

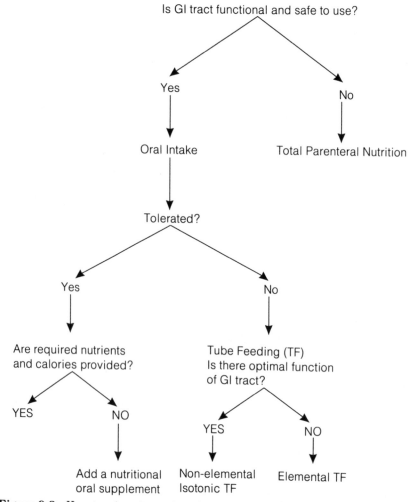

Figure 9-2. How to select the mode and type of feeding.

Calorie Needs

A recent study of practice among registered dietitians and physicians indicated that basal energy expenditure (BEE) as defined by Harris and Benedict was the method most frequently used to calculate caloric needs (Feitelson et al. 1987). (The formulas for calculating BEE in adults were discussed earlier in the chapter.) The following formula is used to calculate total daily energy needs (TDE):

$$TDE = BEE \text{ calories} \times \text{activity factor} \times \text{injury factor} \times \text{infection factor} = \text{total calories/day}$$

To this daily caloric need add or subtract 500 calories/day for weight gain or loss if needed.

Protein Needs

Requirement for protein can be calculated by two methods:

1. Body weight (kg) × protein requirement factor = protein (g/day)
   Protein requirement factors:
   Person with no disease present = 0.8–1.0
   Person with decubiti, fracture, or infection = 1.2–1.5
   To convert pounds to kilograms, divide pounds by 2.2.
2. Calculate nitrogen (N) requirements first and then convert N to protein.
   Anabolic state:
   Total calories per day ÷ 150 = N (g)
   Maintenance state:
   Total calories per day ÷ 300 = N (g)
   To convert N (g) to protein (g):
   N (g) × 6.25 = protein (g/day)

Fluid Needs

If there is no fluid restriction nor reason to force fluids, the requirement can be estimated by the following formula:

$$\text{Body weight (kg)} \times 30 \text{ cc} = \text{total fluid (cc/day)}$$

Restriction of fluid may be necessary with renal or cardiac conditions. Additional fluids (500–1,500 cc/day) may be needed if diarrhea or vomiting exists. A case study with sample calculations is given for illustration.

CASE STUDY

A 60-year-old male patient with desirable body weight of 170 pounds and height of 69 inches is confined to bed in a nursing home with a mild infection. He has normal urine output and no signs of renal or cardiac disease.

Calculations

Calories:

BEE = 66 + (13.7 × 77.2 wt., kg) + (5 × 175 ht., cm) − (6.8 × 60 age)

BEE = 66 + (1057.6) + (875) − (408)

BEE = 1,590.6

TDE − 1,590.6 × 1.2 actual factor × 1.2 infection factor = 2290.4

TDE = 2,290

Protein:

Method 1. 77.2, wt (kg) × 1.2 = 92.6

Method 2. 2,290 ÷ 150 = 15.2 (g) N

15.2 × 6.25 = 95.4

Fluid: 77.2, wt kg × 30 cc = 2,316 cc

In the above formulas pounds and inches must be converted to kilograms and centimeters. To convert pounds to kilograms, divide by 2.2, and to convert inches to centimeters multiply by 2.54.

In evaluating a patient's nutritional status prior to initiation of tube feeding it is valuable to review the following:

1. Any history of weight loss
2. Diet pattern such as eliminating a food group or bizarre eating habits
3. Repeat hospital admissions, surgeries, or pregnancies in a short span of time
4. A disease state that would induce malnutrition
5. Abnormal laboratory data indicative of poor nutritional status
6. Therapy that would affect health status

Weight loss of 5 percent in one month is considered significant, and greater than 5 percent severe. As mentioned, serum albumin is thought to be one of the best indicators of malnutrition since the liver needs a supply of calories and protein to make this visceral protein. Also, measurement of albumin in critically ill patients on tube feeding has been proposed as a reliable predictor of tolerance for enteral feeding (Moss 1988).

To evaluate the severity of malnutrition using serum albumin as an indicator, the following can serve as a guide:

Serum albumin (mg/100 ml): 3.5–3.2 = mild malnutrition

3.2–2.8 = moderate malnutrition

less than 2.8 = severe malnutrition

When there is rapid weight loss and/or serum albumin is low, the feeding formula needs to be high enough in calories and protein to rebuild tissues and promote weight gain.

What Should One Look for When Evaluating Tube Feedings?

An optimal tube feeding, when a special feeding is not required, has the following characteristics:

1. Caloric density equal to 1 calorie/cc
2. Suitable calorie to nitrogen ratio (150 : 1)
3. Relatively low osmolality
4. Balance of nutrients in adequate amounts but not excessive levels
5. Bacteriologic safety
6. Convenience and ease of administration
7. Low cost

Commercial formulas are available for use when gastrointestinal functions of digestion and absorption are present, when digestion and/or absorption is limited, and when specialized feedings are needed for patients with conditions such as renal or hepatic failure.

The registered dietitians responsible for the clinical component of patient care must be aware of the composition of available formulas in order to make the most appropriate choice for individual patient needs.

Table 9-4 lists the most commonly available complete formulas with information on composition and use. This table gives an idea of the great number and types of formulas available. Feedings to use when the gastrointestinal tract is functioning contain intact nutrients such as whole proteins, disaccharides, and triglycerides. These are subdivided into three types: (1) blenderized feedings, (2) milk-based formulas, and (3) lactose-free products. When the mucosa of the gastrointestinal tract cannot perform the functions of digestion or absorption, defined formulas are used. These products have elemental properties and contain simple components such as amino acids, di- and tripeptides, simple sugars, and medium-chain triglycerides to help the body accept the nutrients. When an organ has failed in the body or is not functioning to full capacity, a specialized formula that restricts certain nutrients is needed to prevent the build-up of toxic materials or substances that cells cannot utilize.

It is recommended that commercially available formulas be used rather than feedings prepared in the dietary kitchen. Commercial formulas save time in the preparation process, assure the correct mixture of nutrients to volume each time, and reduce the incidence of contamination through bacterial growth.

Ready-to-use liquid nutritional products are sterile until the container is opened. Numerous factors influence the number and type of microorganisms that might contaminate an enteral feeding product.

Table 9-4. Enteral Feeding Products for Tube Feeding

Product (Supplier)	Calories /ml	Osmolality (mOsm/kg)	Protein (g/l)	Carbohydrates (g/l)	Fats (g/l)	Sodium (mEq/l)	Potassium (mEq/l)	Special Properties
Nonelemental Formulas with Intact Nutrients								
Blenderized enteral feedings								
Complete-Modified (SANDOZ)	1.07	300	43	141	37	29	36	Blenderized, isotonic
Milk-based enteral feedings								
Complete-Regular (SANDOZ)	1.07	405	43	128	43	56	36	Contains lactose, 24 g/l
Lactose-free enteral feedings								
Enrich (Ross)	1.1	480	40	162	37	37	40	Contains fiber
Ensure (Ross)	1.06	450	37	145	37	37	40	
Ensure-HN (Ross)	1.06	470	44	141	35	40	40	
Ensure Plus (Ross)	1.5	600	55	200	53	49	54	Higher calories
Ensure Plus-HN (Ross)	1.5	650	62	200	50	51	46	Higher calories, high protein
Entrition (Biosearch)	1	300	35	136	35	31	31	Isotonic
Isocal (Mead Johnson)	1.06	300	34	133	44	23	34	Isotonic
Isocal-HCN (Mead Johnson)	2	690	75	224	91	35	36	Maximum calories, high protein

Product							
Isotein-HN (Sandoz)	1.2	300	68	156	34	27	27	Isotonic
Jevity (Ross)	1.0	300	44	152	37	40	40	Isotonic with fiber
Magnacal (Sherwood Medical)	2	590	70	250	80	44	32	Maximum calories, high protein
Osmolite (Ross)	1.06	300	37	145	38	24	26	Isotonic
Osmolite-HN (Ross)	1.06	310	44	141	37	40	40	Isotonic
Precision Isotonic Diet (Sandoz)	1	300	29	144	30	20	25	Isotonic
Precision High Nitrogen Diet (Sandoz)	1.05	525	44	216	1.3	43	23	Very low fat
Precision LR Diet (Sandoz)	1.1	530	26	248	1.6	30	23	Very low fat
Resource Instant Crystals (Sandoz)	1.06	450	37	145	37	37	40	
Sustacal (Mead Johnson)	1	625	61	140	23	41	53	Higher Protein

Continued

187

Table 9-4. Enteral Feeding Products for Tube Feeding (*Continued*)

Product (Supplier)	Calories /ml	Osmolality (mOsm/kg)	Protein (g/l)	Carbohydrates (g/l)	Fats (g/l)	Sodium (mEq/l)	Potassium (mEq/l)	Special Properties
Sustacal-HC (Mead Johnson)	1.5	650	61	190	57	37	38	Higher calories, higher protein
Traumacal Fulfil (Mead Johnson)	1.5	550	82	142	68	51	36	Higher calories, higher protein
Twocal-HN (Ross)	2	700	83	217	90	46	59	Maximum calories, high protein
Defined Formulas That Possess Elemental Properties								
Criticare HN (Mead Johnson)	1.06	650	38	222	34	27	34	
Stresstein (Sandoz)	1.2	910	70	173	27	29	23	High BCAA, high protein (for hepatic disease)

Product								Comments
Traum-Aid HBC (McGaw)	1	760	56	166	7	29	30	Low fat content, high BCAA (for hepatic disease)
Vivonex T.E.N. (Norwich Eaton)	1	630	38	206	2.8	20	20	High BCAA, for low fat content (hepatic disease)
Tolerex (Norwich Eaton)	1	550	21	226	1.5	20	30	Low fat content
Specialized Formulas								
Amin-Aid (McGaw)	2	1095	19.4	366	46.2	<15	<6	For renal disease
Haptic Aid II (McGaw)	1.1	560	44.1	169	36.2	< 5	<2	For hepatic disease
Hepatic (Travenol)	1.1	690	28.6	209	14.3	19	29	For hepatic disease
Travasorb-Renal (Travenol)	1.3	590	22.9	271	17.7	0	0	For renal disease
Pulmocare (Ross)	1.5	490	62	105	92	57	49	For decreased lung function

Source: Information furnished by manufacturers of products.

1. The level of care taken when the container is opened and the product is transferred to the feeding container
2. Storage and feeding temperature
3. Time of storage and feeding
4. Additions to formula
5. Environmental microbes
6. Use of sterile or reused feeding paraphernalia

The use of liquid nutrition products requires handwashing with bacteriostatic soap, the use of clean utensils, and simple washing of the container lid before opening.

Before commercial formulas were commonly available, tube feeding formulas were made in the kitchens of health care facilities. Kitchen-made formulas consisted of from 8 to 10 ingredients including milk, juice, pureed vegetables and meats, a starch source, and sometimes raw eggs. Natural foods are subject to a high level of contamination. If not correctly prepared and stored, these products can be very dangerous. When these products were used, a 24-hour supply was prepared and sent to the patient's unit, where it was stored in the refrigerator until use. Feedings were portioned into 200 to 400 meals and the patient fed four to eight times per 24 hours. Administration was by funnel and syringe (bolus feeding) or by a gravity drip delivery system.

Today, because of the emphasis on feeding by continuous drip, pumps have been designed and developed specifically for enteral tube feedings. These pumps feature ranges of controlled delivery rates and assure accurate delivery of formulas of different viscosities through small-diameter tubes. Pump systems that deliver feedings accurately ensure ingestion and adequate nutrients and calories while minimizing associated complications. Most, if not all, pumps have alarm systems that detect empty containers and display the flow rate selected as well as the volume of feeding that has been infused. There are fewer complications when using a pump that regulates the rate of delivery and warns staff of problems.

The facility may choose an open system with refillable feeding containers or bags, or a closed system in which prefilled containers are used. Established guidelines for open systems allow 4 to 8 hours (preferably 4) for hang-time of tube feeding. Closed enteral feeding systems can be safely hung for 24 hours, based on the manufacturer's recommendations, after laboratory analysis shows no bacterial growth in the product. The closed system is more expensive than the open system but saves money by reducing nursing staff time.

What Routes Can Be Used for the Tube?

The placement of the tube for feeding can be in several locations of the gastrointestinal tract. The major types and their use are the following.

Type	Use
Nasogastric (NG) or intragastric	Problems of ingestion such as those related to head or neck surgery
Nasoduodenal	Reduction of vomiting or aspiration of regurgitated material into lungs
Esophagostomy	Long-term feeding; feedings do not require patient to undress; opening is concealed
Gastrostomy	Bypassing the esophagus
Jejunostomy	Bypassing the duodenum and duct system that furnish bile and pancreatic secretion; therefore, to be used with predigested or elemental materials

Feeding via tube is associated with a number of problems. Some common ones, together with possible causes and probable solutions, are listed in Table 9-5.

To keep problems and complications associated with tube feedings to a minimum, patients should be monitored every day. Doctors, nurses, and registered dietitians need to watch for possible signs of complications or malnutrition, by observing physical signs and reviewing appropriate laboratory data.

In summary, enteral feedings via tube require knowledge of *who* needs feeding via tube, *why* feeding via tube is appropriate, *what* to feed, *when* to feed, and *how* to feed. Constant monitoring for complications must be done to correct any problems that are discovered.

SPECIALIZED PROGRAMS

The consultant dietitian may increase his or her clinical effectiveness in the facility by developing specialized programs. Programs targeted toward specific nutrition problems such as weight loss, constipation, pressure sores, and the Alzheimer's patient establish a standardized protocol for treatment of these common areas of concern.

Each program should be developed with the cooperation and assistance of the director of nursing and should be implemented only after sufficient inservice training of appropriate staff.

Specialized programs help the staff to recognize certain nutrition-related problems early and increase understanding of the importance of intervention. Examples of programs targeted toward the problems mentioned above follow:

Weight Loss

Weight loss is a common problem in long-term care facilities today. Established policies and procedures and early intervention make success in reversing it more likely and contribute substantially to the quality of patient care.

Table 9-5. Problems Associated with Tube Feedings

Complications	Possible Cause	Probable Solution
Nausea	Too much volume	Decrease volume
	Excessive rate of feeding	Decrease rate
	Improper tube tip location	Check with physician on replacement of tube
	Anxiety	Reassure patient
Vomiting	Too much volume	Decrease volume
Diarrhea	Excessive rate of feeding	Decrease rate
	Very cold formula	Warm formula to room temperature
	High osmolality in formula	Start formula ¼ then ½ strength full, add anti-diarrhea medication
	Intolerance to lactose	Use lactose-free formula
Vomiting and diarrhea together	Contamination of formula	Check sanitation, equipment, and use only ready-to-use formulas
	Anxiety	Reassure patient
Dehydration	Inadequate fluid intake	Increase fluids
	Excessive protein and/or electrolytes	Reduce protein and/or electrolytes or increase fluids
	Rapid infusion of carbohydrates	Reduce rate of tube feeding May need insulin
Over-hydration	Too much volume in formula or used to clear tubing	Use isotonic solution needing no dilution Clear tubing with less water
Edema	Too much sodium in feeding	Use formula lower in sodium

Documentation is of the utmost importance in protecting the facility when the patient's nutritional needs cannot be met with the conventional diet. Both the dietitian and the director of nursing should work closely to identify, monitor, and treat this problem effectively. Weight loss is one area where success or failure is readily evident; and it becomes part of the medical record. Meeting the nutritional needs of the patient is a significant part of the quality patient care and should be of concern to all health care professionals working together to improve quality of life.

Each facility should have a formal policy and procedure established for patients who have weights that put them at risk.

Many facilities are reducing the use of commercial supplements because of the cost of the products. In-house supplements often taste better and are better accepted as well as far less expensive than their commercial counterparts. Commercial supplements may have a place, however, with patients who are taking less than 30 to 40 percent of their diets consistently, since they are nutritionally complete and can provide 100 percent of the recommended daily allowance if taken in sufficient volume. This question too should be addressed in the policy. The following is a sample policy and procedure for weight loss.

Policy

All patients are evaluated on admission and monthly thereafter for weight loss. Patients presenting with weight 10 percent below ideal weight range for height or patients showing loss of five pounds or greater of total weight within one month or one quarter will be evaluated for placement on a supplement program to promote weight gain.

Procedure

1. Patients are weighed and measured for height on admission. Measurements are recorded on the chart.
2. All patients below ideal body weight range are discussed by the Care Plan Committee, who will formulate individual goals and approaches.
3. Weights are monitored monthly or more frequently, as designated by the Care Plan Committee.
4. Patients determined to be at risk are placed on supplements consisting of 8 oz. of fortified cereal with breakfast and 6 oz. fortified shakes from approved recipes at lunch and bedtime (HS).
5. Intake of meals and supplements is recorded.
6. Patients with consistent intake of less than 40 percent of meals receive fortified cereal each morning with breakfast and the physician is contacted to obtain an order for 8 oz. of commercial supplement on the lunch tray and HS.
7. Progress is evaluated monthly by the dietitian and director of nursing.

Each facility should establish a policy and procedure for weight loss that is suitable for the individual facility. The important aspects of the program are ease of implementation by those individuals responsible and staff awareness of both the program itself and its importance to the patient.

It happens that, despite trying several approaches, some patients simply do not respond. In this instance, it is extremely important that the facility document everything that has been tried with the patient. It might also be beneficial to have the dietitian calculate the patient's intake in kilocalories for several days and report this to the physician along with a summary of the patient's weight history and what the facility has tried to date. At this point, the physician may order a feeding tube if the facility is clearly not able to meet the patient's nutritional needs. His response should be documented in the nursing notes as well as the nutritional progress notes.

Constipation

Commonly related to diminished muscle tone and decreased peristalsis, constipation is one of the most frequent gastrointestinal complaints of the elderly (Pemberton et al. 1988). Treatment of constipation in the elderly must be preceded by identification of the cause or causes. The physician must exclude obstruction as the cause of constipation before any dietary or drug measures are adopted (Roe 1987).

Once obstruction has been ruled out, the dietitian can pursue methods of increasing fiber in the diet as a means of reducing or eliminating episodes of constipation in many elderly patients. Be aware, however, that sudden increases in fiber may be poorly tolerated. Proceed by gradually increasing fiber with the help of the following recipes. Start with small portions and remember to educate nursing aides about the need to encourage more fluids when increasing fiber.

Natural laxative
    2 cups prunes, pureed
    4 cups applesauce
    3 tablespoons unprocessed bran
    Combine in food processor
    Give 2 oz. at HS or supper for constipation
    Give 2 1/2–3 oz. for chronic constipation
    2 oz. = 1/2 fruit for diabetic

Oatmeal with bran
    2 lb. 10 oz. oatmeal
    1 lb. 2 oz. Bran Buds
    Water
    Cook oatmeal according to directions. When cooked, add bran.
    Yield: 28 cups
    Serving size: 1/2 cup
    Total dietary fiber: 8.12 g/cup

Liquid-Fiber Supplement
    1 lb. 2 oz. Bran Buds
    92 oz. prune juice
    Mix bran and juice 24 hours in advance of use. Refrigerate.
    Blenderize until well mixed
    Yield: 12 cups
    Serving size: 1 cup
    Total dietary fiber: 11.4 g/cup

Bran Prune Juice
    1 lb. 2 oz. Bran Buds
    46 oz. prune juice
    2 cups unsweetened applesauce
    Combine all ingredients in large blender. Blenderize until well mixed.

Yield: 64 oz.
Serving size: 1–4 oz.
Total dietary fiber: 2.23 g/oz.

Pressure Sores

It is estimated that 5 to 10 percent of hospitalized patients will develop pressure sores. Once developed, the average pressure sore costs $15,000 to treat with a range of $5,000 to $40,000 for one ulcer (Mead Johnson 1989). In long-term care the incidence of pressure sores can be as high as 24 percent (Moores 1987). Complications arising from the sores can be fatal.

In view of the economic as well as physical impact, it would behoove both the dietitian and nurses to place great emphasis on identification of patients at risk for these lesions and to develop intense treatment protocols for those who do develop pressure sores. The following program was developed by Rhona Thompson (1989):

Treatment Program

The incidence of pressure sores tends to increase with age. As a result, pressure sores tend to be more prevalent among the elderly than among most other groups in the population. The institutionalized elderly may be at increased risk due to lack of mobility. Although there are some variations in the classifications of pressure sores, the following is a useful basic classification system:

Stage   I: A persistent area of skin redness (without a break in the skin) that does not disappear when pressure is relieved.

Stage II: A partial thickness of skin is lost (epidermal layer has been lost, but the dermis is at least partially intact); may present as blistering surrounded by an area of redness and/or induration.

Stage III: A full thickness of skin is lost, exposing the subcutaneous tissues; presents as shallow crater (unless covered by eschar—thick brown, black or yellow crust); may be draining.

Stage IV: A full thickness of skin and subcutaneous tissue is lost, exposing muscle and or bone; at this stage, the sore may be covered with an eschar, draining, necrotic, reddened, and/or indurated.

It is imperative that nutritional intervention be considered at all stages of pressure sore formation. Long-term care facilities tend to focus on cure and place little, if any, emphasis on prevention of diseases. Prevention intervention is in the best interest of the patient and is cost effective for the facility. Early identification of risk factors is essential.

To evaluate the nutritional requirements of the resident with pressure sores, the following may be used:

A. Risk factors to consider
  1. Generally, the overall intake of the diet is inadequate in calories, protein, vitamins, and minerals because of
     a. Chronic illness
     b. Depression
     c. Poor dentition
     d. Anorexia
     e. Dysphagia
  2. Inadequate caloric intake may lead to decrease in cutaneous fat reserves (therefore less "padding").
  3. Inadequate protein intake may lead to increased susceptibility to skin breakdown and delayed tissue healing.
  4. An open, draining pressure sore may result in protein, fluid, and mineral losses.
B. Nutritional therapy
  1. A well-balanced diet, high in calories and high biological value protein is recommended.

    Protein = minimum of 0.8–1.2 g protein/kg present body weight
    Calories = estimated caloric expenditure (ECE)
    ECE (men) = $66.47 + 13.75 W + 5.0 H - 6.76 \times 1.5$
    ECE (women) = $655.10 + 9.56 W + 1.85 H - 4.68 A \times 1.5$
    W = Weight in kg (2.2 kg/lb.)
    H = Height in cm (2.54 cm/in.)
    A = Age in years

  2. Small frequent meals may be necessary to provide adequate calories and protein.
  3. Proper hydration is necessary to maintain skin elasticity. The optimal fluid requirement is 35 ml/kg present body weight. Fruits, fruit/vegetable juices, and soups are recommended.
  4. Vitamin C and zinc supplementation are recommended because of their importance to wound healing (collagen formation and maintenance of good skin integrity).
  5. Nutritional supplements may be recommended to assist in providing the necessary additional protein, vitamins, calories, and minerals.
  6. Multivitamin/mineral supplement may be considered.

For uniformity of care and to ensure that medical, nursing, and rehabilitation therapy staff are aware of the impact made by the food and nutrition services department, the following specific interventions were developed for patients with pressure sores.

Tube-Fed Patients

Stage I: No intervention
Stage II: Liquid vitamin C supplement

Stage III: Liquid vitamin C; allow 0.8–1.2 g protein/kg present body weight
Stage IV: Same as stage III

Diabetic and Weight-Reducing Patients

Stage   I: No intervention
Stage II: 8 oz. high protein supplement
Stage III: Vitamin C and zinc supplements; 8 oz. high-protein supplement
(allow 0.8–1.2 g protein/kg present body weight)
Stage IV: Same as stage III

All Other Orally Fed Patients

Stage   I: 1/2 cup orange juice OD
Stage II: 1/2 cup orange juice BID and 5 oz. of high protein supplement
Stage III: Zinc supplement; 1/2 cup orange juice TID; 2 eggs at breakfast;
5 oz. high-protein supplement (allow 0.8–1.2 g protein/kg present
body weight)
Stage IV: 1/2 cup orange juice TID; 2 eggs at breakfast; 5 oz. high protein
supplement; double portion of meat at lunch

Please note that the above is a general guide and must be adapted to meet each resident's specific needs. For example, for orally fed residents who may not like orange juice or egg or may have a poor appetite, a vitamin C supplement and/or a nutritional formula supplement may be indicated.

Tube-fed residents should be evaluated individually based on the formula specified by the physician and the amount received. For tube-fed residents who receive insufficient amounts of protein or vitamins and minerals, the addition of a multivitamin or protein supplement may be warranted.

Alzheimer's Disease

Alzheimer's disease is a progressive, degenerative condition of the brain that always causes dementia (Roe 1987). In the latter stages of the disease indifference to food, a short attention span, and inability to eat independently may result in weight loss and ultimately malnutrition.

The Alzheimer's patient presents a special challenge to the consultant dietitian. The following program, developed by Monica Lursen, is presented here as an example of a specialized program targeting patients with Alzheimer's.

Treatment Program

All existing foodservice policies and procedures will continue to be in effect in the Alzheimer's Special Care Unit. These policies and procedures include but are not limited to menu planning, nutrition, therapeutic diets, purchasing, receiving, storage, sanitation, food preparation, meal service, staffing, and the care planning process. The following procedures are in addition to and take precedence over pre-existing procedures when functioning in the Special Care Unit.

A. Meal Service
   1. Meals will be served at the following times (example):
      Breakfast 7:40 A.M.
      Dinner 11:40 A.M.
      Supper 5:40 P.M.
   2. Specific between-meal nourishments will be served at the following times (example):
      9:00 A.M.
      1:30 P.M.
      8:00 P.M.
   3. The type and quantity of food served will be determined by the resident's diet order. All therapeutic diets available in the facility will likewise be available in the unit.
   4. Food usually served as between-meal nourishments to increase the protein and/or caloric value of daily intake can include liquid nutritional supplements, malts, ice cream, milk, sandwiches, fruit juice, and cookies, for example. The need for these nourishments will be determined by nutritional assessment.
   5. Caffeine will not be served in these forms: regular coffee, tea, cola beverage, hot cocoa, or chocolate bars. Decaffeinated coffee, tea and other beverages will be allowed, as will the use of cocoa and chocolate in baking; however, residents will be evaluated individually for their tolerance to these low-level caffeine products.
   6. Food will be available 24 hours a day on the unit through the use of a small refrigerator in the nursing chart area. This refrigerator will be supplied daily with orange juice, milk, and other beverages of resident preference. The unit will also have available at all times saltine crackers, cookies and/or fruit.
   7. Family members and/or friends will be discouraged from bringing food into the unit; however, if they insist, the foods will be limited to fresh fruits; baked goods, such as cookies, cake, and breads; and other foods not considered potentially dangerous.
   8. The method of meal service will be as follows: Tray service will be set up in foodservice and delivered to the unit door. The unit nursing assistant will proceed with the trays to the unit dining area.
      The dining area will consist of 4-person tables. All unit residents will use dining room chairs if at all possible. This dining room, which is not used for non-unit residents, functions as the unit's activity area as well.

Tray presentation is critical in the unit to assist with the residents' ability to feed themselves. The following features will be observed:

a. Nonbreakable dishes and glasses

b. Immobile plates with rims to facilitate picking up food

c. A dark tray and light-colored dishes and glasses to aid visual discrimination

d. A minimum amount of tableware utensils to lessen confusion. Knives will be available to residents on an individual basis, but generally will not be set on trays. The type of utensil necessary to eat a meal will depend on the menu; the utensils needed for each meal will be recorded on the menu in foodservice. If there is an individual variation, instruction as to that variance will be on the resident's diet marker card.

e. Adaptive devices for any residents needing special assistance during meals.

9. Meal presentation is also important in a successful self-feeding program. Various techniques will be used in encouraging the unit residents to feed themselves. Those techniques include, but are not limited to the following:

a. Allow use of the fingers, and/or offer more finger type foods. If difficulty with a utensil is noted, use of the fingers allows a continued sense of independence.

b. Food normally needing a knife to be cut or which may be difficult to cut with a fork will be presented to the unit resident already cut. A specific list of these foods will be written for foodservice personnel.

c. Foods may need to be served one at a time, starting with one liquid, an entrée, another liquid, salad, and/or dessert and finishing with a liquid (preferably water to act as a mouthwash). The dessert may be used on a "when nothing else works" basis.

d. Smaller portions may be offered at meals to lessen the time spent eating and to avoid overwhelming the resident with large portions. The number of times this resident is offered food will thus increase to assure an equal amount of food offered throughout the day. The dietitian will be responsible for assessing and planning this meal plan.

e. Cups and glasses should be only half full to lessen the chance of spillage and the resulting upset this may cause.

f. Temperatures will be monitored closely, as food that is too hot could injure a resident or cause a resident to refuse to eat any more. Hot food must be held at 140°F, or above; cold food, at 45°F or below, but may have to be held for a short period (not to exceed 15 minutes) for the food to reach an acceptable temperature for the Alzheimer's patient.

10. Residents of the unit who refuse to eat or allow the staff to feed them will not be force-fed. Every attempt will be made to encourage the resident or to change any of the above variables to promote self-feeding.

11. Nursing service will monitor each resident's meal for intake amounts. This information will be used in determining the need to alter any of the above techniques for meal service or presentation.

B. Care-planning process—the foodservice component: Foodservice will participate in the care-planning process for residents in the Special Care Unit in the same manner as for all other residents. Several additional notes need to be made because of the critical nature of possible weight loss and the importance of documenting individual differences in approach to care.

1. The initial nutritional assessment will begin within 48 hours of admission and will take into consideration the Alzheimer's patient's rating scale when determining any immediate need to alter methods of meal presentation.

2. The dietitian will observe each new resident while eating before completing the initial nutrition assessment to evaluate problems with self-feeding and possible solutions before attending the initial care-planning conference for that resident.

3. Any special techniques for meal service or presentation will be listed on the nutrition assessment/reassessment tool under special concerns/comments.

4. Weekly weights will be monitored by nursing. If any problems (a 6 lb. increase or decrease over the last highest weight) are noted, the unit coordinator will notify foodservice. An immediate reassessment of care may be warranted. The dietitian will then begin the reassessment process.

C. Staffing foodservice: Foodservice staffing requirements will not be changed by the addition of the Special Care Unit. Foodservice personnel will have no direct contact with the unit's residents, with the exception of the dietary manager and the dietitian. Their visits will be to obtain information and observe behavior in relationship to the nutrition assessment.

1. Nourishment and meal service to the Alzheimer's unit does not alter the number of hours staffed in foodservice.

2. Extra food supplies are already being sent to the existing nurses station, so the addition of another refrigerator to stock with specified supplies will be added to the job routine of the P.M. dietary aide. These supplies for the unit will be sent with the supper trays; nursing will be responsible for the storage and care of this food.

3. The dietitian's hours will remain unchanged unless there is an

increased incidence of weight fluctuations, which could trigger a reassessment of care. Any increase in dietitian's hours will be dealt with on a monthly basis until a trend is established.

D. Staff education—the foodservice component: Although food service personnel do not have direct contact with residents of the Special Care Unit, they will need an orientation to the special needs of Alzheimer's patients and residents with related disorders. Foodservice employee training should include, but is not limited to
    1. The disease process, especially its effect on nutritional status.
    2. The basic premise of the Special Care Unit and how it relates to the needs of an Alzheimer's resident.
    3. All areas of meal service and presentation listed under "A meal service." It is especially important to relate the "why" of these procedures to employees, so they may understand the relationship of the disease to what we ask of them.
    4. Subsequent annual inservice training related to the Special Care Unit. This training may include foodservice employees and shall count toward required annual inservice training.
    5. Documentation of orientation and training, which will be part of the employee's permanent file.
E. Staff education—the nursing component. All nursing personnel who have responsibilities in the Special Care Unit will receive inservice training in all areas of meal service and presentation as listed under A. In addition, orientation to the disease and the unit itself will be conducted.

CHOOSING A DIET MANUAL

The dietary consultant is usually responsible for choosing the diet manual used by the facility. While there are many good diet manuals on the market, not all diet manuals are suitable for every facility. If the dietitian consults in several facilities, it may not be appropriate to use the same manual in each.

To match a diet manual with a particular facility, the consultant must first be familiar with the types of therapeutic diets offered in the facility. This depends in part on local physicians—on both their degree of nutrition knowledge and their personal philosophy of treating geriatric patients. Some physicians are not knowledgeable about current nutrition concepts and therapy, while others simply do not believe in restricting geriatric patients unduly unless there is a definite nutrition-related problem such as diabetes or renal failure.

The consultant dietitian must be familiar with the types of diets ordered by local physicians and with their basic philosophies in order to choose a manual consistent with the needs of the facility. It would be neither necessary nor practical to choose a 400-page diet manual that offers every obscure diet that might be encountered when local physicians are only prescribing three or four types of therapeutic diets. Keep it simple!

It is also important to remember that many residents of long-term care facilities are there for extended periods of time—perhaps for the remainder of their lives—and to keep this in mind when choosing a diet manual. A manual with a liberal approach may be better accepted by these residents than a manual that takes a stricter approach to diet therapy.

Another consideration is whether dietitians from the local hospital have developed a diet manual. If so, chances are the manual might be well suited to surrounding long-term institutions since these facilities usually share the same physicians as the hospital. By the same token, the dietary consultant could work with the local hospital dietitians to develop a diet manual suitable for both the hospital and the long-term care facilities in the area. The result would be a diet manual very specific to the needs of local patients.

When choosing a diet manual, remember that it must be from a reputable source. It must also be updated regularly and be current. The rule of thumb is an update every five years. Because diet therapy is constantly being revaluated and revised, a manual over five years old is considered outdated. Check to see if the manual being considered is a revision of an earlier edition. In general, the state dietetic association, the American Dietetic Association, many health care institutions, and a number of universities publish diet manuals. It may be helpful to talk with local dietary consultants and dietitians to determine what manual they are using and to review a copy.

Last but not least, the diet manual should have a good format, one that is easily read and with information readily accessible. Dietary employees should be able to read the manual and understand the instructions. If they cannot, they will not use the manual. While it is nice and necessary to have a complete and thorough clinical reference, keep the facility diet manual simple. Very technical manuals can and should be part of your reference library, but probably are not the best choice for the dietary department of a long-term care facility.

Once a potential diet manual has been selected, allow the administrator and director of nursing to review it and consider their input. If the facility is fortunate enough to have an interested, active medical director, allow him or her to review it as well. Once a manual is chosen, it should be approved by the medical staff or the medical director.

When adopting a diet manual, remember that the manual will in effect become part of the policies and procedures of the dietary department. All therapeutic diets should be written in accordance with the principles in the manual. After choosing a manual appropriate to the needs of each individual facility, train the dietary staff on the use of the manual and adherence to its principles. The diet manual is a valuable tool if used properly and should be familiar to all dietary employees.

REFERENCES

Appalachian Regional Healthcare. 1988. Physicians' handbook for nutritional care, Supplement I, *Manual of clinical dietetics.* Lexington, Ky. Appalachian Regional Healthcare.

Barness, Coble, MacDonald, and G. Christakis. 1981. *Nutrition in medical practice.* Westport Conn.: AVI Publishing.

Blackburn, G. L., B. R. Bistrian, B. S. Maini, et al. 1977. Nutritional and metabolic assessment of the hospitalized patient. *Journal of Parenteral and Enteral Nutrition* 1:11.

Brunnstrom, S. 1972. *Clinical kinesiology.* Philadelphia: F.A. Davis Co.

Chernoff, R., C. Mitchell, and D. Lipschlitz. 1987. Assessment of the nutritional status of the geriatric patient. In *Nutrition in long term care facilities: A handbook for dietitians.* Chicago: American Dietetic Association.

Chicago Dietetic Association and the South Suburban Dietetic Association. 1988. *Manual of clinical dietetics.* Chicago: American Dietetic Association.

Christakis, G. 1973. Nutritional assessment in health programs. *American Journal of Public Health* 63, supplement no. 1 (November).

Chumlea, W. Cameron., Alex F. Roche, and Debabrata Mukherjee. 1987. *Nutritional assessment of the elderly through anthropometry.* Columbus, Ohio: Ross Laboratories.

Feitelson, M., P. Fitz, S. Rovezzi-Carrol, and L. H. Bernstein. 1987. Enteral nutrition practices: Similarities and differences between dietitians and physicians in Connecticut. *Journal of American Dietetic Association* (October) 87(10):1363.

Harris, J., and F. Benedict. 1919. *A biometric study of basal metabolism in man.* Washington, D.C.: Carnegie Institute of Washington.

Hunter, A., and F. Rogers. 1988. Assessment in LTC: A cooperative venture. *Topics in Clinical Nutrition* 3, no. 4, 40–45.

Jernigan, Anna K. 1987. *Nutrition in long term care facilities: A handbook for dietitians.* Chicago: American Dietetic Association.

Kittelberger, Sherry, Mary B. Foltz, and Eldonna Shields. 1984. *Nutrition support in the long term care institution.* Columbus, Ohio: Ross Laboratories.

Long, C., N. Schaffel, J. Geiger, W. R. Schiller, and W. S. Blackmore. 1979. Metabolic response to injury and illness: Estimation of energy and protein needs from indirect calorimetry and nitrogen balance. *Journal of Parenteral and Enteral Nutrition.* 3:452.

Lursen, Monica. 1989. Alzheimer's special care unit foodservice procedures. *The Consultant Dietitian in Health Care Facilities* 14, no. 4: 1–11.

Mead Johnson. 1989. Prevention and treatment of pressure sores. Evansville, Ind.: Bristol-Meyers Company.

Moores, S. 1987. Nutrition and pressure sores. *Today's Nursing Home* (October) 8(10):41–44.

Moss, G. 1988. The role of albumin in nutrition supplements. *Journal of American College of Nutrition* 7:441.

Pemberton, Cecilia, Karen Moxness, Mary German, Jennifer Nelson, and Clifford Gastineau. 1988. *Mayo Clinic diet manual.* Philadelphia: B. C. Decker Inc.

Powers, Dorothy E., and Ann O. Moore. 1988. *Food medication interactions.* Phoenix, AZ.

Roe, Daphne. 1983. Geriatric nutrition. Englewood Cliffs, N.J.: Prentice-Hall, Inc.

———. 1987. Geriatric Nutrition. Englewood Cliffs, NJ: Prentice-Hall, Inc.

Thompson, Rhona, 1989. Nutritional care of residents with pressure sores. *The Consultant Dietitian in Health Care Facilities* 14, no. 4:1–9.

Weinsier, R., C. Heimburger, and C. Butleworth. 1989. Handbook of clinical nutrition, 2d ed. St. Louis, Mo.: C. V. Mosby Co.

10

Documentation

"NOTHING DOCUMENTED, NOTHING DONE"

Health care professionals often jokingly remind one another, "Nothing documented, nothing done!" Simply put, this means there must be documentation to support every significant observation made or action taken. This is particularly true in the field of health care today where legal repercussions of lax documentation abound. The medical record or chart is considered a legal document and must be accurate.

The consulting dietitian should also consider another aspect of documentation. Good documentation is a marketing tool for the dietetic profession. The medical record is shared by all health care professionals involved in the care of each patient and so affords the dietary consultant the opportunity to communicate both information and an impression to other professionals. In reading the nutrition documentation, practitioners in other disciplines form an impression of both the dietary consultant and the dietetic profession as a whole.

A third and final consideration for good documentation of nutrition services is cost justification:

> Documentation of nutrition services is especially important in the current atmosphere of health care cost reduction. Many health care professionals believe that nutrition services, such as nutritional assessments, consultations, and patient education will be cut in an effort to reduce hospital costs unless the value of these services can be clearly demonstrated. [Zeman and Ney 1988]

This chapter will discuss the various types of documentation for which the dietary department and/or the dietary consultant are responsible and will offer guidelines in each area.

THE INITIAL VISIT

The initial visit is the first made to the patient by a representative of the dietary department. Since dietary consultants are not usually full-time employees and may not be in the facility at the time of each admission, this visit is often made by the dietary manager.

Documentation of the initial visit should be done within the first several days of admission and is important for several reasons. The initial visit

1. Establishes prompt attention to the patient by the dietary department
2. Affords the dietary manager an opportunity to meet the patient, to establish rapport with him or her, and to open a line of communication between the patient and the dietary department
3. Is an excellent opportunity to gather pertinent data on food allergies, individual likes and dislikes, food intolerances, problems with chewing or swallowing, and any other areas of concern the patient may wish to address or the manager may wish to observe
4. Provides the consultant dietitian with additional information to be considered in developing the initial nutritional assessment

Observations made and information obtained should be summarized in a note in the medical record. The placement of dietary notes in the chart should be determined by facility policy. Some facilities designate a section of the chart for all dietary records. Others may combine the notes of several disciplines under a common heading such as "Consults," "Special Services," or "Progress Notes."

If no form has been developed for documentation of the initial visit, the dietary progress note form may be used. An example of documentation of an initial visit is as follows:

12-4-89. 84-year-old W/F on a 2 g Na diet. Talked with patient about food preferences and dislikes. She states no food dislikes or intolerances. Prefers cereal and juice only for breakfast. Complains of difficulty chewing meats unless they are very tender but does not want her meats chopped or ground. When asked about her current weight of 120 lb., she reported a gradual loss of 10 lb over the past year. Will report findings to the dietitian for consideration in the nutrition assessment. Signature of dietary manager.

Obviously the content of the initial visit summary will depend on both the mental status of the patient being interviewed and the competency and ability of the dietary manager writing the note. In general, documentation of the visit should include any data obtained from the patient or from visiting family members as well as any observations made by the manager during the visit (for example, "Patient appears to choke easily on thin liquids"). As with all documentation, it should be written in ink (black is easiest to read), dated, and signed by the author.

The consulting dietitian should evaluate the manager's competency in this area and—based on the manager's level of expertise—should advise the manager concerning the content of the note. If the dietary manager's charting ability is limited, it is best to keep the note simple, perhaps addressing only patient likes and dislikes. If, however, the manager has good documentation skills, the note can be expanded to include more information such as ideal body weight range, skin status, and so forth.

THE INITIAL ASSESSMENT

Content of the nutrition assessment is addressed thoroughly in the previous chapter and need not be discussed in depth here other than to note the following:

1. Federal regulations state: "Each assessment must be conducted or coordinated with the appropriate participation of health professionals" (HCFA 1989). This can and should be interpreted to mean that the nutrition assessment should be completed by a qualified dietitian, not by the dietary manager. Do not allow the dietary manager to do your work. If assessments can be done by the manager, there is no need for a consulting dietitian. The registered dietitian is the appropriate health care professional to analyze the data contained on the nutrition assessment and to make recommendations concerning the patient's nutritional care. Although teamwork is vital for the well-being of the patient, responsibility for the assessment rests with the consulting dietitian.

2. Federal regulations also state: "Each individual who completes a portion of the assessment must sign and certify the accuracy of that portion of the assessment" (HCFA 1989). The dietitian is legally liable for any information or recommendations documented on the assessment. This is not to be taken lightly. Remember this statement each time the temptation arises to rush through an assessment or simply to cosign the manager's work.

The nutrition assessment serves as documentation that the dietary consultant has visited the patient, assessed his or her nutritional needs, and made appropriate recommendations. The initial assessment establishes baseline data from which to make future comparisons and so must be accurate. If the assessment is not accurate, future comparisons will be inaccurate as well.

Information obtained during the assessment process should be discussed with the care plan committee in order to formulate interdisciplinary approaches to nutrition problems and to demonstrate each discipline's awareness of problems identified by other disciplines. Most problems require the cooperation of several branches of the health care team before resolution can be achieved.

PROGRESS NOTES

The purpose of dietary progress notes is to provide a documented update of the patient's nutritional status. Theoretically these notes are best made by the consulting dietitian. In reality, time and cost constraints imposed on the consultant may rule out that option. Here again the consultant must assess the dietary manager's ability to document and, based on this assessment, develop a system of documentation that is appropriate for each situation. At the very least, the consultant should be responsible for progress notes on patients with acute or serious nutrition problems.

In addition to updating the patient's nutrition status, progress notes should address nutrition problems identified on the interdisciplinary care plan, evaluate the success or failure of planned interventions, and suggest new interventions if appropriate.

Content

In updating the patient's nutritional status, the progress note should contain the following information (as applicable to the individual patient):

1. Current weight: Always use an up-to-date weight, not one from a previous month. If a current weight is not available, request one.
2. Any significant laboratory values: Examples include hemoglobin, albumin, glucose, and electrolytes as well as any value pertinent to individual patient nutrition status.
3. Intake summary: A summary of the patient's average percentage of intake, should be included, together with information relative to the patient's ability to eat independently.
4. Any change in diet or food consistency since the previous review.
5. Any change in patient status or diagnosis that might affect nutrition status: Examples are skin breakdown, deterioration of mental status, or a change in drug therapy such as the addition of a diuretic.

As mentioned previously the progress note must also address all nutrition-related problems identified by the care plan committee and answer the following questions:

1. Is the problem listed still current?
2. Has the goal been met? If not, is it still reasonable?
3. Are approaches listed being carried out? Are they accomplishing what the committee hoped for?
4. Is the intervention successful? If so, should it continue? If not, what else can be tried?

Writing a Progress Note

In order to write a good progress note, it is important to visit the patient, review problems and goals established on the nutrition assessment, and review the interdisciplinary care plan.

Visiting the patient allows the dietitian to discuss any real or perceived dietary problems with the patient. If the patient is nonverbal or unable to communicate, the dietitian can observe the patient to evaluate changes in physical appearance or status that may reflect nutritional status.

Reviewing problems and goals established on the nutrition assessment and on the care plan is essential in determining progress or lack of progress in these areas. Continued reports on these problems and goals establishes the revaluation process and provides documentation that is truly ongoing and not merely "paperwork compliance."

Progress notes should be written no less often than quarterly or whenever there is a significant change in patient status, for example, when a patient has a stroke and is no longer capable of eating independently. Another example of significant change would be insertion or removal of a feeding tube.

The charting format may be a matter of personal choice or of facility policy. Generally, progress notes are written in narrative style or in the standardized "SOAP" format: "subjective," "objective," "assessment," and "plan." Elements of the SOAP format are summarized below (Zeman and Ney 1988).

Subjective: Information that is pertinent to a listed problem and that is obtained from the patient or patient's family or significant others. Information may be recorded as a direct quote or it may be paraphrased. The key characteristic of the subjective data is that it expresses the patient's perception of a problem.

Objective: Factual information relevant to the problem that can be confirmed by others, including laboratory and physical findings and observations by health care professionals. Factual nutrition information often found in this section of a progress note includes prescribed diet (diet Rx), height (ht.), weight (wt.), ideal body weight (IBW), pertinent laboratory values, results of measured food intake, calculation of nutrient needs, and observed difficulties with eating. At a minimum, initial chart notes should state diet Rx, ht., wt., and IBW under "O."

Assessment: The health care team member's evaluation or interpretation of subjective and objective data. In this section the nutritional care specialist's judgment about a particular problem, based on patient provided and factual information, is presented.

Plan: The specific course of action to be taken, based on S, O, and A, to resolve the patient's problem. The plan may include all or part of the following components:

1. Dx (diagnosis): Further workup needed, such as nutrition history, calorie count, lactose tolerance test, or serum albumin or lipid measurement
2. Rx (therapy): Suggested diet or diet changes (the diet order would have to be written by the physician), supplemental feedings, request for and eating aid
3. Pt Ed (patient education): Plans for future individual or group instruction and notation of teaching just completed, including major instructional materials provided and plans for follow-up

Examples of a progress note written in two different formats follow.

12-7-89. 84-year-old white female on a regular puréed diet. Fed by staff and consumes 80–100 percent of breakfast and 20–40 percent of lunch and dinner with encouragement. Recent labs include hgb 10.7, Na 136, K+ 4.2, albumin 2.8. Skin remains intact. Height 65 in. Weight loss continues to be a problem. Current weight of 107 lb. represents a 5-lb. loss in one month. Ideal body weight range 120–130 lb. Patient complains of lack of appetite. Rarely accepts substitutes for foods refused and usually refuses commercial supplement. Will try increasing portions of cereal and eggs at breakfast and will offer 1/2 cup ice cream each HS in place of supplement. Weight will be monitored every 2 weeks and patient will be reviewed again in 1 month to assess weight status. [Signature of registered dietitian]

Alternative format:

12-7-89
S—Patient complains of lack of appetite and usually refuses commercial supplement.
O—Receives regular puréed diet. Fed by staff and consumes 80–100 percent breakfast and 20–40 percent lunch and dinner. Hgb 10.7, albumin 2.8, Na 136, K+ 4.2; ht. 65 in., wt. 107 lb., ideal body weight range 120–130 lb.
A—Patient intake inadequate to maintain weight or achieve weight gain. She does not like the commercial supplement and is uncooperative with all meals except breakfast.
P—1. Offer larger portions cereal and eggs at breakfast.
   2. Offer 1/2 cup ice cream at HS
   3. Monitor weight every 2 weeks.
   4. Reassess in 1 month.
[Signature of registered dietitian]

Progress notes provide documentation that nutrition status has been correctly assessed and addressed. As stated previously, the progress note should ideally be written by the consulting dietitian. If time constraints prevent this, the dietitian must work with the manager to determine what the manager is reasonably capable of charting. If charting ability is limited, teach the manager to keep the note simple and concise. Never expect the manager to exceed his or her capabilities. The result may be an embarrassment to both the facility and the manager. For the patient discussed in the examples above, a simple yet adequate progress note might be:

12-7-89. Weight 107 lb. Patient has lost 5 lb. since previous review. No change in regular puréed diet. Appetite poor for lunch and dinner and patient does not accept supplement well. Will provide larger servings at breakfast, 1/2 cup of ice cream for evening snack, and ask nursing staff to weigh her every 2 weeks. [Signature of dietary manager]

In summary, evaluate each situation individually based on facility policy, consultant time available, and the ability of the dietary manager. Do not lose sight of the fact that dietary progress notes establish correct identification, intervention, and monitoring of nutrition-related problems and should always be treated with respect.

REASSESSMENT

Progress notes are needed to provide a continual update of the nutrition status of the patient. They must be made at least quarterly or after any significant change in the patient's condition—whichever occurs first. In addition to this documentation, it is necessary to do a complete reassessment of the nutrition status of the patient periodically.

How often is periodically? Federal regulations call for reassessment of the patient annually or more frequently if there is significant change in the patient's condition. Annual reassessment is a straightforward requirement, but deciding when a progress note would be appropriate or when an additional reassessment is necessary is a matter of judgment. Written standards should be developed to cover this area.

In general, it is first necessary to evaluate the "significant change" being considered. For example, if the patient has been transferred to the hospital for pneumonia but returns to the facility on the same diet as prescribed before the transfer and has no major changes in nutrition status, a progress note will suffice. If, on the other hand, the patient returns to the facility with a stage III pressure sore or a nasogastric tube, reassessment is usually necessary. The nature of the change must be evaluated for its potential impact on nutrition status. The decision concerning the type of charting to be done should be made by the consulting dietitian rather than the dietary manager, since it will be based on interpretation of medical data. It is helpful to have the manager keep a list of all patients who may require reassessment so that each can be evaluated for the appropriate documentation.

A reassessment need not be quite as detailed as the initial assessment and should basically be a tool for comparison to the original assessment or to the most recent reassessment. In this way changes in nutrition status can be readily identified. A sample reassessment form is shown in Figure 10-1. Note that the form allows the dietary consultant to compare the patient's current nutrition status with that recorded at the time of admission.

The following is a good system for organizing the timetable for routine reassessment:

1. When a patient is admitted to the facility, fill out a 5 × 7 in. index card with the patient's name and the date of admission.
2. File the card by the month of admission in a box provided for this purpose. The card box should be divided by months of the year.
3. As new admissions occur, add these cards to the box according to the month of admission.
4. After keeping this record for a year, the consultant need only check the cards each month to determine which patients are due for an annual reassessment.

Nutrition Reassessment

Name _____ Date _____

Age _____ Physician _____

Date of Admission _____ Diagnosis _____

DIET/INTAKE

Admission diet: _____ Ability to feed self: _____

Current diet: _____ Degree of assistance: _____

Supplements: _____ Assistive devices: _____

% intake of diet _____ % intake supplements _____

WEIGHT HISTORY

Admission Weight: _____ Current weight: _____

Height: _____ % loss or gain _____

Ideal weight range: _____ % ideal weight range: _____

Weight history: _____

LAB VALUES

Glucose: _____ Na: _____ Albumin: _____

Hgb: _____ Kt: _____ Other: _____

Hct: _____ Bun: _____ Other: _____

ROUTINE MEDICATIONS

_____

_____

ADDITIONAL INFORMATION

Mental status: _____ Activity level: _____

Skin condition: _____ Dentition _____

Other: _____

_____

ESTIMATED BASAL ENERGY EXPENDITURES

Base kcal: _____ Injury factor: _____ Protein _____

Activity factor: _____ Total kcal: _____ Fluid _____

SUMMARY/RECOMMENDATIONS

_____

_____

_____

_____

_____

_____

Figure 10-1. Sample form for reassessing nutrition status.

DOCUMENTATION OF SPECIAL NUTRITION PROBLEMS

As stated previously, documentation serves as the legal record that the dietary consultant has properly identified and addressed the nutritional needs of the patient. Patients with acute or serious chronic nutrition problems require more intensive documentation on the part of the consultant in order to establish that appropriate monitoring has occurred. Examples of common problems requiring more frequent documentation include, but are not limited to, weight loss, skin breakdown, refusal of food or fluids due to dysphagia, dementia, or eating assistance, and noncompliance with a prescribed diet.

Weight Loss

Weight loss can be either acute or chronic and should always be considered significant unless it has been a goal of the health care team, as in the case of an obese diabetic. Once acute weight loss has occurred, or a chronic weight loss trend is identified, the problem should be added to the interdisciplinary care plan and monitoring should begin. Although medical records may normally be revised quarterly, the records of patients with special concerns should be reviewed more frequently. In the case of weight loss, charting should probably be done monthly until the patient has stabilized. Weight may also be measured every two weeks rather than monthly. It is important to monitor the patient's condition frequently enough to be current with the problem at all times so that other approaches may be tried if those established initially do not work. For example, if the patient was placed on a commercial supplement to increase calorie and protein intake, the dietitian must monitor the patient's acceptance of the sup-plement and change it if necessary. This is something that needs to be deter-mined in a relatively short period of time—not three months after the fact. Two examples of documentation of weight loss follow:

Patient is an 85-year-old white female on a regular diet with ground meat. She has lost 12 lb. in the past 2 months. Current weight 100 lb. Ideal body weight range 120–130 lb. Consumes 30–40 percent of meals and complains of lack of appetite. Nursing will encourage patient at mealtime and offer to feed her any foods left on her plate at the end of the meal. Physician has been contacted and has ordered 8 oz. commercial supplement at 2 and 8 P.M. [Signature of registered dietitian]

Alternative format:

S—Patient complains of lack of appetite.
O—Receives regular diet with ground meat. Consumes 30–40 percent, wt. 100 lb.; ideal body wt. range 120–130 lb.
A—Present intake inadequate for nutritional needs. Patient appears weak and may need more assistance with meals.
P—1. Offer encouragement at mealtime.
   2. Offer assistance with feeding if patient does not eat well independently.
   3. Offer 8 oz. commercial supplement at 2 and 8 P.M.

Inadequate oral intake can also be the result of a patient experiencing difficulty in eating independently and is essentially passive in the eating process. Even though the consultant dietitian is not solely responsible for identifying residents with eating skill difficulties, it is important to evaluate this area and its relationship to weight loss and inadequate intake during the nutrition assessment process.

The consultant dietitian should work with the nursing staff, speech therapist, and/or occupational therapist in developing a rehabilitative eating program. By addressing the actual eating process as the problem, often the related nutritional problems can be resolved.

When establishing a rehabilitative eating program, the target patient population must be realistically evaluated. The target population includes patients who are experiencing difficulty eating and are essentially passive in the eating process, requiring one to one assistance, but have the potential to eat independently if supervised, encouraged, and given the necessary self-help feeding device.

Suggested patient criteria method, equipment, and staffing to establish a rehabilitative eating program are as outlined:

Criteria for Target Population

1. Tolerates sitting up in a chair at least 30 minutes.
2. Upper body function (range-of-motion, strength, coordination) adequate to transport food to mouth with adaptive utensils, if needed.
3. Responsive for 15–20 minutes and consistently able to perform one-step, repetitive task.
4. Shows interest in food. This should be tested in a group setting as interest may improve when others are also eating.

Method

1. Group patients together in a semicircle around a feeding table or small oval table.
2. Provide proper seating and mirror for improved feedback.
3. Provide appropriate feeding devices.
4. Utilize the back of the dietary tray card (or other convenient method) for technique summaries.

Equipment

1. Proper seating requirements include
   A. Mobile "chair" in order for resident to be moved easily out of room and to a central location.
   B. "Chair" with adequate support to trunk and feet (adjustable leg rests).
   C. Wedge cushions—for prevention of patient slipping out of chair, and promotes upright position. To be used as cushion for sitting.
2. High/low table to accommodate various armrests or chairs with desk arms. May use lap boards, preferably with rim around edge.
3. Adaptive utensils to include built-up handles and a rocker knife.

4. Pycem for nonslip surface under dishes.
5. Plate guards or plates with built-up edges.
6. Drinking aides to include long straws, mug with lid, and nose cut-out glass.

Staff Requirements

1. Speech therapist and/or occupational therapist (consultative basis).
2. Trained nurses' aides.
3. Consultant dietitian/dietary manager.

The progress of a patient in the rehabilitative eating program must be documented in the dietary progress notes as well as in the nursing and consultative services section. It is important to document the patient's acceptance and use of self-help feeding devices to show the facility's effort in rehabilitating the patient to their maximum level of functioning. Good rehabilitative eating programs can prevent further nutritional-related problems associated with poor oral intake and weight loss.

Skin Breakdown

Although not exclusively a nutrition problem, skin breakdown should be monitored by the dietitian more often than quarterly. This is especially true of stage III and IV pressure sores. (See "Specialized Programs" in Chapter 9 for an example of dietary protocol for pressure sores and other specialized nutrition problems.) Here again, frequent documentation establishes the consulting dietitian's awareness of the problem and records nutrition intervention efforts. Examples of documentation follow:

75-year-old W/M with stage III pressure sore on coccyx. Wt. 150 lb., ideal body wt. range 150–160 lb. Receives regular diet, is fed by staff, and consumes 50–100 percent. Appears to have difficulty chewing meats. Will try to increase patient's protein consumption by serving an additional egg each A.M., modifying consistency of meats to puréed and offering 8 oz. commercial supplement at HS (with physician's approval). Fruit juices high in vitamin C will be offered on each tray. Reassess in 1 month.

Alternative format:

O—Pt. has stage III pressure sore on coccyx. Wt. 150 lb, ideal body wt. range 150–160 lb. Consumes 50–100 percent of regular diet but appears to have difficulty chewing meats.
A—Pt. may benefit from additional protein and vitamin C to heal pressure sore.
P—1. Modify consistency of meats to puréed
    2. Monitor protein intake
    3. Offer additional egg each A.M.

4. Offer 4 oz. juice high in vitamin C on each tray
5. Offer 8 oz. commercial supplement at HS

The patient's response to these approaches should be evaluated and documented monthly until resolution is achieved or until the consultant feels frequent documentation is no longer warranted.

Poor Intake

Acute or chronic changes in appetite can be overlooked if intake is not monitored carefully or accurately. If poor intake continues unchecked over a period of time, the patient may become malnourished to the point where repletion is difficult if not impossible. It is important to take action early to have the best chance of success with this problem.

For patients who cannot take adequate nourishment because of problems with chewing or swallowing or as a result of dementia, maintenance of adequate nutritional status becomes the responsibility of the staff. The approaches taken to provide nutrition must be thoroughly documented since the facility is legally liable to do everything possible to maintain adequate hydration and nutrition. If, despite the best efforts of the facility staff, the patient does not respond to these efforts, a recommendation to provide nutrition and hydration by tube may be appropriate.

If this recommendation is made, it is helpful to provide the physician with an estimate of calorie and protein intake. A two- or three-day food intake record should provide sufficient information for this calculation.

The decision as to whether or not to begin feeding may rest with the physican, the family, or may be determined by facility policy in this area. Regardless of how the decision is made, it is the responsibility of the consulting dietitian and the dietary manager to identify these patients, make every effort to meet their nutritional needs, and carefully document how or why it can or cannot be done. For example;

> Pt. is a 97-year-old W/M on regular puréed diet. Fed by staff and has been refusing all but small amounts of food for the past six weeks. Weight is 90 lb., a loss of 20 lb. in the past two months and of 40 lb. since admission one year ago. Staff attempts to encourage pt. to eat more of meals have been unsuccessful. Pt. has refused all supplements offered as well as between-meal snacks of ice cream. A three-day calorie count revealed that this pt. is consuming less than 500 calories per day. The physician has been contacted but states that both the family and the patient refuse to consider tube feeding. Dietary is continuing to send high calorie supplements three times per day and to visit the pt. daily to offer other foods. [Signature of registered dietitian]

This documentation summarizes the problem, states what has been done, and basically reports that there are no further options to consider. It is important never to criticize any other department and to write objectively at all times.

Dietary documentation should substantiate that the dietitian and dietary manager have assessed the problem and acted appropriately.

Refusal To Follow a Prescribed Diet

Most consulting dietitians deal with this problem at one time or another. A diabetic patient who visits the vending machines daily or whose family brings in restricted foods is a perfect example in this category. In this instance the consulting dietitian should document;

1. What counseling has been done with the patient or family to alleviate the problem
2. Patient or family response to counseling
3. The physician's response (if any) when notified of the problem

If the patient continues to refuse to comply with the diet, it is, finally, his or her right to refuse. This assumes mental competency to make this decision. Documentation should show the consulting dietitian's efforts to steer the patient in the right direction and the patient's refusal to comply.

If, however, a patient is not mentally competent the facility must take responsibility for his or her actions and follow the course of action most beneficial to the patient. For example, this may mean confiscating food purchased from the vending machine when that food is contrary to the diet order. Here again, it is best to notify the physician about the problem and obtain a documented response. Examples of documentation in each instance follow.

Competent Patient

Mr. Smith is an alert, oriented insulin-dependent diabetic on a 1,500 calorie ADA diet who refuses to comply with his prescribed diet. He visits the vending machines once or twice daily to purchase cola and snacks contraindicated on his restricted diet. His most recent blood sugar was 354. This patient has been counseled twice about the importance of dietary compliance to blood sugar control but stated: "I ate what I wanted to at home and I intend to continue to do so here!" The physician was notified of Mr. Smith's behavior and talked with him about his diet, again with no result. Dietary will continue to send the prescribed diet but at this point is unable to prevent Mr. Smith from eating additional foods. [Signature of registered dietitian]

Incompetent Patient

Mr. Smith is an insulin-dependent diabetic on a 1,500 calorie diabetic diet who refuses to comply with his diet. His diagnosis includes Alzheimer's. He visits the vending machines once or twice daily to purchase cola and snacks contraindicated on his diet. His most recent blood sugar was 354. Since he is unable to comprehend the importance of dietary compliance to blood sugar control, the staff has contacted his family and asked that they no longer bring in money for the machines. In addition, snacks recently purchased have been confiscated and returned to family members. The physician has been made aware of the problem and is in agreement with actions taken. [Signature of Registered Dietitian]

DISCHARGE PLANNING

Dietary discharge planning is important for a number of reasons:

1. When a patient is discharged to home, written diet instructions are easily referred to and can reinforce previous diet instructions.

2. When a patient is discharged to a hospital or a nursing home, the discharge summary is a valuable source of dietary information on nutrition status, what has been tried, and the patient's response to nutrition intervention efforts. This information can save the admitting facility time and avoid the likelihood of trying approaches that were previously unsuccessful. It can also highlight a problem such as weight loss that might not be readily apparent to the admitting institution. Figure 10-2 illustrates a sample discharge referral record.

3. Good dietary discharge planning can serve as an excellent marketing tool. Patients returning to the home setting have a written reminder of the nutrition services offered by the facility. Good discharge information also makes an impression on other health care institutions and enhances the facility's image in the medical community.

Discharge summaries can be developed to include a variety of information to suit each individual facility. Spending time to develop attractive handouts neatly packaged in a folder with the facility logo makes an excellent marketing tool and a handy reference for the patient discharged to the home setting. A good summary of the patient's nutrition status and problems while in the facility is invaluable information for another facility receiving the patient and will aid it in developing an effective nutrition care plan much sooner than otherwise possible. An example of information that might be included in a discharge summary is shown in Figure 10-2.

CARE PLANS

Nutrition Input in the Care-Planning Process

Care plans have received a bad reputation in recent years as being yet another form of "paper work compliance." This is regrettable since the care-planning process can be a learning process for the entire health care team. It can also be an important tool for achieving quality patient care.

On the other hand, care plans have gained importance in the last few years as federal regulation of health care have mandated increasingly sophisticated care

NUTRITIONAL DISCHARGE REFERRAL RECORD

Date ______

Resident name ______ Age ______ Sex ______

Facility transferred from ______ To ______

Current diet order ______

Admission weight ______ Admission date ______ Discharge weight ______

FOOD PREFERENCES	FOOD DISLIKES

Food allergies ______ Usual food intake ______

Diet compliance ______

Current lab work (include dates) ______

Routine medications ______

Nutrition supplements ______

Nutrition status summary ______

Dietitian or dietary manager ______ Phone number ______

Figure 10-2. Sample form for discharge referral.

planning by placing more emphasis on both the written care plan and evidence (documentation) that it is being implemented by the staff.

As the importance and sophistication of the interdisciplinary care plan has grown, so has the opportunity for input by the consultant dietitian. Nutrition has become recognized as an integral part of quality patient care and an important component of treatment in many disease states.

The dietitian should look upon the care-planning process as an opportunity for real impact in patient care as well as an opportunity for marketing nutrition services in the facility.

It should also be noted that care plans serve as documentation that patients' needs have been properly identified and assessed and are a permanent part of the legal medical record. Failure to identify a patient's nutritional needs may imply professional neglect or lack of expertise on the part of the consultant.

The Increasing Need for Good Patient Care Planning

Various trends in health and health policy have increased the need for good patient care planning. First of all, greater longevity has often resulted in multiple disease processes. Dealing with these problems requires careful planning by the health care team as well as awareness of all health concerns by all disciplines involved in patient care. The interdisciplinary care plan conference can provide valuable insight into the "total picture" of each patient.

Shorter hospitalizations resulting from reimbursement based on diagnostic-related grouping have resulted in patients being admitted to long-term care facilities in a subacute state. Need for staff expertise in long-term care has grown accordingly. The skills of the dietitian in long-term care have been challenged as well.

Financial constraints of Medicare and Medicaid encourage facilities to become more cost effective. Good patient care planning can reduce patients' length of stay and, in some cases, reduce costly complications that may arise from poor planning or from failure to recognize all the patients' needs.

Increasing public awareness of health care liability as well as the increasing liability of each individual discipline involved in patient care encourages a careful, thorough consideration of each individual patient's needs and an effort by all disciplines to work together to define and meet these needs to the best of their ability.

In long-term care physicians depend on the health care team to coordinate the overall plan of care with the medical care plan. The physician is the head of the health care plan team but often leaves the formulation of the plan to the director of nursing and the interdisciplinary care planning team. The increasing awareness of need for input by all disciplines has provided an excellent opportunity for dietitians to display their expertise.

Consideration of the trends mentioned above should encourage dietitians to take care plans seriously and to see them as blueprints for quality patient care as well as marketing opportunities for the dietetic profession and the individual consultant.

THE CARE-PLANNING PROCESS

Since many consultant dietitians are not allotted sufficient time to attend all care plan meetings, a system must be devised to transmit information to the care-planning team for inclusion in the interdisciplinary care plan. If it is not possible to be present at care plan meetings, the following process can be effective.

- The dietary manager visits soon after admission (preferably one to two days). A list of food preferences and dislikes is obtained. The patient is observed for difficulty in chewing and self-feeding.
- Information is passed on to the registered dietitian on the first consulting visit following admission. The registered dietitian completes the nutrition assessment. The assessment identifies patient strengths, weaknesses, and possible risk factors, which may in turn need to be addressed on the care plan.
- The nutrition assessment is taken to the care plan meeting and any significant areas are incorporated into the overall (interdisciplinary) plan of care. All disciplines are made aware of problems identified and goals set for each patient by each discipline.

- The care plan is formulated from input from all disciplines. Team members make others (nursing aides, dietary aides, and so on) aware of the risk factors, problems, goals, and approaches being addressed for each individual.
- Risk factors, problems, approaches, and goals are reviewed regularly and progress, or lack of progress, is discussed and revaluations are made if necessary.

The nutrition assessment is crucial to the formulation of a good nutrition care plan. If the assessment is inaccurate, the care plan will be inaccurate as well. Take care to review the medical record thoroughly and interview the patient and family members carefully before devising a plan for resolving any nutrition problems identified. (Chapter 9 deals with this process in more detail.)

Components of the Care-Planning Process

In writing the care plan, several areas must be addressed. A good care plan addresses patient strengths, weaknesses, potential for improvement, and anticipated decline. (A method of indicating these components on the care plan is shown in Table 10-1) Once these areas are identified, goals and approaches are established. The specific discipline or disciplines responsible for the approach are specified and a time frame established for resolution or evaluation.

Patient Strengths

With the advent of regulations resulting from the Omnibus Budget Reconciliation Act of 1987 (OBRA), there has been a shift of emphasis to patient strengths as well as weaknesses. The role of the care planning team is to identify strengths and devise a plan of care for maintenance or improvement. The consultant must learn to recognize patient strengths as they relate to the nutrition assessment and care plan.

Examples of patient strengths include

- Ability to feed self
- Ability to chew and swallow without difficulty
- Intact skin
- Normal visceral protein status
- Good appetite
- Ability to understand and willingness to comply with dietary restrictions
- Body weight within ideal range or within average range for the individual

Patient Weaknesses

The consultant must next address the patient's weaknesses (also defined as problems or needs). Examples of weaknesses to be addressed by the dietitian include but are not limited to the following:

- Refusal to eat
- Inability to feed self
- Significant weight loss or gain
- Weight below or above ideal body weight
- Routine refusal of foods in a specific food group
- Fluid loss as a result of diarrhea or vomiting
- Pressure sores
- Low hemoglobin or hematocrit
- Inability to make wants or needs known
- Medications causing possible food/drug interactions
- Constipation, prolonged or recurring
- Acute illness or infection
- Need for enteral nutrition such as tube feeding
- Unstable blood sugars
- Chronic or acute renal failure
- Epigastric distress
- Ascites

These examples are some of the problems that may be experienced by elderly patients.

Once the weakness or problem is identified, it should be stated simply and specifically. If possible include an explanation of why the problem might occur, such as poor appetite secondary to disease process (metastatic cancer) or poor appetite related to difficulty chewing or swallowing. Making the etiology of the problem as specific as possible will facilitate establishing goals and approaches that are specific to the problem.

Potential for Improvement or Anticipated Decline

The potential for improvement or anticipated decline is used to assess the patient's prognosis when change is anticipated.

Potential for improvement (PI) is indicated when the patient may have the ability to improve or to be rehabilitated in a specific area. For example, a patient admitted after suffering a stroke may be unable to eat independently at the time of admission but with proper rehabilitation and access to assistive devices may eventually be able to do so.

Anticipated decline (AD) can be used to indicate instances when decline in a certain area is nearly inevitable. A good illustration is the patient with terminal cancer who is admitted with a weight within ideal range but will almost certainly begin to lose weight as the disease progresses.

Goals

Goals should be defined as objectives for the patient, not the dietitian. They should be specific and measurable so progress can be evaluated. Consider these examples of goals:

Table 10-1. Care Plan Format with Sample Nutritional Problems, Goals, and Approaches

Code[a]	Strength/Weakness	When To Address	Goals	Approaches	Discipline
W	Pressure sores (May be secondary to immobility, malnutrition, or wasting due to disease process, etc.)	Skin is reddened or broken particularly stages II, III, and IV	Correlate with nursing goals	1. Provide nutrient-dense foods	D
				2. Place on a supplement program (If appropriate.)	N, D
				3. Monitor intake	N, D
				4. Recommend MVI with zinc	N, RD
				5. Increase sources of vitamin C	D
W	Dry or sore mouth (May be secondary to drug therapy or ill-fitting dentures, etc.)	Patient voices complaints (ask during assessment phase), or these problems are observed	Patient will receive foods more easily tolerated (1 month)	1. Modify consistency of the diet if necessary	D
				2. Evaluate drug regime for drugs contributing to these disorders	RD
				3. Avoid spicy, rough, highly acidic foods	D
				4. Add sauces, gravies to moisten food	D
				5. Incorporate cold foods or beverages—ice cream, etc.	D

	Nursing Diagnosis/Risk Factor	Goal/Outcome	Interventions	
W	Patient has difficulty chewing secondary to ill-fitting dentures	Patient will receive foods they can tolerate (ongoing)	6. Counsel patient to swallow foods with a beverage	D
	Dentures no longer fit. Patient has difficulty chewing all or part of meals (such as meats)		7. Decrease dry, salty foods	D
			1. Modify consistency of meats to ground	D
	Risk Factor: May choke easily		2. Avoid foods patient does not tolerate	D
			3. Observe for choking	N
			4. Talk with family about dental consult	N
W	Poor appetite (May be secondary to depression, chronic illness, drug therapy or chemotherapy, etc.)	Patient will consume 50–75% of all meals	1. Assist with meals as necessary	N
		Maintain weight range of _____ lb. (3 months)	2. Avoid foods patient will not eat	D
	Consistent consumption of less than 50% of meals		3. Provide substitutes for foods refused	N, D
			4. Monitor weight and intake	N, D
	Risk Factor: Skin breakdown		5. Assess tolerance to consistency of food	N, D
			6. Inform the physican of significant weight loss	N
			7. Calculate calories, protein etc, consumed	D
			8. Monitor skin status	N, D

Continued

Table 10-1. Care Plan Format with Sample Nutritional Problems, Goals, and Approaches (*Continued*)

Code[a]	Strength/Weakness	When To Address	Goals	Approaches	Discipline
W or AD	Weight loss (may be secondary to disease process, poor appetite, unexplained etiology)	5-lb. decrease per month when below IBW and edema not a problem Trend of weight loss over a over a period of time Weight loss can be anticipated when secondary to a disease process such as terminal cancer	Patient will gain 2 lb. per month to achieve a range of ——— lb. (6 months) If decline is anticipated: Patient will receive measures to stabilize weight and halt weight loss (ongoing)	1. Assist with meals as necessary 2. Monitor weight and intake 3. Avoid foods patient will not eat 4. Provide substitutes for foods refused 5. Assess tolerance to consistency of food 6. Place on supplement program 7. Inform the physican of weight status 8. Encourage the family to bring in favorite foods 9. Offer small amounts of foods frequently	N N, D D D N, D N, D N, D N, D
W	Patient is diabetic Risk factor: At risk for increased blood sugar levels	Patient has a diagnosis of diabetes	Patient will achieve FBS of ——— (3 months)	1. Monitor labs as ordered by the physican 2. Counsel the patient about the importance of compliance	N, RD D, RD

Code	Problem	Assessment	Goal	Intervention	Responsible
				3. Counsel the family about bringing in foods	D
				4. Visit the patient to obtain list of food preferences and dislikes	D
				5. Substitute for food dislikes	D
PI	Patient is unable to feed self	Patient does not eat independently	Patient will progress to eating independently by —— (date)	1. Evaluate for occupational therapy and use of assistive devices	OT
				2. Assist with meals as necessary	N
				3. Praise efforts to eat independently	N, D
				4. Allow sufficient time to feed self; then have staff assist	N
W	Epigastric Distress	Patient complains of stomach discomfort, heartburn or indigestion	Patient will experience no episodes of discomfort (1 month)	1. Review drug regime for drugs with these side effects	RD
				2. Question the patient about specific foods causing discomfort	RD
				3. Offer small, more frequent meals	D
				4. Elevate the head of	N

Continued

Table 10-1. Care Plan Format with Sample Nutritional Problems, Goals, and Approaches (*Continued*)

Code[a]	Strength/Weakness	When To Address	Goals	Approaches	Discipline
				the bed and advise the patient to maintain an upright posture for about 1 hour after meals	
W	Low hemoglobin (May be secondary to malnutrition, blood loss, end-stage renal disease, cirrhosis, cancer, etc.)	Levels more than 1.0 below normal range (unless this is by history a chronic problem or in presence of a disease such as leukemia)	Hemoglobin will increase to within normal range (3 months)	1. Consult with the physican about appropriate supplementation	N, RD
				2. Monitor intake of foods high in iron	D
				3. Increase portions of meats	D
				4. Increase consumption of vitamin C	D
S	Patient feeds self without difficulty and consumes 75–100% of meals	No problems are observed in ability to feed self or intake	Patient will continue to eat independently and to consume 75–100% of meals (3 months)	1. Monitor intake	N, D
				2. Monitor ability to eat independently	N, D
				3. Give resident positive feedback for efforts	N, D
W	Diarrhea Risk factor: Dehydration	Continuous or chronic problem	Patient will have normal bowel movements (2 weeks)	1. Monitor fluid intake; encourage more fluids	N, D
				2. Higher fiber in foods	D

			3. Evaluate prescribed medications for possible side effects	RD
			4. Recommend dietary restrictions such as clear liquids for 24 hours	RD
			5. Small, frequent meals	D
W	Vomiting/nausea Risk factor: Dehydration	Patient will have fewer episodes of vomiting (2 weeks)	1. Visit the patient to obtain a list of tolerated foods	D
			2. Offer small quantities of foods at frequent intervals	D
			3. Serve liquids after meals	N, D
			4. Suggest intake of crackers, toast, etc.	D
			5. Serve cold, clear, or carbonated beverages (avoid lukewarm)	N, D
			6. Avoid fried, greasy foods	D
W	Obesity	Patient will lose 2 lb. per month to achieve a range of _____ lb. (1 year) When patient also is diabetic, has elevated	1. Assess patterns of intake for problems	D
			2. Provide diet counseling	D

Continued

Table 10-1. Care Plan Format with Sample Nutritional Problems, Goals, and Approaches (*Continued*)

Code[a]	Strength/Weakness	When To Address	Goals	Approaches	Discipline
		serum cholesterol, is hypertensive, or has hiatal hernia		3. Discourage between-meal snacks	N, D
				4. Discourage foods brought in by family	N, D
				5. Monitor weight and intake	N, D
				6. Diet as ordered	D
W	Consistently refuses foods from ____ food group(s) (may be meat, vegetable, milk, etc.)	Regular refusal of foods within a major food group	Patient will consume an appropriate amount of recommended daily allowances for all food groups (3 months)	1. Provide appropriate substitute for foods refused	D
				2. Recommend MVI (or calcium or high-protein supplement)	RD
				3. Provide diet counseling	RD
S	Patient appears well nourished as evidenced by appropriate weight and lab values and absence of clinical signs of malnutrition	There is no problem or weakness identified with the patient's nutritional status	The patient will maintain present status as evidenced by weight and normal lab values	1. Monitor weight and intake	N, D
				2. Monitor lab values	N, D
				3. Review medical record quarterly or more frequently if appropriate	N, D

Codes:/[a]S = strength, W = weakness, PI = potential for improvement, AD = anticipated decline.

The patient will consume 75–100 percent of meals,
not
Provide the patient with adequate nutrition.

The first example establishes a goal for the patient and is specific as to what is trying to be achieved. Progress can be easily evaluated. The second example is a dietitian's goal, not the patient's, and is vague and difficult to define and measure. When establishing goals, the consultant should determine the highest practical level of functioning possible to achieve. In many instances it is no longer acceptable simply to maintain. If the goal proves unrealistic or unattainable, it can be revised during subsequent reviews. Examples of possible goals established by the dietitian are listed in Appendix H.

Approaches

The approach, the means by which the goal is achieved, should also be very specific. If the problem, for example, is identified as poor appetite related to difficulty chewing or swallowing, some appropriate approaches would include the following:

- Modify the consistency of the food to puréed.
- Assist the patient with eating as necessary.
- Avoid any specific foods the patient does not tolerate.
- Monitor food intake at each meal.
- Talk with family members about the possiblity of a dental consult.

With the advent of regulations based on OBRA 1987, more aggressive approaches to patient problems and needs are mandated for long-term care professionals. As mentioned above, the consultant dietitian must determine the highest practical level of functioning possible to obtain and plan approaches accordingly.

Dentition provides a good example of the recent change in approach. In past years plans for a patient with ill-fitting dentures might include modification of food consistency and elimination of foods such as raw fruits and vegetables that are difficult to chew. With the increased emphasis today on achieving the highest practical level of functioning, the approach should include the option of a dental consult to improve the underlying condition, rather than simply addressing the "symptoms."

It should be indicated which discipline is responsible for carrying out the approach, by writing in either the initial or the title of the responsible discipline, as follows:

Modify the consistency of the food to puréed—D
Modify the consistency of the food to puréed—Dietary

An approach may be carried out by more than one discipline. For example, the approach "monitor intake" may be taken by both nursing and dietary and both disciplines will be responsible for evaluating progress in this area. Further examples of dietary approaches are included in Appendix H.

Time Frames

The estimated time frame needed to accomplish the goals can be noted in parenthesis following the goal:

Patient will consume 75–100 percent of meals (3 mos.)

The time frame given indicates when the problem and goal need to be revaluated. If the goal is not met but still appears to be reasonable, a new time frame may be established and the goal continued as stated. If met, that fact needs to be noted in the review, for example by highlighting the goal with a magic marker and writing "resolved" and the date of resolution by the mark.

An appropriate time frame is established according to the type of problem and a reasonable time of resolution. For example, chronic weight loss may take a year or more to resolve. On the other hand, a problem with chewing may be resolved quickly by a simple modification of food consistency.

Problems Frequently Identified with Care Plans

Although care planning is actually a simple process based, to a great extent, on common sense, certain problems frequently arise in connection with care plans. Being aware of the following pitfalls may make them easier to avoid.

- Care plan goals stated are not realistic or measurable.
- There is confusion between the definition of goals and approaches. (A goal is the desired result, the approach is the method used to achieve the result.)
- Time frames established are unrealistic.
- Other employees such as nursing assistants, who are important to the success of the plan, are not made aware of goals and approaches established by the care-planning team.
- Important information from the assessment is not included in the overall plan of care.
- The care plan is not properly revaluated and revised in a timely manner. (If an approach is unsuccessful, change it!)
- Some disciplines may not "take credit" for approaches already in place. For example, the facility may be monitoring patient weight and intake routinely, but not listing these actions as "approaches."
- Stated approaches do not always match goals.
- Care plan participants do not state problems clearly—often using broad, nonspecific terms.

- Participants do not take a common-sense approach to solving problems.
- Team members come to care plan meetings unprepared.
- Knowledge of care plan goals and approaches is not reflected in nursing notes or dietary progress notes.

Using Care Plans Wisely

Once the care plan has been written, it should be be followed conscientiously. The dietitian or dietary manager should review the plan before writing any progress notes or updates. Problems addressed on the care plan should be reviewed in these notes and progress or lack of progress reviewed and evaluated. If a goal cannot be met in an appropriate amount of time, the reason should be thoroughly documented in the progress notes. The goal may then be removed from the care plan as unrealistic.

Table 10-1 shows a format for a care plan with sample nutritional problems, goals, approaches, and the responsible discipline noted.

NURSING DOCUMENTATION OF NUTRITION STATUS

The consulting dietitian and the dietary manager are responsible for documentation of nutrition status. Nevertheless, the dietary department and the nursing department share responsibility for meeting the nutritional needs of the patient and a team approach must be reflected in both the nursing and dietary sections of the chart.

It is the responsibility of the consulting dietitian to work closely with the director of nursing to establish a basis for appropriate documentation of nutritional problems and needs. This task might be accomplished through inservice, policies and procedures, or a combination of the two.

Nursing documentation of nutrition status is important for two reasons: (1) to provide an accurate record base for evaluation of patients at nutritional risk and for appropriate intervention, and (2) to verify that the facility has correctly identified and addressed nutrition problems and needs. From a liability standpoint the latter is crucial.

Necessary Areas of Documentation

Nursing documentation of nutrition status should begin at the time of admission and continue throughout the entire length of the patient's stay. It encompasses documentation of anthropometric data on admission, maintenance of accurate food intake records, evaluation of weight status, and recording of acute or chronic problems affecting nutritional status.

Height and weight should be taken and recorded as part of the admission process. This information establishes a base from which to evaluate changes in nutrition status if, for example, the patient loses or gains weight after admission. It also establishes weight status at the time of admission, an important factor in liability. Since future evaluations, including the nutritional assessment, hinge on these values, accuracy is a must and the need for accuracy must be understood by the nursing staff.

The admission nursing assessment should also note the presence or absence of dentures, any assistance needed in eating and any condition related to the diagnosis that might compromise nutrition status, such as hiatal hernia, skin breakdown, the tremors of Parkinson's disease, or the short attention span often seen in Alzheimer's patients. In short, admission information should comprise a thoughtful assessment of present and potential problem areas that will require observation.

Once the patient has been admitted, food intake should be monitored. In the past, documentation of intake was done primarily on patients with established problems such as weight loss or diabetes. It is now becoming common practice at many facilities to document food intake on all patients in order to establish that proper intake monitoring is being done and to identify potential problems early, when intervention may be most effective.

Intake cannot be properly documented until degrees of intake have been defined and a method of evaluation established. For example, consumption of less than 50 percent would be rated poor; 50 percent to 74 percent, fair; 75 percent, good; greater than 75 percent, excellent. The consulting dietitian should work with the director of nursing to establish a rating scale and teach staff members to use it.

Food intake must be recorded in measurable amounts or percentages. Nursing assistants should be trained to record intake at the time of observation to ensure accuracy. A small pocket notepad or intake sheets attached to the food cart or the patient's door may be helpful for this purpose. In addition, assistants should note any significant aspect of intake such as the inability to chew meats or avoidance of particular food groups and report these findings to the nurse. The nurse can pass the information on to the dietitian, who will evaluate the problem and suggest a plan for resolution. Many plans for resolution involve input from both dietary and nursing and will be documented by both departments.

An intake record might consist of a sheet devised for this purpose or may be part of the daily nursing notes. Examples of intake record forms can be found in Appendix A. The intake sheet can be part of the patient chart or may be attached to a clipboard at the nursing station. If not part of the chart, the record may be summarized in a weekly or monthly nursing note. For example, "Patient takes 75 percent of most meals per self with some assist, occasionally less in the evening." Wherever they are placed, these records provide evidence that the patient's intake is indeed being monitored and observed.

Weight has become recognized as one of the most important indicators of nutrition status and so must be carefully monitored. The dietitian should establish ideal body weight range in the initial nutrition assessment during the first consulting visit following admission. The ideal weight range, along with information obtained from the patient or family concerning historical weight and weight loss or gain, will be used in the nursing evaluation of current weight status.

Once again, in order to document appropriately in this area, a means must be established to evaluate weight change. The table below is often used to establish a framework for evaluating weight change (see also Chapter 9).

Time Interval	Significant Weight Loss (%)	Severe Weight Loss (%)
1 week	1.0–2.0	Greater than 2.0
1 month	5.0	Greater than 5.0
3 months	7.5	Greater than 7.5
6 months	10.0	Greater than 10.0

By the standards defined in this table, a significant weight loss for a 120-lb. woman would be a loss of 2.5 lb. or more in 1 week, 6 lb. or more in 1 month, 9 lb. or more in 3 months, or 12 lb. or more in 1 year.

Weight loss should also be noted in patients above ideal body weight range, even though intervention may not be necessary or planned at the time, to establish recognition and monitoring of a potential problem. A weight graph is an excellent means of documenting monthly weight because a graph makes loss or gain readily apparent. The graph should be placed on the chart as part of the permanent record. The graph results in increased awareness of weight status by all departments.

In case of serious weight loss, nursing documentation should record notification of the physician and the physician's response or lack of response to the notification. Until the physician has been notified, the facility has not done all that should be done. The physician should share responsibility for evaluating the problem and planning intervention or documenting that current intervention is appropriate.

Acute or chronic problems should also be documented by nursing. Examples of problems of this nature include diarrhea, nausea and vomiting, dysphagia, skin breakout, dental problems, and noncompliance with dietary instructions. Documentation in this area can sometimes provide clarification as to why a patient may be losing weight or may not be responding to diet therapy. The patient on a weight reduction diet who fails to lose weight because family members bring in special meals each evening is a good illustration of this.

Where To Document

Nursing documentation of nutrition problems should be concentrated in two areas: (1) care plans and updates and (2) the monthly nursing summary. Care plans should address the nutrition problems and needs of each patient and should establish goals for resolution of these problems as well as methods of intervention. The consulting dietitian should have input in establishing the initial care plan whenever possible. The care plan should provide a blueprint for patient care and cover all significant dietary problems. This document serves as proof that the nursing and dietary staff have correctly assessed the patient's nutritional needs and are planning an intervention.

Updates to the care plan should be done quarterly or as needed. Patients with significant weight loss or with acute nutrition problems should be reviewed more frequently. Updates should address each problem identified on the care plan and summarize progress or lack of progress in each area. Once again, updating is important in establishing that the facility is monitoring the patient appropriately. The monthly nursing summary is also an important instrument for documenting nutrition problems and needs. Information that should be included in the summary routinely includes:

1. Percentage of intake for the month
2. Whether the patient is fed or eats independently and any self-help devices provided by the facility
3. Weight and an evaluation of loss/gain status (For example: "Weight is 114 lb., a loss of 3 lb. for the month and 10 lb. since admission one year ago. Patient remains within ideal body weight range.)
4. Any other significant information as noted in the paragraph addressing acute or chronic problems such as dysphagia or diarrhea
5. Intervention and progress reports (If the patient is losing weight or has been identified as at nutritional risk, the summary should include what the facility is doing to resolve the problem and how the patient is responding to the therapy.)

In general the monthly summary should always address nutrition problems noted in the care plan and should summarize and evaluate intervention efforts. The summary should provide an accurate picture of the patient and his or her nutrition status at the time of the summary and should substantiate facility efforts to resolve the nutritional problems identified by the care plan. Neither record is totally effective without the other. The nursing summary should also substantiate nursing awareness of nutrition problems and needs and the team approach to their resolution.

As mentioned previously, the consulting dietitian must have a strong working relationship with the director of nursing to accomplish optimal results with nutrition problems. The rewards of this team approach are a better quality of life for patients and, as a byproduct, good surveys!

SUMMARY

In summary, documentation should not be viewed from a single perspective. Remember that all documentation reflects on the department or person responsible for it and do not ignore the opportunities documentation presents for the dietary department. The following guidelines for documenting data in a patient's chart were offered by James C. Zimmerly, MD, JD, Chairman, Department of Legal Medicine, Armed Forces Institute of Pathology, Washington, DC. when speaking at the 1984 Annual Meeting of the American Dietetic Association.

1. Use black ink; colored ink can fade.
2. Direct quotes from the patient may be helpful, but must be identified as such.
3. Place only facts on medical records. Impressions should be so identified since that type of information might be questioned later.
4. When entering data on a form with blocks or spaces for specific data, complete all such spaces. N/A may be used for data that is not applicable.
5. Use standard abbreviations, which save time and are legally valid.
6. Be certain to date all entries; when appropriate, insert time. This procedure is important in case the pages from the medical record get out of order.
7. If your signature cannot be deciphered, print your name or use a stamp in addition to signature.
8. Do not obliterate anything on the record. If a mistake is made, line out the incorrect entry (without rendering it illegible), initial and date the correction, then write in the correct data. This is important because the medical record may be used as legal evidence of what you have done or have not done.
9. Document well the indications for diagnostic procedures and therapy that pose a risk of serious side effects or complications.
10. When noting a referral or a return visit on a specific day, note the date, not the day of the week.
11. Execute reports in a timely fashion and place them on the medical record.
12. Do not go back to the medical record and insert an entry that was drafted at a later date but purports to have been recorded earlier.
13. Document missed appointments and all other lack of patient compliance.
14. Do not make uncomplimentary comments about the patient or a member of the patient's family in the medical record. Patients have access to the chart.
15. Do not place anything in the medical record that has no bearing on the patient's care.
16. Do not use the medical record to criticize prior care or the incompleteness of the record keeping of other health care professionals.
17. Be complete, accurate, legible, and informative.

REFERENCES

Health Care Financing Administration (HCFA). 1989. Medicare and Medicaid: Requirements for long term care facilities. *Federal Register* 54, no. 21.

Jernigan, Anna K. 1987. Nutrition in long term care facilities. The American Dietetic Association.

Maryland Dietetic Association. 1984. ADA Convention Highlights. *Maryland Dietetic Association Bulletin* 37, no. 4: 56.

Zeman, Frances, and Denise Ney. 1988. *Applications of clinical nutrition.* Englewood Cliffs, N.J.: Prentice-Hall, Inc.

11

Regulations and
the Consultant

On October 1, 1990, the Health Care Financing Administration's (HCFA) Office of Survey and Certification, through its regional offices and the state survey and certification agencies, implemented a revised survey and certification process to assess nursing facilities' compliance with statutory and regulatory requirements for participation in the Medicare and Medicaid programs. This survey process responds to regulatory changes in requirements for participation first proposed by HCFA in October 1987 and to Congressional mandates for nursing home reform found in the Omnibus Budget Reconciliation Act of 1987 (OBRA) (Friedlob et al. 1989).

CURRENT LONG-TERM CARE REQUIREMENTS FOR DIETARY DEPARTMENTS

Although it may not seem "fair," the consulting dietitian is often judged by the survey records of the dietary departments with which he or she consults. With the implementation of the new long-term care requirements, deficiencies are taking on a new significance as the emphasis on punitive corrective action grows. Public availability of state and federal survey results also increases pressure to minimize deficiencies to enhance the public image of long-term care facilities. In addition, there is growing public interest in care of the elderly as the population of the United States ages steadily. "The graying of America" is resulting in an increase in a major national expense—the care of the growing number of geriatric patients requiring institutionalization.

In order to comply with federal regulations governing the dietary department, the dietary consultant must have firsthand knowledge of both the regulations and the published interpretive guidelines relating to the regulations. Although these guidelines are not regulations, they establish parameters of compliance and offer insight into how the regulation will be interpreted by surveyors. There is no substitute for time spent studying each regulation that relates to the dietary department. The dietitian must take the time to become an expert in this area in order to provide expert advice to dietary managers and administrators. It is impossible to assess a dietary department accurately without this knowledge. Copies of the regulations and interpretive guidelines may be obtained from the

American Health Care Association, 1201 L Street N.W., Washington, D.C. 20005; phone, 202-842-4444.

THE SURVEY PROCESS

In order to understand the regulations, the consultant should review the survey process itself. A complete survey of a nursing facility consists of two components: the life safety code and the standard survey of resident care.

The standard survey process is the one of concern to the consultant dietitian. This process assesses compliance with resident's rights, accuracy of resident assessment and care planning, and quality of services furnished by the facility. The process is designed to focus on outcomes rather than policies and procedures or "paperwork compliance." If, however, negative outcomes are observed, the survey can be extended to review these areas as they may relate to the negative outcomes.

The OBRA regulations mandate that surveys should be unannounced and that the facility should not know when the survey will be expected. In order to comply with this regulation, surveyors will no longer inspect facilities approximately every 12 months. Instead, the time frame will vary. For example, a survey may be repeated in 6 months or may not be repeated for 18 months.

The standard survey process consists of 12 tasks:

1. Offsite survey preparation
2. Entrance conference
3. Orientation tour
4. Resident sampling
5. Environmental quality assessment
6. Quality of care assessment
7. Resident rights
8. Dietary services and dining
9. Medication pass
10. Closed record review of discharges
11. Forming a deficiency statement
12. Exit conference

These tasks and the objectives of each, as they relate to the dietary department, are reviewed below.

Task 1: Offsite Survey Preparation

During this phase, the facility file is reviewed for basic information such as bed capacity, staffing information, and previous deficiencies. Areas in which past problems have been identified may receive closer inspection during the current survey. The consultant dietitian should review survey results from previous years and take a close look at any area of dietary services that has been cited for deficiencies.

Task 2: Entrance Conference

The term coordinator introduces the survey team members to the facility staff, explains the survey process, and answers questions. At this time, the administrator is asked to arrange for test trays to be sent out during a designated meal according to instructions outlined in task 9.

Task 3: Orientation Tour

The survey team tours the facility and seeks to identify interviewable and noninterviewable residents and potential areas of poor care that may require in-depth investigation. The following areas are observed closely at this time:

- Skin conditions
- Dehydration risk factors including availability of bedside water
- Resident grooming and dress
- Clinical signs such as edema, emaciation, and contractures
- Functional risk factors such as poor positioning, use of physical restraints, and the need for assistive devices
- Staff-resident interaction
- The level of activity among physically independent residents

Task 4: Resident Sampling

The purpose of this task is to select a sample of residents for quality of care and resident rights interview assessments. Surveyors have been told to "oversample" residents who require total assistance or who require special care treatments, such as residents fed by tube or suffering from pressure sores.

Task 5: Environmental Quality Assessment Objectives

The purposes of this task are

1. To observe physical features in the facility's environment that affect residents' quality of life, health, and safety
2. To determine the impact of a nursing facility's environment on resident outcomes (maintenance of function, comfort, and infection control)

Task 6: Quality of Care Assessment

Assessment of this area determines how resident outcomes are related to the provision of care by the facility. Surveyors are to note changes in the resident's status—improvement, maintenance, or decline—and relate these changes to facility performance. Areas of review in terms of outcome include

- Maintaining or improving functional abilities in performing activities of daily living
- Maintaining psychosocial status (activities, social services assessments, and care planning)
- Preventing pressure sores
- Monitoring nutritional status and hydration
- Maintaining or improving range of motion
- Maintaining urinary continence or effectively managing incontinence
- Preventing accidents, principally falls
- Monitoring drug use, including the use of psychoactive drugs
- Monitoring potential or actual abuse or neglect
- Preventing and managing infectious disease
- Monitoring the accuracy and adequacy of the comprehensive assessment and care plan
- Assessing how staff have implemented the care plan, and if care plan objectives are being met
- Assessing how staff-resident interaction and communication fosters residents' maintaining or attaining their physical, mental, and psychosocial wellbeing.

For each quality of care requirement reviewed, if observations are inconsistent with the clinical record, a quality of care problem may exist.

Task 7: Closed Record Review

Appropriateness of transfers and the quality of discharge planning are reviewed.

Task 8: Individual and Group Resident Rights Interviews

Interviews are conducted with residents, family members, and legal representatives to determine how the facility protects and promotes residents' rights and quality of life.

Task 9: Dietary Services System Assessment

The objectives of this task are

- To evaluate food preparation techniques and sanitation
- To determine nutritional adequacy of the menu and accuracy of therapeutic diets and to confirm the availability of substitutes

It is during this part of the survey that tests will be requested if concerns and/or complaints regarding food quality and temperature have been expressed by the residents during the interview process. The test tray is sent to the unit or wing from which the complaint arose. Food temperatures are taken in the kitchen prior to tray preparation and at the point of service, after the last resident on the designated unit is served and begins eating. The surveyor is also instructed to taste the food and evaluate palatability.

Quality of life as related to the dining experience and the basic dining room environment are also evaluated at this point.

Observations of residents made at this time are compared to information gathered from the medical record. If discrepancies are noted, a problem may exist. For example, if the medical record indicates that the resident feeds himself and has an excellent appetite, yet the surveyor observes the resident sitting during mealtime, eating little, staring into space and the resident appears underweight, a discrepancy may exist that will require a more in-depth investigation.

Task 10: Medication Pass

Preparation and administration of medication is observed to evaluate accuracy of the pass.

Task 11: Information Analysis and Decision Making

Surveyors review and analyze all observations and findings to determine whether the facility meets requirements or whether deficiencies exist in any area. If problems exist, the survey can be extended for further investigation of problem areas. Deficiency statements are written. These statements should be clearly written and include tag numbers of problem areas.

Task 12: Exit Conference

During the exit conference, the facility is informed of the survey team's observations and findings. The facility should be given the opportunity to discuss and supply additional information if appropriate, and to resolve differences regarding deficiencies.

Regulations impacting on or directly pertaining to dietary and nutrition services are listed below along with a detailed list of actions necessary to comply with each regulation. Where applicable, timetables and relevant definitions are also included.

RESIDENTS' RIGHTS

Level A requirement: Residents' rights

F150   The resident has a right to a dignified existence, self-determination, and communication with and access to persons and services inside and outside the facility. A facility must protect and promote the rights of each resident, including each of the following rights:

F157   The resident has a right to refuse treatment.

Facility responsibilities:

A resident's refusal of treatment must be persistent and consistently documented in the resident's record. Refusals of treatment should also be countered by discussions with the resident of the health and safety consequences of the refusal and the availability of any therapeutic alternatives that might exist. If a resident consistently refuses all treatment, discharge on the grounds that the resident's welfare cannot be met in the facility may be the ultimate outcome. Transfer and discharge rights are dealt with under 483.12.

Level B requirement: Self-determination and participation

The resident has the right to:

F213   Choose activities, schedules, and health care consistent with his or her interests, assessments and plans of care;

F214   Interact with members of the community both inside and outside the facility; and

F215   Make choices about aspects of his or her life in the facility that are significant to the resident;

Survey procedure and probes pertaining to these rights

- (Individual) Do you usually get up in the morning and go to bed at night at time of your choosing?
- (Individual) Is your sleep interrupted by anyone during the night? Why?
- (Individual) Can you eat other than during scheduled meal times?
- (Individual) Can you choose what you wear? How are you groomed?
- (Individual) With whom do you eat? Is that your choice?
- (Individual) If you want to visit somebody here, can you do it? If you need help getting there, do you get it?
- (Individual) If you want to leave the facility for short periods of time, can you do so?
- (Individual) Can you spend your time around here pretty much the way you like?

Level A requirement: Resident assessment

F239   The facility must conduct initially and periodically a comprehensive, accurate, standardized, reproducible assessment of each resident's functional capacity.

A. Level B requirement: Admission orders

F240   At the time each resident is admitted, the facility must have physician orders for the resident's immediate care

B. Level B requirement: Comprehensive assessments

F240   The facility must make a comprehensive assessment of a resident's needs, which;

F241   (1) Describes the resident's capability to perform daily life functions and significant impairments in functional capacity

(2) The comprehensive assessment must include at least the following information:

Content:

F242   Medically defined condition and prior medical history

F243   Medical status measurement—objective measurements of a resident's physical and mental abilities

F244   Functional status

F245   Sensory and physical impairments

F246   Nutritional status and requirements

F247   Special treatments or procedures—treatment for pressure sores, N-6 feedings, etc.

F248   Psychosocial status

F249   Discharge potential

F250   Dental condition—condition of teeth, gums, and other structures of the oral cavity that may affect nutritional status, communication abilities or quality of life. Assessment should include need for and use of dentures and other dental appliances.

F251   Activities potential

F252   Rehabilitation potential

F253   Cognitive status

F254   Drug therapy—includes potential side effects. Need not appear in the assessment but must be in the resident's clinical record.

Level B requirement: Accuracy of assessment

F260   Each assessment must be conducted or coordinated with the appropriate participation of health professionals.

F261   Each individual who completes a portion of the assessment must sign and certify the accuracy of that portion of the assessment.

Timetable

F255   Residents residing in an intermediate or skilled care facility prior to the effective date of the requirements must receive a comprehensive assessment no later than October 1, 1991. For individuals admitted on or after (effective date of regulation) no later than 14 days after the date of admission.

Purpose/scope

F259   The results of the assessment are used to develop, review, and revise the resident's comprehensive plan of care.

The assessment is used to determine the resident's highest practicable level of physical, mental, and psychosocial well-being and to plan aggressive, competent approaches to meet goals.

Persons responsible

F260   Each assessment must be conducted or coordinated with the appropriate participation of health professional (i.e., a registered nurse, a dietitian, an activities director, etc. The assessment should be multidisciplinary in nature).

F261   Each individual who completes a portion of the assessment must sign and certify the accuracy of that portion of the assessment.

Revision of the assessment

The resident assessment should be revised:

F256   Promptly after a significant change in physical or mental condition.

As appropriate to assure accuracy of the assessment.

After hospitalization if the hospital stay is likely to affect preadmission functional or cognitive status.

F257   No less often than once (1) every twelve (12) months.

F258   The facility must examine each resident no less often than once (1) every 3 months and as appropriate and revise the assessment to assure continued accuracy.

Relevant definitions

"Comprehensive" means that the information in the assessment enables facility staff to plan care that allows the resident to reach his/her highest paracticable level of physical and mental functioning. At a minimum, the assessment describes the resident's physical and mental deficits and strengths and the equipment and staff assistance with resident needs, It should also identify risk factors associated with possible functional decline and describe the resident's objections for maintaining or improving functional abilities.

"Promptly" means as soon as the resident stabilizes at a new functional or cognitive level or within 2 weeks—whichever is earlier.

The accuracy of the assessment means that the appropriate health professionals, taking into account their clinical knowledge and expertise, correctly document the resident's medical, functional, and psychosocial problems and identify resident strengths to maintain or improve medical status, functional abilities, and psychosocial status. The initial comprehensive assessment is the baseline data for ongoing assessments of resident progress.

"After a significant change" means a major improvement or decline in the resident's physical, mental, or psychosocial status. The assessment must address all aspects of the resident's condition that are affected by the change. Acute conditions such as a stroke or broken hip, life-threatening conditions such as heart disease or cancer, or clinical complications such as advanced skin breakdown or recurrent urinary tract infections can trigger a reassessment.

The facility should consider hospitalization a significant change requiring the resident's reassessment if the hospital stay is likely to affect the resident's pre-admission functional or cognitive status.

"Nutrition status and requirements" means weight, hematological and biochemical assessments; clinical observations of nutrition; nutritional intake, resident eating habits and preferences; and dietary restrictions.

CARE PLANS

Level B requirement: Comprehensive care plans

F262   The facility must develop a comprehensive care plan for each resident that includes measurable objectives and timetables to meet a resident's medical, nursing, and psychosocial needs that are identified in the comprehensive assessment.

Timetable

The care plan:

F263   Must be developed within 7 days after the completion of the comprehensive assessment.

F266   Should be periodically reviewed and revised by a team of qualified persons after each assessment.

Must be consistently implemented.

Purpose/use

Care plans should show an interdisciplinary treatment approach to maintain or improve functional abilities.

Persons responsible

F264

F265   Each care plan should be prepared by an interdisciplinary team that, effective October 1, 1990, includes the attending physician, an RN with responsibility for the resident, and other appropriate staff in disciplines as determined by the resident's needs, and with participation of the resident, the resident's family, or legal representative, to the extent practicable.

F267   The services provided or arranged by the facility must meet professional standards of quality and be provided by qualified individuals in accordance with each resident's written plan of care.

Content

F262   An interdisciplinary team, in conjunction with the resident, resident's family, or legal representative as appropriate, should develop quantifiable objectives for the highest level of functioning the resident may be expected to attain, based on the comprehensive assessment. The care plan must reflect intermediate steps for each outcome objective. The facility staff will use these objectives to follow resident progress.

The care plan should:

- Reflect resident assessment
- Attempt to manage risk factors identified for each resident
- Identify and build on resident strengths
- Reflect standards of current professional practice
- State treatment objectives with measurable outcomes
- Reflect intermediate steps for each outcome objective
- Show an interdisciplinary approach to maintain or improve functional abilities

EATING

Level A requirement: Quality of care

F272   Each resident must receive and the facility must provide the necessary care and services to attain or maintain the highest practicable physical, mental, and psychosocial well-being, in accordance with the comprehensive assessment and plan of care.

Level B requirement: Activities of daily living

Based on the comprehensive assessment of a resident, the facility must ensure that,

1. A resident's abilities in activities of daily living do not diminish unless circumstances of the resident's clinical condition demonstrate that diminution was unavoidable. This includes the resident's ability to:

F273   (A) Bathe, dress, and groom;

F274   (B) Transfer and ambulate;

F275   (C) Toilet;

F276   (D) Eat; and

F277   (E) To use speech, language or other functional communication systems.

F278   2. A resident is given the appropriate treatment and services to maintain or improve his or her abilities specified in paragraph (1)(A) of this section.

F279   3. A resident who is unable to carry out activities of daily living receives the necessary services to maintain good nutrition, grooming and personal and oral hygiene.

Facility responsibilities

- Identification of risk factors during assessment/care planning process (example: decreased ability to chew and swallow, confusion interfering with resident's ability or desire to consume food).
- Documentation of facility efforts to address individual needs to maintain eating abilities (use of assistive devices, seating arrangements to improve sociability, seating in calm, quiet setting for residents with dementia).
- Provision of sufficient staff to assist resident to maintain abilities (allowing sufficient time to eat independently).
- Consistent implementation of care plan objectives in this area.
- Periodical evaluation of care plan objectives in this area and development of alternative approaches when necessary.
- Maintenance of good nutrition status which may include feeding of foods served on dishes; syringe feeding, tube feeding provided through naso-gastric, gastrostomy, or other external tubes; or total parenteral nutrition provided through a central intravenous line.
- Demonstration that any decline in eating ability was unavoidable.

Relevant definitions

"Necessary care" means services and treatment that enable the resident to reach his/her highest practicable physical, mental, or psychosocial well-being. Highest practicable physical, mental, or psychosocial well-being is the highest level of functioning and well-being possible, limited by the individual's presenting functional status and potential for improvement or reduced rate of degeneration. "Highest practicable" is not a diagnostic, prospective, delineating determination made without aggressive, competent efforts to halt degenerative processes and to achieve or restore independent free choice functioning. It is determined through functional assessment and aggressive, competent addressing of the physical, mental, or psychosocial needs of the individual.

"Eating" means nourishing and hydrating oneself (regardless of skill) once the meal is prepared.

"Unable to carry out activities of daily living" means residents need extensive or total assistance with maintenance of nutrition, grooming, and personal and oral hygiene.

"Highest practicable" is the highest level of functioning and well-being possible, limited by the individual's presenting functional status and potential for improvement or reduced rate of functional decline. Highest practicable is determined through functional assessment and aggressive, competent addressing of the physical, mental, or psychosocial needs of the individual.

PRESSURE SORES

Level B requirement: Pressure sores

Based on the comprehensive assessment of a resident, the facility must ensure that:

F283 A resident who enters the facility without pressure sores does not develop pressure sores unless the individual's clinical condition demonstrates they were unavoidable; and

F284   A resident having pressures sores receives necessary treatment and services to promote healing, prevent infection and prevent new sores from developing.

Facility responsibilities

Identification of residents at risk for development of pressure sores (if the resident does not have one at the time of admission). Specific risk factors include:

1. The resident has two (2) or more of the following diseases:
   - Severe chronic pulmonary obstructive disease
   - Diabetes
   - Severe peripheral vascular disease
   - Chronic bowel incontinence
   - Paraplegia
   - Sepsis
   - Terminal cancer
   - Chronic or end stage renal, liver, and/or heart disease
   - Disease- or drug-related immunosuppression
   - Fully body cast
2. The resident receives two (2) or more of the following treatments:
   - Steroid therapy
   - Radiation therapy
   - Chemotherapy
   - Renal dialysis
   - Head of the bed elevated most of the day due to medical necessity
3. The resident shows evidence of malnutrition/dehydration as indicated by decreased albumin, weight loss of more than 10 percent of body weight over the previous month, serum transferrin below 170 mg/dl, hemoglobin less than 12 mg/dl. Clinical signs include pale skin; dull eyes; red, swollen lips; swollen and/or dry tongue with scarlet or magenta hue; poor skin turgor; cachexia; bilateral edema, muscle wasting; calf tenderness; and reduced urinary output.
   - Provision of routine preventative measures specific to the resident. (For example: if serum albumin is below 3.4 mg/dl, additional protein may be added to the diet.)
   - If pressure sores are present at the time of admission, documentation is made of measures taken to promote healing (for example: turning every hour, relieving pressure, medicated dressings, etc.).
   - Observation of measures to prevent infection of the sore (for example: use of aseptic techniques, good handwashing before treatment, etc.).
   - Evaluation of care plan objectives in this area and selection of alternative approaches when applicable.

Exceptions

If, despite, adequate preventative care, pressure sore still develop, the following conditions may demonstrate that the sores were unavoidable:

"The resident is moribund" (e.g., has less than 8 weeks to live; is semicomatose or comatose; life sustaining measures have been withdrawn or discouraged).

Relevant definitions

"Pressure sore" means an area where the skin and underlying tissues are eroded as a result of lack of blood flow caused by pressure of friction, commonly described in four (4) stages:

Stage   I: A persistent area of skin redness (without a break in the skin) that does not disappear when pressure is relieved.

Stage   II: A partial thickness of skin is lost (epidermal layer has been lost, but the dermis is at least partially intact); may present as blistering surrounded by an area of redness and/or induration.

Stage   III: A full thickness of skin is lost, exposing the subcutaneous tissues; presents as shallow crater (unless covered by eschar—thick brown, black or yellow crust); may be draining.

Stage   IV: A full thickness of skin and subcutaneous tissue is lost, exposing muscle and/or bone; at this stage, the sore may be covered with an eschar, draining, necrotic, reddened, and/or indurated.

TUBE FEEDING

Level B requirement: Naso-gastric tubes

Based on the comprehensive assessment of a resident, the facility must ensure that:

F292   A resident who has been able to eat enough alone or with assistance is not fed by naso-gastric tube unless the resident's clinical condition demonstrates that use of a naso-gastric tube was unavoidable; and

F293   A resident who is fed by a naso-gastric or gastrostomy tube receives the appropriate treatment and services to prevent aspiration pneumonia, diarrhea, vomiting, dehydration, metabolic abnormalities, and nasal-pharyngeal ulcers and to restore, if possible, normal feeding function.

Facility responsibilities

If the tube was initiated by the facility, the facility is responsible for:

- Demonstration that the resident was at risk for malnutrition unless fed non-orally (for example: documentation of poor/inadequate intake).
- Documentation of efforts made to maintain oral feeding prior to inserting the tube (for example: supplement program, modification of diet to puréed, assistance with meals).

Responsibility for all tube fed residents includes:

- Verification that the NG tube is properly placed.
- Clear delineation of staff responsibilities for all aspects of tube feeding (example: who administers the feeding, type of formula used, flow rate, etc.).
- Documentation that staff is knowledgeable of/and monitors possible complications of tube feeding (example: diarrhea, aspiration) and administers corrective actions when necessary (example: changing flow rate, changing formula).

Minimization of potential for complications of tube feeding by:

1. Use of small bore, flexible naso-gastric tube, unless contraindicated
2. Securely attaching the tube to the nose/face
3. Checking for correct tube placement prior to feeding

4. Checking a resident with a newly inserted gastric tube for gastric residual volume every 2–4 hours until the resident has demonstrated an ability to empty the stomach
5. Properly elevating the resident's head
6. Providing the type, rate and volume of feeding as ordered
7. Using aseptic or clean technique as per facility/manufacturer's directions, when starting and stopping the feeding
8. Using a pump equipped with a functional alarm (if a pump is used)

• Establishment of criteria for determining when a resident may be able to return to eating by mouth (example: a stroke victim whose ability to swallow may be returning).
• Documentation that substantiates efforts to return appropriate residents to oral feeding.

Exceptions
Clinical conditions demonstrating that feeding via enteral tube is unavoidable include:

• The inability of the resident to swallow without choking or aspiration such as in cases of Parkinson's disease, pseudobulbar palsy or esophageal diverticulum.
• Lack of sufficient alertness for oral nutrition (i.e., the resident is comatose).
• Malnutrition not attributable to a single cause or causes that can be isolated and reversed. There is documented evidence that the facility has not been able to maintain or improve the resident's nutritional status through oral intake.

Relevant definitions
This requirement includes all feeding introduced into the enteral tract via tube, (e.g., gastrostomy, jejunostomy). It does not include parenteral feedings.

NUTRITION

Level B requirement: Nutrition
Based on a resident's comprehensive assessment, the facility must ensure that a resident:
F296 Maintains acceptable parameters of nutritional status, such as body weight and protein levels, unless the resident's clinical condition demonstrates that this is not possible; and
F297 Receives a therapeutic diet when there is a nutritional problem.
Facility responsibilities
Evaluation of nutritional status parameters such as weight loss or gain, hematological and biological assessments, and clinical observations. Suggested parameters for evaluating significance of weight loss are:

Interval	Significant Loss	Severe Loss
1 week	1–2%	Greater than 2%
1 month	5%	Greater than 5%
3 months	7.5%	Greater than 7.5%
6 months	10%	Greater than 10%

The following formula will determine percentage of loss:

Percentage of body weight loss = (usual weight − actual weight × 100) ÷ usual weight

Evaluation of clinical observations such as: dull, dry, brittle hair; pale, dull eyes; swollen lips; swollen and/or dry tongue with scarlet or magenta hue; poor skin turgor; goiter; cachexia; bilateral edema; muscle wasting; tenderness and reduced urinary output.

Identification and evaluation of factors which may place the resident at risk of malnutrition, including, but not limited to:

1. Taking drugs that may contribute to nutritional deficiencies, such as:
   A. Cardiac glycosides
   B. Diuretics
   C. Anti-inflammatory drugs
   D. Antacids (antacid abuse)
   E. Laxatives (laxative abuse)
   F. Psychotropic drug overuse
2. Poor oral health status
3. Depression
4. Lack of access to culturally acceptable foods
5. Being a slow eater resulting in food becoming unpalatable, or in removal of tray before resident has finished eating
6. Provision of clinically appropriate therapeutic diets when indicated (example: a restricted sodium diet for a resident with edema)
7. Provision of routine preventative measures and care (example: assistance with meals, modification of diet consistency)
8. Clear delineation of staff responsibilities for maintenance of nutrition status (example: who is to feed the resident, who evaluates residents for a diet supplement)
9. Evaluation of care plan goals for this area and development of alternative approaches as necessary

Exceptions

Clinical conditions demonstrating that the maintenance of acceptable nutritional status is not possible include, but are not limited to:

- Refusal to eat and refusal of other methods of nourishment
- Advanced disease (i.e., cancer, malabsorption syndrome)
- Increased nutritonal/caloric needs associated with pressure sores and wound healing (e.g., fractures, burns); receiving radiation or chemotherapy
- Kidney disease, alcohol/drug abuse, chronic blood loss, hyperthyroidism
- Gastrointestinal surgery
- Prolonged nausea, vomiting, diarrhea not relieved by treatment given according to accepted standards of practice

Relevant definitions

"Nutritional status and requirements" means weight, hematological and biochemical assessments; clinical observations of nutrition; nutritional intake, resident eating habits and preferences; and dietary restrictions.

"Therapeutic diet" means a diet ordered by a physician because of nutritional deficiency, a disease, or to eliminate or decrease certain substances in the diet (e.g., cholesterol).

HYDRATION

Level B requirement: Hydration
F298 The facility must ensure that each resident is provided with sufficient fluid intake to maintain proper hydration.
Facility responsibilities

1. Identification and evaluation of risk factors for a resident becoming dehydrated including:
   - Coma/decreased sensorium
   - Fluid loss and increased fluid needs (e.g., diarrhea, fever, uncontrolled diabetes)
   - Functional impairments making it difficult to drink or communicate fluid needs (e.g., aphasia)
   - Refusal of fluids
   - Dementia in which the resident forgets to drink
2. Observation for clinical signs of possible insufficient fluid intake such as dry skin and mucous membranes, poor skin turgor, thirst, abnormal laboratory values.
3. Development of plan to assure adequate fluid intake (examples: offer fluids every hour; give popsicles between meals; add foods high in water content)
4. Calculation of approximate daily fluid needs (example: 30 cc fluid per kilogram of body weight or other accepted formula)
5. Evaluation of the resident for extraordinary measures to assure hydration (example: IV's)
6. Assurance of staff awareness of fluid needs

Exceptions
Despite proper identification of and efforts to address risk factors associated with dehydration, the facility is unable to improve the resident's fluid status.
Relevant definitions
"Sufficient fluid" means the amount of fluid needed to prevent dehydration and maintain health. The amount needed is specific for each resident, and fluctuates as the resident's condition fluctuates (e.g., increase fluids if resident has fever or diarrhea).

DIETARY SERVICES

Level A requirement
F323 The facility must provide each resident with a nourishing, palatable, well-balanced diet that meets the daily nutritional and special dietary needs of each resident.

A. Level B requirement: Staffing
F324 The facility must employ a qualified dietitian either full-time, part-time, or on a consultant basis.

1. If a qualified dietitian is not employed full-time, the facility must designate a person to serve as the director of food services.

2. A qualified dietitian is one who is qualified based upon either registration by the Commission on Dietetic Registration of the American Dietetic Association, or on the basis of education, training, or experience in identification of dietary needs, planning and implementation of dietary programs.

Interpretive guideline
The Dietitian should have experience or training in the following areas:

- Assessing nutritional needs of geriatric and physically impaired persons
- Developing therapeutic diets
- Developing "regular diets" to meet the specialized needs of geriatric and physically impaired persons
- Counseling geriatric and physically impaired persons in nutrition
- Developing and implementing continuing education programs for dietary services and nursing personnel
- Participating in interdisciplinary care planning
- Budgeting and purchasing food and supplies, including budget and purchasing experience or knowledge
- Supervising institutional food preparation

[Author's note: Although these federal regulations do not actually require a registered dietitian or a qualified dietary manager, many problems noted in the facility dietary services could be referenced back to lack of a qualified manager or consultant dietitian. Also, as of October, 1990, Congress passed a bill which requires the Secretary to establish requirements for social workers, dietitians, and activities professionals employed in a nursing facility that are at least as strict as the requirements applicable to such professionals prior to the enactment of OBRA '87. It remains to be seen how this will be interpreted by HCFA.]

B. Level B requirement: Sufficient staff
F325   The facility must employ sufficient support personnel competent to carry out the functions of the dietary service. Sufficient support personnel means enough cooks, dishwashers, and food servers to prepare and serve food on time. Nursing aides helping residents eat are not support personnel.

Interpretive guidelines

- Sufficient support personnel means enough staff to prepare and serve palatable, attractive, nutritionally adequate meals at proper temperatures and appropriate times.
- Food is prepared in scheduled time frames
- Food leaves the kitchen in scheduled time frames

[Author's note: Surveyors will not review staffing patterns unless a problem or "negative outcome" is traced to possible insufficient staffing.]

C. Level B requirement: Menus and nutritional adequacy
        Menus must:
F326   (1) Meet the nutritional needs of residents in accordance with the recommended dietary allowance of the Food and Nutrition Board of National Research Council, National Academy of Sciences

Interpretive guidelines

1. Menus should allow residents to maintain usual body weight and acceptable nutrition values: i.e., menus should meet the calorie and nutrient needs of residents.
2. If dairy foods, vegetables, and fruit are missing from the residents' daily diet, the facility should have an alternative means of satisfying the resident's nutrient needs.
3. The menu should supply at least 4 ounces of edible meat, 2 cups fruit/vegetables, 4 servings bread/cereal, and 2 cups of milk.

[Author's note: If the facility has a large number of patients below ideal body weight, the surveyor will probably review the menu carefully to determine nutritional adequacy.]

F327   (2) Be prepared in advance
Interpretive guideline
   Cycle menus are dated for both regular and modified diets.

[Author's note: The manager should record the date the cycle is implemented. The consultant dietitian should sign the menu cycle as proof of review or approval.]

F328   (3) Be followed.
Interpretive guideline
   The facility follows the menu as written.
D. Level B requirement: Food each resident receives and the facility provides
F329   (1) Food prepared by methods that conserve nutritive value, flavor, and appearances;
Interpretive guideline
   Food preparation that conserves nutritive value does not destroy vitamins because of prolonged food storage, light exposure, prolonged cooking of foods in a large volume of water, addition of baking soda, and overcooking for soft texture.
RE: 1. Food has a distinctively appetizing aroma and/or appearance such as attractive use of garnishes and variety in color as plated.
   2. Food is generally well seasoned.
   3. Food preparation does not destroy vitamins.
F330   (2) Food is palatable, attractive, and at the proper temperature.

[Author's Note: There is no interpretive guideline for the acceptable temperature range of food at the point of service. The consultant dietitian should develop an in-house policy on this and monitor foods accordingly. For example, the house policy for the temperature of vegetables at the point of service may be 120°F ± 5°F. Be sure to include cold foods in the policy as well.]

Interpretive guideline
   Food is served at appropriate temperatures (hot foods are served hot and cold foods are served cold).

F331   (3) Food prepared in a form designed to meet individual needs:
Interpretive guideline
   Food is cut, chopped, or ground for individual residents' needs.
F332   (4)Substitutes offered of similar nutritive value to residents who refuse food served.
Interpretive guideline
   Residents who refuse food are offered a substitute of similar nutritive value.

[Author's note: This may be handled by obtaining a detailed list of patient preferences and dislikes at the time of admission and making the dietary staff aware of this information.]

E. Level B requirement: Therapeutic diets
F333   Therapeutic diets must be prescribed by the attending physician.
Interpretive guideline
   Meal served conforms with the physician's order.
F. Level B requirement: Frequency of meals.
F334   (1) Each resident receives and the facility provides at least three (3) meals daily, at regular times comparable to normal mealtimes in the community.
F335   (2) There must be no more than 14 hours between a substantial evening meal and breakfast the following day, except as provided in (4) below.
Interpretive guideline
   A "substantial evening meal" is defined to mean an offering of three (3) or more menu items at one time, one of which includes a high quality protein such as meat, fish, eggs, or cheese. The meal represents no less than 20 percent of the day's total nutritional requirements.
F336   (3) The facility must offer snacks at bedtime daily.
Interpretive guideline
   "Nourishing snack" is an offering of items, single or in combination, from the daily food guide.
F337   (4) When a nourishing snack is provided at bedtime, up to 16 hours may elapse between a substantial evening meal and breakfast the following day if a resident group agrees to this meal span and a nourishing snack is served.
G. Level B requirement: Assistive devices
F338   The facility must provide special eating equipment and utensils for residents who need them.
Interpretive guideline

1. Assistive devices maintain or improve resident's ability to eat independently, for example, improving poor grasp by enlarging silverware handles with foam padding, aiding residents with impaired coordination or tremor by plate guards, or providing postural supports for head, trunk, and arms.
2. Effective adaptive utensils are used to promote maximum resident independence in dining.

[Author's note: The facility needs to establish a policy concerning who evaluates a resident for need for an assistive device—one suggestion is the care plan committee.]

H. Level B requirements: Sanitary conditions
>The facility must:

F339 (1) Procure food from sources approved or considered satisfactory by Federal, State, or local authorities.

Interpretive guideline
>All foods are obtained from sources approved or considered satisfactory by Federal, State, or local authorities.

F340 (2) Store, prepare, distribute, and serve food under sanitary conditions;

Interpretive guideline

1. "Sanitary conditions" means storing, preparing, distributing, and serving food to properly prevent food borne illness. Prevention of food borne illness focuses on potentially hazardous food; foods subject to continuous time/temperature controls in order to prevent either the rapid and progressive growth of infectious or toxigenic microorganisms. Potentially hazardous food tends to focus on animal products (milk, eggs, poultry, fish, and synthetic food ingredients).
2. Hot foods should leave the kitchen (or steam table) above 140 degrees and cold foods below 45 degrees. Temperatures within 3 degrees are acceptable. Refrigerator temperatures should be maintained at less than 45 degrees.
3. Containers of food should be stored off the floor and on clean surfaces in a manner protecting it from contamination.
4. Potentially hazardous foods should be stored at 45 degrees or below and frozen foods kept at 0–20 degrees.
5. Leftovers should be handled properly.
6. Frozen foods should be thawed properly.
7. The staff should handle and cook potentially hazardous foods properly. No risk of food borne illness should be evident.
8. Potentially hazardous foods should be kept at an internal temperature of 45 degrees or below in cold storage facility or at an internal temperature of 140 degrees or above in a hot food storage facility during display and service.
9. Food is transported in a way that protects it against contamination (covered containers, wrapped, or packaged).
10. There is no sign of rodent or insect infestation.
11. The water source is safe; sufficient hot and cold water is available under sufficient pressure.
12. Food preparation equipment, dishes, and utensils are effectively sanitized to destroy potential disease carrying organisms.
13. All sewage, including liquid waste, is properly disposed of by a public sewege system or by a sewage disposal system constructed and operated in accordance with state and local laws.
14. Potable and nonpotable water systems are connected in accordance with state and local laws.
15. Handwashing facilities are convenient and properly equipped for dietary services staff use.
16. Toxic items (such as insecticides, detergent, polishes) are properly stored, labeled, and used.

F341 (3) Dispose of garbage and refuse properly.

Interpretive guideline
> Garbage and refuse containers are in good condition (no leaks) and waste is properly contained in dumpsters and compactors.

Level B requirement: Space and equipment
> The facility must:

F389 (1) Provide sufficient space and equipment in dining, health services, recreation, and program areas to enable staff to provide residents with needed services as required by these standards and as identified in each resident's plan of care; and

Interpretive guideline
> Dining, health services, recreation, and program areas should be large enough to accommodate comfortably the maximum number of persons who usually occupy that space, including wheelchairs, walkers, and other ambulation aids used by many residents who require more than standard circulation spaces. The facility must use space to promote the resident's full physical and social participation. Sufficient space means the resident can access the area, it is not functionally off-limits, and the resident's functioning is not restricted once access to the space is gained.

F390 (2) Maintain all essential mechanical, electrical, and patient care equipment in safe operating condition.

Interpretive guideline
> All essential equipment is in safe operating condition, for example, kitchen refrigerator and freezer.

G. Level B requirement: Dining and resident activities

F406 The facility must provide one or more rooms designated for resident dining and activities. These rooms must:

F407 (1) Be well lighted.

Interpretive guideline

1. "Well lighted" means levels of illumination are suitable to tasks performed by a resident.
2. There is little glare, no sharp contrasts of light and dark, and lighting supports independent functioning.

F408 (2) Be well ventilated with non-smoking areas identified.

[Author's note: It may be easier to prohibit smoking during meals.]

Interpretive guideline

1. "Well ventilated" means good air circulation, avoidance of drafts at floor level, and adequate smoke exhaust removal.
2. "Non-smoking areas identified" means signage in accordance with state law regulating indoor smoking policy and/or facility policy.
3. The area must have good air movement with acceptable temperature, humidity, and odor levels.

F409 (3) Be adequately furnished.

Interpretive guideline

1. An adequately furnished dining area demonstrably accommodates different residents' physical and social needs, including those in wheelchairs.
2. Furnishings are structurally sound and functional (e.g., chairs of varying sizes to meet varying needs of residents and tables wheelchairs can fit under).

F410   (4) Have sufficient space to accommodate all activities

Interpretive guideline

1. "Sufficient space to accommodate all activities" means that the space available is adaptable to a variety of uses and residents' needs.
2. Space adaptable to a variety of uses and residents' needs. Residents and staff have a maximum flexibility in arranging furniture to accommodate residents who use walkers, wheelchairs, and other mobility aids. There is no crowding evident. Space does not limit resident access.

WORKING WITH SURVEYORS

If possible, the consulting dietitian should try to be present for the annual survey by licensure and regulation. Reasons for this include

1. Being available to answer any questions the surveyors may have or to clarify existing facility policies and procedures. There are often numerous ways to accomplish a goal or to comply with a regulation. Most surveyors will be receptive to new ways of achieving objectives or maintaining compliance with regulations if the desired outcome is achieved. The presence of the dietitian may ultimately reduce the number of deficiencies in situations where questions arise.
2. Being present for the survey assures that the consultant will hear firsthand any problems noted by the dietary surveyor and so will understand what is necessary to achieve compliance.
3. Using the survey as an opportunity to meet the state surveyors and to establish a rapport with the survey team. This contact can be useful when questions arise that make it necessary to call a member of the survey team for information or clarification of a regulation or interpretive guideline.

As stated earlier, it is necessary to know and understand all regulations pertaining to the dietary department in order to work most effectively with the survey team. Once having demonstrated an in-depth knowledge of the regulations and a personal concern for excellence, the consultant will begin to build a relationship of trust with the survey team. This relationship may prove valuable when a consultant accepts a new facility that has not had a good survey record in the past. In this instance the survey team may allow the facility "the benefit of the doubt" until the dietary consultant has had time to implement new policies and procedures. Ultimately, however, the consultant will be judged by the facilities with which he or she becomes involved and by the survey records these facilities achieve.

JOINT COMMISSION

The Joint Commission on Accreditation of Healthcare Organizations (JCAHO) was established in 1951 as a voluntary accreditation agency for acute care facilities. The Accreditation Program for Long-Term Care was initiated in 1967. Even though the majority of acute area facilities participate in the JCAHO accreditation process, few long-term care facilities presently participate in this agency's accreditation process.

Unlike annual licensure surveys conducted by a state's licensure and regulations department, surveys conducted by JCAHO occur every three years. Visits are preplanned and usually last two to four days, depending on the size of the facility.

The responsibility of the Joint Commission is to develop standards that will assure high quality care to the patients by the health care organization. JCAHO develops "Quality Assurance" standards with a corresponding systematic monitoring and evaluation tool. This tool identifies important aspects of patient care and service within the context of a facility-wide program for ongoing quality assurance activities.

Currently, JCAHO is developing new clinical indicators for specific areas (oncology, surgery, and cardiovascular) of acute and long-term care. The American Dietetic Association is assisting JCAHO with the nutrition components of these areas.

Copies of JCAHO current standards can be obtained by writing to:

Joint Commission on Accreditation of Healthcare Organizations
875 North Michigan Avenue
Chicago, IL 60611

REFERENCES

Friedlob, Alan, Lois Steinfort, Santoro Vittorio and Emma Luten. 1990. Meeting the OBRA Mandate. *Provider* 16(4):14.

Health Care Financing Administration. 1989. Medicare and Medicaid; Requirements for long-term care facilities. *Federal Register* 54, no. 21.

House of Representatives, 100th Congress. 1987. Omnibus Budget Reconciliation Act of 1987, Report no. 100-391. Washington, D.C.: U.S. Government Printing Office.

12

Developing a Quality Assurance Program

What is quality assurance? Why is it important in today's health care institution? Quality assurance has evolved into its present sophisticated form as a result of the Joint Commission of the Hospital Accreditation Organization's (JCAHO) focus on quality patient care and its effort to define an objective and systematic approach to the evaluation of care. In 1983, the JCAHO developed standards for the purpose of defining quality patient care. These standards have become the accepted goal for every health care institution accredited by the JCAHO. In the Omnibus Budget Reconciliation Act of 1987, ongoing quality assurance programs in Medicaid- and Medicare-reimbursed facilities were mandated by the federal government for implementation by October, 1990. Quality assurance programs in long term care facilities emphasize the importance of standardized care guidelines for the total healthcare delivery systems. Health care facilities and practitioners must comply with the regulatory agencies by developing their own quality assurance programs. Today, quality assurance has moved beyond simple paperwork compliance and is emerging as a major force in health care.

Quality assurance is defined by JCAHO as a planned, systematic procedure that monitors, evaluates, and corrects activities in order to achieve agreed-upon standards for quality and appropriateness of patient care services that are provided. The purpose of quality assurance is to help health care providers and professionals identify their internal problems before they become problems to the patient. It protects the patient and the facility. In today's political and legal climate, it is the wise administrator or board of trustees who has a quality assurance program that validates the level of patient care being provided.

"THE TEN-STEP MONITORING AND EVALUATION PROCESS"

How does one implement a quality assurance program? The Joint Commission of the Hospital Accreditation Organization has published the following guidelines for developing a quality assurance plan.[1]

1. *Assign Responsibility*—The chairman, chief, or director of the department or service is responsible for its monitoring and evaluation activities. This person identifies and assigns the responsibilities of others in the department and ensures that these responsibilities are fulfilled. Joint Commission standards to not require individual departments to have written Quality Assurance plans; however, department heads often find that a working outline of the departmental monitoring and evaluation process provides focus and direction for departmental activities.

2. *Delineate the Scope of Care*—Delineating the scope of care involves identifying the diagnostic and therapeutic modalities used (e.g., procedures performed, medications frequently used, rehabilitative services provided), as well as ascertaining the types of patients served (e.g., major age or disability groups, diseases treated). Health care professionals in the department identify the patient care services they provide and the clinical activities they perform. Monitoring and evaluation activities should encompass the major diagnostic, therapeutic, and/or preventive functions in the department or service.

3. *Identify Important Aspects of Care*—After the scope of patient care is defined, the next task is to identify the diagnostic and therapeutic modalities that are considered most important in providing these services. Priority should be given to those aspects of care for which one of more of the following is true:
   - The aspect of care occurs frequently or affects large numbers of patients.
   - Patients are at risk of serious consequences or are deprived of substantial benefit if care is not provided correctly and in timely fashion or on proper indication; and
   - The aspect of care has tended to produce problems for staff or patients in the past.

   High-volume, high risk, or problem prone aspects of care should be the highest priority for monitoring and evaluation.

4. *Identify Indicators*—An indicator is a defined, measurable dimension of the quality or appropriateness of an important aspect of patient care. Indicators describe measurable care processes, clinical events, complications, or outcomes for which data should be collected to allow comparison with the threshold for evaluation related to each indicator. Indicators should relate to patient care rather than administrative procedures and should address aspects of care that have the greatest effect on quality. For example, if personnel responsible for monitoring and evaluation of anesthesia services have identified management of patients during anesthesia as an important aspect of care, the following are possible indicators:
   - Neurological deficit not present prior to surgery.
   - Need to reintubate trachea during anesthesia.
   - Heart rate less than 40 or greater than 140 during anesthesia.

5. *Establish Thresholds for Evaluation*—The data collected for each indicator

cannot alone lead to conclusions about the quality and/or appropriateness of care. The indicator can, however, direct attention to those areas in which a problem or other opportunity to improve care may be found. To conclude that there is an actual problem requires intensive evaluation of the care provided. As data is collected over a series of cases or events being monitored, there should be a pre-established level or point in the cumulative data that triggers this intensive evaluation. When reached, this *threshold for evaluation* initiates the evaluation to determine whether an actual problem or opportunity to improve care exists. For the indicator related to measuring blood pressure of potentially hypertensive patients, the threshold for evaluation might be set at 98%. That is, intensive evaluation of the quality and appropriateness of this aspect of care would be undertaken if this indicator is not fulfilled for over 2 percent of such patients. The indicator in this example is an established standard of care that practitioners should strive to meet 100 percent of the time. Rare instances of noncompliance, however, may not indicate a systematic or continuing problem and may be justified. Therefore, a department may deem the investment of professional resources in intensive evaluation unnecessary for only rare instances of noncompliance (in this case, under 2 percent).

Using another example, the threshold for evaluation relating to the wound infection rate indicator may be set for 2.5 percent. Because a certain percentage of wound infections are not preventable even with the best of care, professionals may find it unproductive to intensively evaluate each instance of infection.

Although many thresholds will be set at levels other than 0 percent or 100 percent, some events or occurrences are so serious that every case must be evaluated or are so rare that it is not appropriate to accumulate a series of instances before evaluating. An example of such an indicator is failure to type a patient's blood before a transfusion. The thresholds for evaluation pertaining to such indicators would be 0 percent or 100 percent.

6. *Collect and Analyze Data*—To collect and organize data, appropriate staff members must determine the following for each indicator: the data sources, data-collection method, appropriateness of sampling, time frame for data collection, and process for comparing cumulative data with the thresholds for evaluation.

Data Sources—Rather than create all new data sources and data-collection methods for monitoring and evaluation, staff should first attempt to use existing sources and methods. Existing sources of potentially useful data include patient records, laboratory reports, medication sheets, incident reports, and department logs. The specific indicator will help determine the appropriate data sources.

Data Collection—The individual responsible for monitoring and evaluation activities must determine the data collection method and who will collect the data. In some organizations, the department staff, either clinical or clerical, collect data. Other organizations may have an individual or group from outside the department (such as medical records or quality assurance personnel) collect data.

Sampling—For each indicator, staff members should decide whether sampling is appropriate for data collection. Sampling would not be correct for an indicator that describes an infrequent but serious complication. It may be appropriate to use sampling in data collection for an indicator pertaining to a high volume occurrence.

Time Frame—The frequency with which data will be collected and tabulated should be sufficient to accumulate the necessary data to compare with thresholds for evaluation. The frequency should be based on the number of patients affected by the care being monitored, the risk involved in the care, and the regularity with which the aspect of care is performed.

Comparing Cumulative Data with Thresholds for Evaluation—After data is tabulated, the cumulative data for each indicator should be compared with its corresponding threshold for evaluation. This comparison is used to determine whether further evaluation is necessary.

7. *Evaluate Care*—When the cumulative data reaches the threshold for evaluation, staff members qualified in the particular area should evaluate the care provided to determine if a problem exists. The evaluation may include analysis of patterns or trends in the care. When it is appropriate to conduct an intensive review of care provided by an individual practitioner and/or to an individual patient, peer review is undertaken.

8. *Take Actions to Solve Identified Problems*—The evaluation may conclude that the care is acceptable and no further action is necessary. If the evaluation identifies a problem, department staff should decide what action is necessary to solve the problem. A plan of corrective action identifies *who* or *what* is expected to change; *who* is responsible for implementing action; *what* action is appropriate in view of the problem's cause, scope, and severity; and *when* change is expected to occur. If a needed action exceeds the department's authority, recommendations are forwarded to the body that has the authority to act.

To be effective, corrective action must be appropriate to the problem's cause. Three common causes of problems are insufficient knowledge, defects in systems, and deficient behavior or performance. Insufficient knowledge often is addressed by (1) adding or developing training classes or other activities, (2) providing additional reference sources, or restructuring existing educational procedures. Defects in systems often are addressed by changing policies and procedures, redistributing staff, altering use of equipment and supplies, or correcting any communication problems. Behavior or performance deficiencies often are addressed by counseling, increasing supervision, changing duties, transferring, or withdrawing certain privileges of the individuals involved.

9. *Assess the Action and Document Improvement*—Next, the staff must ask themselves whether the action was successful. Continuous monitoring and evaluation should provide the information to answer this question. For

example, if the level of performance for the given indicator is unchanged, the problem likely persists. If the level of performance improves notably, the action was probably successful in solving the problem. Even if the problem appears to be solved, monitoring and evaluation are continued to assure that care remains at a high level of quality and any additional problems are identified and solved.

10. *Communicate Relevant Information to the Appropriate Organizational Quality Assurance Committee.*

In summary, the critical indicators are the foundation of monitoring and the evaluation of patient care services. Indicators define the expected performance of the patient care services. Indicators must include all important aspects of a department, and standards must be written by which the criteria is judged. A data collection system is established to evaluate the department's service and a course of action for follow-up is determined. Further review decides whether or not the follow-up or action was appropriate. The effectiveness of actions must be documented.

PLANNING A QUALITY ASSURANCE PROGRAM

In evaluating a dietary service there are two basic components: nutritional care of patients and quality control of food preparation and service. When writing the indicators of the quality assurance plan for your department, start small. Do not overwhelm yourself or your staff with the burden of too much documentation. Do not attempt to solve all problems at once. Choose three or four areas in the department where you suspect there might be a problem. For example, is there a problem with weight loss or food intake? How many patients consume 50 percent or better of the meal served? How many residents have lost more than 10 lb. since admission? Are nourishments passed out by nursing and consumed by the residents in the evening? Obviously, nutritional intake is an important factor in quality patient care. Choose indicators that tell you if patients' needs are being met and how well the food is accepted. If your clientele are not consuming the food prepared, what course of action can be taken in order to solve the problem? Do you need to make changes on the menu? Is the appearance of the food colorful and appealing? Is food served in a texture that patients are able to eat? Are the cultural habits of the area considered? Is the food served in the facility familiar to patients? These are only a few examples of clinical indicators. Some others might include

1. Inappropriate diet order for diagnosis
2. Therapeutic diets not in compliance with the approved diet manual
3. Error in therapeutic diets served
4. Patient NPO or on clear liquids longer than three days
5. Diet order not received within 24 hours of admission
6. Nutrition assessments incomplete or inaccurate

7. No weight or height history
8. Change in diet order not received by dietary department
9. Nutritional supplement ordered but not given
10. Wrong diet served

The areas of quality control for food preparation and service that should be monitored include food temperatures, cooling equipment temperatures, labeling and dating of food, sanitation inspection reports, number of trays served per minute, patient survey questionnaires, and food cart delivery times.

Effective quality assurance programs have other benefits in addition to improvement in patient care. Once the departmental quality assurance plan is implemented, it enables the supervisor to manage his or her department more effectively. By providing focus and direction for the department, managers are able to pinpoint specific problem areas and prioritize goals. Another benefit of quality assurance planning is increased interdepartmental communication. Many problems in patient care involve more than one department. When this overlap occurs, departments are forced to develop action plans that hopefully will result in solutions. It becomes evident in interdepartmental quality assurance meetings that provision of quality patient care is impossible without the cooperation of every department involved in direct patient care. Cooperation results in improved working relationships within the health care facility, a heightened sense of accomplishment for all those involved, and improved patient care.

Quality Assurance Self-Assessment Checklist

A comprehensive quality control program must include indicators for all important aspects of the dietary department. Look closely at what you are evaluating and include topics that are representative of the services the department provides. The following sample quality assessment checklist may assist you in prioritizing problem areas. Keep in mind that you will need to indicate whether or not the criteria are met and to specify any variances.

Clinical Documentation

1. A physician's diet order is a part of the admitting and subsequent orders. Special orders, such as for salt substitute and commercial supplements need to be part of the physician's order.
2. A complete written diet requisition is sent to the dietary department prior to serving the first meal to the resident and as physician's orders are updated—whether diet order change or not.
3. The foodservice manager or designee visits the new resident within 24 hours after admission to obtain food preferences and objections and other pertinent information. Documentation of visit, date, time, and signature is noted on the Resident Assessment Form.

4. The nutritional assessment is initiated within 24 hours of admission and all items are completed within 7 days of admission. Data include
   a. Initial weight
   b. Ideal or acceptable body weight
   c. Laboratory data (hemoglobin, hematocrit, FBS, electrolytes, BUN, cholesterol, triglycerides, albumin, and creatinine)
   d. Medication affecting nutrition status (such as diuretics, phenobarbitol, antibiotics, insulin, and potassium supplements)
   e. Nutritional physical assessment (dentition, edema, nausea, bowel and bladder functions, and the condition of the face, eyes, lips, gums, and skin)
   f. Fluid consumption
   g. Food intake
   h. Documentation of recommendations by the dietitian, signature, and date
5. Nutritional progress notes are charted on each resident in a timely manner according to resident's level of care and/or nutrition status.
6. Each resident has a current Dietary Plan of Care that is integrated into the overall plan of care. A copy of the Dietary Plan of Care is filed within the dietary department; there is evidence that all dietary employees are aware of the care plan.
7. Each resident has a pertinent discharge plan in relation to nutritional needs in preparation for discharge.
8. Daily meal and snack intake are recorded.
9. Each resident has an information file within the dietary department. Information includes:
   a. The resident's name, room number, and admission date
   b. The current diet requisition (current with physician's orders on medical chart)
   c. Food preferences and objections
   d. Allergies/intolerances
   e. Monthly weights, IBW range, and height
   f. The location of meal service
   g. Nourishment, if applicable
   h. Self-help devices, if applicable
10. Each resident has a planned daily diet that includes three meals and HS snack in accordance with the physician's diet order.
11. Each resident has a clean, legible tray card that is used for meal service. Information on the card includes
   a. The resident's name and room number
   b. The location of meal service
   c. Diet
   d. Food and beverage preferences and objections
   e. Allergies/intolerances
   f. Special information (self-help devices, salt substitute, extra fluids, and so on)

Foodservice Documentation

1. Each prepared menu item is made from a legible recipe that yields the correct number of portions for the facility.
2. The recipe filing system is organized either by categories in a recipe box or by categories or menu cycles in a binder.
3. All meat items have been prepared and portioned correctly to equal the amount of edible protein specified on the menu.
4. The menu cycle will be in use. The menu spreadsheets will be clean, legible, and dated correctly on the face sheet with the month, day, and year. The menus shall be posted to be visually accessible in the preparation and service areas.
5. All diets (including combinations) not planned on the menu will have the daily meal plan extended onto the menu and approved by the dietitian.
6. Daily substitutions are recorded on the front of the day's menu with the date and foodservice manager's initials. The reason for the substitution shall be recorded on the back of the menu. Permanent substitutions are made on the appropriate cover and spreadsheet and approved by the dietitian.
7. HS snacks are outlined on the daily spreadsheet and are prepared and distributed to all residents.
8. Production sheets are correct with correct items and amounts to be prepared each day as specified on the menu, with census. Additional information required includes frozen items to be transferred, items to be pre-prepared, and the use of leftovers.
9. The cleaning schedule is posted in kitchen area and covers all equipment and dietary areas. There is evidence that the cleaning schedule is in use.
10. Temperatures of all refrigeration equipment and dishmachines are recorded daily on a temperature chart.
11. Line temperatures of all menu items served at each meal are recorded daily on a temperature chart.

Foodservice Delivery

1. Each menu item is prepared in proper baking pans and using proper utensils (for example, correct steamtable pan size, meat thermometer for roasts). Accuracy is checked during review.
2. Each food product has a satisfying color and is uniform in size. The meal presents a pleasing combination of shapes and sizes.
3. Each food product is properly cooked and has an identifiable texture and the proper moisture content. There is a variety of texture in the menus and on the trays.
4. Each food product has a desirable flavor and pleasing aroma and is seasoned adequately. All food items for regular diets are well seasoned. Food items are separated as needed for modified diets.

5. Food temperatures on the line and at the bedside are within the proper range:
   a. Trayline temperatures
      Hot foods—160° to 180°F
      Cold foods—35° to 42°F
      Pureed foods (hot)—140°F
   b. Bedside temperatures
      Hot foods—130° to 140°F
      Cold foods—40° to 50°F
      Pureed foods—120° to 130°F
6. Trayline assembly system: An average of 2.5 to 3.0 trays per minute are produced on the trayline with two persons on the line. An average of 3.5 to 4.0 trays per minute are produced on the trayline with three persons on the line.
7. Overall tray/plate appearance is neat and correct. All items are in good condition.
   a. Trays are clean, in good condition, and matched.
   b. The china is clean, in good condition, and matched.
   c. Glassware is clean, in good condition, and matched.
   d. Flatware is clean, in good condition, and matched.
   e. A specific tray "setup" pattern is followed.
   f. Plate covers and bases are clean, and in good condition.
8. Food is attractively served with no spills, garnished, and properly arranged.
9. Tray accuracy includes correct menu items, utensils, condiments, and observance of the resident's preferences.
   a. All food items specified on the menu are present on the tray and in correct portions depending on diet modification.
   b. All utensils needed for eating the meal are provided on the tray.
   c. Correct condiments are served.
   d. Food likes and dislikes of the particular resident are observed.
10. All meals are served according to the time schedule posted in the dietary department and listed in the policies and procedures manual. Breakfast is scheduled no more than 14 hours after the evening meal.
11. Room service trays are delivered in an efficient and orderly manner.
    a. All foods are covered for room service delivery. If an enclosed cart is used, trays need not be individually covered unless they will be carried more than 15 feet.
    b. Trays are placed in the cart in order of room numbers.
    c. The food cart is moved down the hall as trays are delivered.
    d. Plate covers and bases are used.
    e. Used trays are not placed back on cart with clean, unserved trays.
    f. Tray cards remain on the tray until the meal is set before the resident.
    g. All trays are distributed within 20 minutes of food cart arrival on the floor.

    h. The meal tray is on the bedside table and positioned at an appropriate distance from the resident. Residents are positioned in a bedside chair or upright position in bed.

    i. Sufficient time is allowed for residents to eat—at least 20–30 minutes.

    j. Asepto feeding syringes are sanitized after each use.

12. The dining room is clean, attractive, properly set up, and well attended.
13. Leftovers are minimal (3–4 servings) and all are properly stored in durable, plastic containers with tight-fitting lids, labeled, and dated.

Organization

1. The policies and procedures manual is current, accurate, and in use. There shall be policies for all systems in operation and all are typed and dated. The manual must be updated annually and signed by the dietitian, foodservice manager, and administrator.
2. The manual shall contain policies on
   a. Admissions
   b. Discharges
   c. Patient care planning
   d. Meal times
   e. The tray delivery system
   f. Nourishments
   g. Food consumption records
   h. Meal replacement
   i. Food handling
   j. Temperature charts
   k. Meal substitutions
   l. Food tasting
   m. Food storage
   n. Security
   o. Self-help feeding devices
   p. The isolation system
   q. Pitcher sanitation
   r. Pot and pan washing
   s. Emergency and disaster planning
   t. Organization and training
3. A current diet manual (less than five years old) is available in the dietary office, kitchen, director of nursing office, and each nursing station. The diet manual shall be reviewed and signed by the medical director or other physician and the dietitian.
4. There is an annual dietary inservice schedule and documentation of compliance on file. Topic changes shall be noted on the schedule. Documentation of inservices contains names of participants and proof of skills learned or information comprehended and is filed in chronological order.

5. The dietary manager's office is clean and well organized and provides adequate space for a desk, chair, bookshelf, and filing cabinet.
6. A food-tasting panel of residents/employees is formed and meets monthly to conduct taste tests of particular meals or food items. Documentation of results and subsequent actions are filed in the dietary office.

Employees

1. Dietary employees are properly attired and well groomed in the kitchen area. Uniforms are free of soil, pressed, and in good repair and fit properly. White butcher-style aprons are worn in the kitchen prep area. Clean stockings and clean closed-toe protective shoes are worn. Hairnets or approved hair restraints are worn. Men with haircuts above the ears wear foodservice hats. Hairnets or hats are worn in all areas of the dietary department. Hands and fingernails are clean and free of nail polish. No jewelry other than wedding rings and watches are worn.
2. Job descriptions are current and available for each dietary position. Each job description is neatly typed, in use, and part of the policies and procedures manual. Job descriptions are posted in the kitchen area.
3. Proper food-handling techniques are practiced by all dietary employees. Unprotected food items are handled with tongs, utensils, or plastic gloves as efficiently as possible.
4. All dietary employees involved in food preparation and actual meal service to residents have a thorough understanding of the menus. Dietary employees are familiar with preparation techniques of specific diet modifications; this knowledge is verified by the reviewer.

Environmental Status

1. Each piece of equipment within the dietary department is clean and sanitized, free of rust and chipped paint, and operable.
   a. Refrigerators
      i. Reach-in: temperature 35° to 40°F; thermometer is inside the unit.
      ii. Walk-in: temperature 35° to 40° F; thermometer is inside the unit.
   b. Freezers
      i. Reach-in: temperature 0°F or below; thermometer is inside the unit.
      ii. Walk-in: temperature 0°F or below; thermometer is inside the unit.
      iii. Ice cream: temperature 0°F or below; thermometer is inside the unit.
   c. Milk dispenser: temperature 35° to 42°F; thermometer is inside the unit.

     d. Range top, grill

     e. Ovens

          i. Conventional

          ii. Convection

          iii. Microwave

     f. Steamer

     g. Deep fat fryer

     h. Ingredient processing equipment

          i. Mixer

          ii. Meat slicer

          iii. Blender

          iv. Food processor

     i. Steamtable, tray rail

     j. Toaster

     k. Can opener

     l. Cutting boards

     m. Ice machine

     n. Coffee urn, servers

     o. Worktables and drawers

     p. Utility carts, bussing equipment

     q. Diet cards

     r. Dish dollies and dispensers

     s. Dish tables and booster heater

     t. Disposals

     u. Sinks

          i. Hand (towels, soap, and waste container)

          ii. Food preparation

          iii. Pot and pan (final rinse 170° to 180°F. Chemicals used for sanitation are 100 ppm.)

     v. Dishwasher: wash temperature 150° to 160°F; final rinse 180°F.

     w. Areas behind equipment

2. Smallware is clean, dry, and organized.

     a. Food preparation utensils—all handles stored in same direction

     b. Pots and pans

     c. China

     d. Glassware

     e. Flatware

3. All storage areas are clean, dust free, rust free, and organized.

     a. The food storage area is clean, dust free, rust free, and organized with like items together. No cleaning items are stored here! Items are stored at least 6 in. off the floor. Containers are labeled correctly; open boxes are stored in plastic bags or closed containers. All products are dated with the month, day, and year. Items are stored at least 18 in. away from the sprinkler system. Food bins are labeled correctly; no scoops are stored inside.

    b. The refrigerator/freezer storage area is: clean and rust free; foods are organized, covered or completely wrapped, and labeled. Items are off the floor in walk-in areas, door gaskets fit properly and are clean. There is no evidence of condensation in walk-in storage areas.

    c. The chemical and cleaning storage area is clean, dust and rust free, organized, with items stored off the floor. Mops and brooms are in good condition and hung for storage.

4. The general physical plant is clean and free of the need for repairs or painting.

    a. Cabinets are clean and in good repair.

    b. Walls are clean with no evidence of grease, or grime buildup.

    c. Ceilings are in good repair.

    d. Floors are in good repair with no chips or cracks.

    e. Baseboards are clean and tightly attached to wall area.

    f. Lights are clean; all bulbs are functioning and have protective covers.

    g. Drains/floor sinks are clean, free of debris, and emptying properly.

    h. Doors are clean, not scarred, and opening and closing properly.

    i. Windows are clean and free from cracks; screens fit tightly.

    j. Hoods and filters are clean and free of excessive grease.

5. A nourishment pantry at each nursing station is available with specified equipment: refrigerator storage; hot cabinets; a warmer plate, burner, a microwave; handwashing lavatory with soap and disposable towels; disposable eating utensils. Food supply is as specified in policies and procedures manual.

REFERENCES

Graham, Nancy O. 1982. Quality assurance in hospitals. Rockville Md.:Aspen Systems Corp.

Hopkins, Julie. 1989. Numbers, numbers. *QRC Advisor* 5, no. 9: 1–2.

Joint Commission. 1984. *Quality assurance in support services: Advanced approaches.* Chicago: Joint Commission on Accreditation of Hospitals.

Joint Commission Forum. 1986. Monitoring and evaluation of the quality and appropriateness of care: A hospital example. *QRA Advisor* (September):326–30.

Meisenheimer, Claire G. 1985. *Quality assurance: A complete guide to effective programs.* Rockville, Md.: Aspen Publishers, Inc.

Rose, James C. 1986a. Quality assurance: Part 1. *Hospital Food and Nutrition Focus* 2, no. 8:1–7.

———. 1986b. Quality assurance. Part 2. *Hospital Food and Nutrition Focus* 2, no. 9:1–8.

13

Marketing the Foodservice Department

In recent years, the American Dietetic Association has encouraged, educated, and trained its members to market themselves as "the nutrition experts." The concept is simple. If we do not market ourselves as nutrition experts, other health care professionals (less qualified) will assume our roles in the future.

This same concept is true for marketing health care facilities. The health care industry has become competitive in recent years, forcing each operation to develop an unique quality that can be marketed to the consumer in order to preserve or increase its share in the market. Foodservice can be that unique quality! The foodservice element should be recognized by individuals and regional and national health care providers as a resident/patient amenity as well as a marketing tool (Smith 1986). Foodservice departments are no longer obscure corners in a health care operation but a vital component of any facility's total image and marketing effort.

A dietary consultant must assume the role of a "marketing specialist" when working with the foodservice manager and staff to achieve visible foodservice marketing efforts within the facility and the community.

THE DEPARTMENT'S "IMAGE"

Prior to initiating a department marketing program, attention must be given to the image of the foodservice department. Does the foodservice department project "a professional image"? Do the appearance and behavior of each foodservice employee reflect the marketing program philosophy? If positive responses cannot be made to these questions, two basic image enhancement steps must be initiated prior to implementation of a marketing program.

Employee Appearance and Personal Hygiene

We must remind ourselves of the old adage, "The first impression is lasting." The first step in creating a favorable impression is to see that foodservice workers are dressed in clean, matched uniforms daily to project a professional image. Policies and procedures developed to emphasize the importance of personal appearance and hygiene will enhance compliance of the program. An example of policy and guidelines is shown below.

EXAMPLE 1: PERSONAL APPEARANCE AND HYGIENE

Policy

Dietary employees shall wear clean uniforms in accordance with the facility uniform policy when reporting to work. Hair restraints must be worn and personal grooming standards practiced.

Procedure

A. Uniforms
   1. Each employee shall report to work in a clean, standard uniform. No T-shirts, jeans, blouses, or smocks will be acceptable.
   2. Closed-toe, rubber-soled uniform shoes shall be worn. No sneakers or sandals are accepted.
   3. Ripped, stained, or worn uniforms must be repaired or replaced at the employee's expense.
   4. Employees failing to report to work in accordance with the uniform policy will not be permitted to work until the appropriate uniform is worn.
   5. Colored cotton aprons shall be worn for serving purposes only.
   6. White butcher's aprons shall be worn for production and cleaning use. Butcher's aprons are to be worn within the dietary department only.
B. Hair restraints
   1. Dietary employees shall wear the following hair restraints during work hours:
      Men—white paper cap (or white hairnet) depending on the length of hair
      Women—white, waitress style hairnet
   2. White paper caps and hairnets will be supplied by the facility.
   3. Sheer hairnets may also be worn, but must be supplied by the employee.
   4. Unacceptable hair restraints include scarves, baseball caps, scrub caps, and shower caps.
C. Personal grooming
   1. Employees shall appear clean and free of odor when reporting to work. Daily bathing or showering is a must!
   2. Fingernails shall be clean, trimmed, and free of nail polish.
   3. Excessive use of cologne or perfume is prohibited.
   4. No rings other than wedding rings may be worn.
   5. Bracelets, necklaces, and earrings that dangle or extend beyond the lobes of the ear are prohibited.

6. Employees failing to demonstrate good personal grooming shall not be permitted to work until appropriate grooming is practiced.

Employee Attitudes

The second step in setting up an effective marketing program is "selling the concept" or developing appropriate attitudes in all personnel involved in preparation and service of the facility's food. The theory that "the customer is always right" should be stressed throughout the training process because meal time is considered a special event by many residents in long-term care facilities. Training programs should involve nursing personnel as well as dietary staff and should address topics ranging from correct table settings and place presentation of menu items to actual dining room and room service techniques. Written guidelines for each of these topics should be provided to the trainee and incorporated into the dietary services policy and procedure manual. The following examples offer sample policies and guidelines for both dining room service and room service.

EXAMPLE 2: DINING ROOM SERVICE

Policy

Residents shall be served in a timely, efficient manner in the dining room area.

Specific Guidelines

1. The server (nursing or dietary) shall pick up the filled tray from the serving window or cart and deliver it to the specific resident.
2. All plates and utensils shall be removed from the tray and placed in front of the resident.
3. Each menu item is to be served from the left, using the left hand, except those containing beverages, which are to be placed from the right with the right hand.
4. Desserts shall be served after residents are finished with the main course.
5. If time permits and personnel are available, soiled plates shall be removed prior to dessert service.
6. Beverage service and special requests will be handled by the designated hostesses and/or service personnel.
7. Residents will be served by table, allowing all at one table to eat simultaneously.
8. Soiled dishes shall be removed by tables when all residents have finished eating.
9. Dishes will be stacked according to similar type and placed in a bussing tub.
10. The bussing tub will be transported on a bussing or utility cart to the dietary

department. Tubs shall not be carried by employees due to the risk of back strain and the possibility of accidents.

EXAMPLE 3: ROOM SERVICE

Policy

Residents shall be served in a timely, efficient manner in their respective rooms.

Specific Guidelines

1. Covered, filled trays should be delivered by dietary to specific halls and wings.
2. Nursing personnel will serve meal trays by rooms, transporting the cart as meals are served.
3. Trays will be delivered within 20 minutes of their arrival on the hall or wing.
4. Trays will be delivered to residents requiring minimal assistance with tray preparation first, followed by those requiring total assistance in the feeding process.
5. Nursing personnel will be responsible for communicating special requests or substitutions desired by residents to dietary services.
6. Soiled dishes shall be removed from rooms on the original tray on which the meal was served.
7. Trays with soiled dishes will be returned to the enclosed carts (void of undelivered meals) and transported to the dietary department.
8. No trays may be transported on top of the enclosed cart or stacked on top of another tray.

MENU PLANNING AND PRESENTATION

In addition to initiating foodservice training programs for dietary and nursing personnel, menu planning and preparation is a vital aspect of the total marketing effort. Health care professionals are realizing that aesthetically pleasing meals will aid in stimulating the geriatric resident's appetite, as well as favorably impressing the resident's families and friends. As dietitians, we must ensure that menus reflect the marketing philosophy, emphasizing garnishment and plate appearance. Menus should incorporate the basic elements of menu planning—taste, texture, shape, size, and temperature—along with the use of garnishes. Garnishes can be quite simple but can change an "institutionalized" plate into a "gourmet" meal. Development of plate arrangement guides will assist dietary staff in arranging foods for the most attractive plate presentation and ensure consistent quality control. Inservices and workshops on plate presentation and garnishment help reinforce awareness of the visual aspect of meal preparation. Use of local chefs to help train dietary staff has been quite successful.

Effective menu planning also includes the written description of menu items. Describing menu items with "a touch of gourmet appeal" tends to heighten interest in the presentation of the meal for residents as well as residents' families and employees. A menu consisting of Roast Beef, New Potatoes, Green Beans, Rolls, and Pie sounds more exciting when presented as Roast Beef Au Jus, Parsleyed New Potatoes, Green Beans Almondine, Homemade Rolls with Butter, and Fresh Apple Pie.

Plate presentation and garnishment emphasis should not stop with regular menus. Increased emphasis needs to be directed to the preparation and presentation of diet-modified menus, from sodium-restricted and diabetic diets to texture-modified meals. Presenting these meals with flair will definitely enhance the marketing effort of dietary services, as well as enhancing resident acceptance of the food.

THE DINING ENVIRONMENT

As consultant dietitians, we need to be involved in planning the "total dining experience." Enhancing the dining environment by utilizing knowledge of the physiological sensory changes and cultural backgrounds of the residents can revitalize "ho-hum" institutional dining areas (Smith 1986).

Attractive meals are enhanced by the dishware on which they are arranged and the atmosphere in which they are served. Meals presented on stained, green nonbreakable dishes in a noisy, institutionalized dining room are less attractive to residents, families, and employees.

Using china and glassware improves the marketing image of any facility, but when choosing china, it is important to consider the visual loss experienced by the aged individual. Decreased muscle strength of the eye reduces one's ability to focus clearly and minimize glare from clear tablecoverings or sunlight reflecting from an unshaded window. White or neutral colored china with a contrasting border creates a definite boundary between the plate and the table. Placing the china on nonglare vinyl or a fabric tablecloth with contrasting placemats visually enhances individual table settings as well the total dining room appearance.

Consideration needs to be given to glassware, too. Selecting a pattern with an uneven texture rather than a smooth surface allows an older person to hold a glass more securely. Also, a glass with a smaller base (that is, a footed glass) allows the resident to grasp it more securely. Total weight of the glassware is another factor in manageability. To complete the table setting an appropriate stainless flatware pattern and attractive placecards and centerpieces need to be selected.

Creating a positive dining environment requires giving attention to the physical plant of the dining area. Soft pastel or earthtone colors for the wallcovering, preferably wallpaper, are perceived as restful, intimate, and warm, especially by the geriatric resident. Use of plants or free-standing cloth screens can change a large open dining area into smaller, "intimate" dining areas. Coordinating window treatments, lighting, and appropriate paintings or prints will complete the creation of a dining room atmosphere.

Dining area appearance may be an excellent marketing tool for the facility initially, but without excellent service at mealtimes, the "glitter" will start to fade. Restaurant-style service is becoming an accepted concept in health care facilities, especially for long-term care and retirement facilities. Residents are being served at tables, off trays and per course. Tables are set with silverware, napkins, water goblets, and coffee service before residents enter the dining room.

To maintain a restaurant-style image throughout mealtime, meal servers' appearance and manner of responding to requests need to be considered. If nursing personnel are responsible for serving the residents in the dining room, an option is to use color-coordinated chef-type aprons for them during mealtimes. In facilities employing enough dietary staff to serve in addition to preparing meals, consider the use of restaurant-style uniforms. These uniforms can consist of black slacks or skirt with a white shirt, black tie, and black cobbler apron or color-coordinated pants or skirt with a white shirt and corresponding print tie or bow. It is also desirable to have a designated hostess (the department head or a nursing employee) present at mealtimes to assist residents to their seats, pour beverages, and respond to residents' requests.

MARKETING THROUGH EXPANDED SERVICES AND PROGRAMS

The most successful marketable dining programs exist in facilities where mealtime is a priority with all staff. Once the basic principles of food marketing have been accomplished by the facility's employees, the initiation of "image-building" services can begin.

Selective Menus and Meal Options

The use of selective menus has traditionally been associated more with hospitals than with long-term care facilities. In recent years, however, restaurant-style meal service, including the provision of alternative meal plans and selections, has become an accepted concept in long-term care facilities. In many facilities the traditional three-meal per day plan based on a four-week menu cycle is now augmented with selective options.

As consultant dietitians, we must assist facilities in selecting options that will meet their budgetary guidelines for food and labor while enhancing their "marketing" image. Selective menus are not only the three meals per day with multi-options per menu item. Current innovative selective meal service programs offer:

- Entrées using selected frozen dishes as options
- Selective breakfast programs—juice, egg preparation, bread and cereal op-

tions in addition to "specials of the day" printed checklist style for the resident's selection prior to mealtime

- "Open breakfast" service or breakfast buffet, allowing residents to eat during a designated period rather than at a set time (especially applicable for retirement facilities)
- A dessert cart in the dining room for serving fresh fruits, sherbets or ice cream, in addition to the planned dessert of the day

In addition to daily meal options, other special touches that can entertain residents as well as enhance the facility's reputation with families include

- Monthly or weekly theme meals selected and planned by the resident food committee with assistance from the dietary manager or registered dietitian. (Themes can revolve around holidays, special occasions, or travel. Working with the activity department to obtain decorations, travel posters, and costumes makes the meal a festive occasion. One nursing home used the theme "Around the World in 80 Days" with stops in China, India, Hawaii, Mexico, and Europe. Decorations and meals highlighted each stop. Local people who had visited these areas presented a talk and/or slide show during the meal period.)
- Wine and cheese social hour or "happy hour" prior to the evening meal
- Gourmet meals for families and residents at a special price for birthdays, anniversaries, and other events. (One nursing facility developed a brochure highlighting three gourmet meals available to families for entertaining their family member resident. The meal cost was $5.00 per family member with a complimentary glass of wine. No additional cost was charged to the resident. The facility requested three-days' advance notice to prepare the meals and special dining area. To announce this service, a brochure was sent with the facility's monthly newsletter.)
- Sunday buffets for residents and families
- "High Tea" as a special event for families and residents, offering tea, coffee, pastries, and fruit

Community Events

Successful foodservice marketing events can enhance the facility's image within the community and result in referrals, admissions, and increased private pay census. Community events include

- Monthly breakfasts for discharge planners, doctors, and key business leaders together with facility department heads and resident representatives
- Luncheons for medical auxiliaries and professional organizations (Using the facility's china service and menus as originally planned enhances the image of the facility's foodservice to community leaders.)

- Open houses highlighting special events such as Grandparents' Day and National Nursing Home Week
- Health fairs, offering free blood pressure checks, cholesterol testing, educational seminars on nutrition and medications, and so forth
- Seminars for the community relating to the caregiver and the geriatric person, for example, the patient with Alzheimer's disease
- Political forums for local and state candidates, with a reception for candidates and residents following the forum

Guidelines for Dietary Marketing Activities

Community and family events require advance planning. Duties and responsibilities need to be listed and delegated one to three weeks in advance of the event. Written guidelines such as those given in this section are helpful in planning these marketing events.

EXAMPLE 4: DIETARY MARKETING ACTIVITIES

Policy

Dietary marketing events are considered to be any food-related activity other than a routine resident meal, including but not limited to theme meals, resident parties, buffets, open houses, professional luncheons and teas, and medical auxiliary luncheons.

Procedure

A. Planning
   Special functions should be planned well in advance (4–6 weeks for large functions, 2–3 weeks for smaller or regularly scheduled functions) to allow for
   1. Menu planning
   2. Food ordering and advance preparation
   3. Staff scheduling and assignments
   4. Decoration and setup arrangements
B. Recommended planning timetable
   1. Three weeks in advance
      a. Reconfirm menu with administrator.
      b. Set up a log for the event to document menu, cost, procedure, and attendance. This information will be helpful for similar events in the future.
      c. Make sure sufficient doilies, napkins, and dishes are available.
   2. Two weeks in advance
      a. Place all nonperishable food orders.

      b. Place orders for floral arrangements.

      c. Test any unfamiliar recipes with staff.

      d. Review decoration and setup arrangements with other involved departments.

  3. One week in advance

      a. Reorder or change any nonperishable orders that were "stock-out."

      b. Review staffing needs and make necessary changes in the work schedule.

      c. Place produce, meat, and special dairy products order to arrive two days prior to the event.

      d. Review the regular menu and the marketing event menu. Rearrange production to equalize work flow.

      e. Revise production sheets to include marketing event production that may be done in advance.

      f. Develop special work assignments/time activities sheet for each employee, outlining specific assignments and time frames.

      g. Conduct a dietary staff meeting, reviewing the menu, performance expectations, and work assignments.

      h. Check on dietary apron supply, to assure that sufficient clean aprons will be laundered and available by the scheduled function date.

      i. Make sure all table service equipment and table cloths are available and in good condition.

  4. One day in advance

      a. Clean all produce items.

      b. Arrange platters appropriately.

      c. Complete all unfinished baking.

      d. Complete any advance decorating if possible.

  5. Same day

      a. Hold a brief meeting with staff, reviewing all work assignments and the menu.

      b. Supervise the layout of all items and table set-ups.

      c. Greet guests.

      d. Circulate among employees to assure that food is replenished, tables are cleared, and so on.

C. Theme meal ideas

Hawaiian Day	*Indy 500*
Hula Ham Salad on Lettuce	Racey Ravioli
Leaf with Sandy Saltines	Speedway Green Beans
Surf's Up Strawberries, Polynesian	Go-Go Garlic Bread
Pineapple, Beach Blanket Bananas	Revved-up Garden Cottage Cheese
Don Ho's Hawaiian Salad	Checkered Flag Cupcakes
Aloha Punch	Victory Punch

Back to the Fifties
Drive-in Coneys
Neat-O Potato Chips
Cool Cat Coleslaw
Howdy Doody Apple Pie
Big Al's Brown Cow

Oktoberfest
German Beer
Beef Cubes (German style)
Spaetzle
Pickled Red Cabbage
Rye Toast
Black Forest Pie

Halloween Party
Orange Spiced Love Potion
Pumpkin Cauldron Soup
Beef Goulash Over Weird Noodles
Ghostly Green Beans

Beastly Biscuits
Monster Mousse
Thanksgiving Dinner
Iced Orange Spice Tea
Cream of Tomato Soup
Sliced Breast of Turkey
Dressing and Gravy
Sweet Potatoes and Apples
Green Beans
Homemade Rolls
Pumpkin Pie
Christmas Dinner
Spicy Cranberry Tea
Corn Chowder
Sliced Ham with Pineapple Ring
Au Gratin Potatoes
Broccoli
Homemade Rolls
Pecan Pie

Employee Programs

Effective marketing events can also enhance the image of the foodservice department within the facility. Employees can be the most difficult audience to impress! Successful employee-oriented meal programs can be beneficial to the foodservice department in two ways: (1) Positive attitudes about the meals served in the facility will be reflected in conversations with residents and families; and (2) endorsement of the meal programs will be reflected in increased participation and revenue.

Employee meals can generate revenue and satisfy an assortment of personal preferences when a "pinch" of creativity is added. A variety of employee meal programs can be offered (even when an employees' cafeteria is not available) without increasing labor hours or reducing the quality and/or level of service of residents' meals. Meal programs can include:

Full Meal Deal

The complete menu as planned for the residents is sold for the lunch and evening meals. The price needs to reflect a small percentage of profit. Even with a price of $2.00 per meal, revenue can be realized and employees can have a well-balanced, nutritious meal as an alternative to a sandwich, fries, and a drink at the local fast food establishment.

Soup, Sandwich, Salad Combinations

Combinations of soup and sandwich, soup and salad, or sandwich and salad are usually popular with employees. These variations can be offered without increasing dietary labor hours by using prechopped produce items and coordinating the sandwich or soup menus with existing resident meals.

Breakfast Programs

Although offering a complete breakfast meal may not be feasible because of the usual reduced dietary staffing at this time, convenience items such as donuts, muffins, French toast, waffles, sausage, and biscuits can be purchased in the frozen state and prepared in minutes. Preparation from "scratch" of items such as muffins and biscuits is relatively easy, and the smell of fresh bakery products will produce sales.

Selling these items at 100 to 150 percent markup generates revenue for the facility, but is still economical for the employee who would pay higher prices at a fast food establishment or vending machine.

All or a combination of these employee meal ideas can be implemented successfully in long-term care facilities as well as acute care facilities by establishing the following basic guidelines:

- Offer meal options in which employees express interest.
- Evaluate dietary work schedules and provide inservice training to dietary employees prior to implementation.
- Establish a meal sales system that avoids the need for the dietary department to accept money.
- Use a daily meal census form to ensure accurate counts.
- Develop definite time periods for employees to sign up for meals offered.

In addition to meal program options, health care facilities are offering educational events in conjunction with meals served. These events promote sales, enhance the employee's personal image and create a positive image of the foodservice department with employees. Planning events during National Nutrition Month (March) can highlight good nutrition amongst employees. One hospital in Illinois sponsored a wellness program called "All Aboard the Nutrition Express." Employees participating in this program joined the "4-30" Club, agreeing to limit each of their daily meals to 400 calories or less, with fat content of no more than 30 percent of total calories per meal. Each participant was asked to keep a daily log of their diet and exercise habits. Hospital dietitians monitored the program by making themselves available in the cafeteria to answer employees' questions about fat and cholesterol and checking each participant's log. "Heart" stickers were awarded to those who met the specified guidelines.

Another National Nutrition Month activity included a 5-kilometer/1 mile "fun" race sponsored by a midwestern nursing home chain. This event was for employees as well as the public. Ribbons were presented to all participants in the run while T-shirts and trophies were awarded for five age categories of each sex. Awards were also given to the company's facility with the largest percentage of employees participating in the event.

Staging special promotions in conjunction with the seasonal availability of food items can also generate revenue and increase customer satisfaction. A 460-bed hospital in Baltimore promoted the arrival of the "fresh fruit" season by setting up a "typical old fashioned fruit stand" in the cafeteria area. The area was decorated with crates of various fruits and vegetables. Hanging scales added charm to the display, and paper bags were available for bulk purchases. Over four cases of fruit were sold daily from this display.

Developing educational, customer-appealing meal programs for the health care employee is limited only by the dietary staff's imagination and creativity. As a consultant dietitian, one must promote development and implementation of these types of programs.

Other Revenue-producing Programs

Revenue-generating ideas are not limited to employee meal programs. Over the past few years, hospitals have been generating considerable revenue by augmenting their foodservice. As reimbursement rates decrease in relationship to escalating health care costs, hospitals are attacking the economic challenge aggressively and creatively. Revenues as high as $500,000 annually have been reported by some hospitals. Projects include an in-house bakery, gourmet meal programs, room service, catering, gift shop ideas (meal gift certificates, gift food baskets), and take-out service.

Even though long-term care facilities may not be able to implement as elaborate programs as hospitals can, modified small-scale programs can be successful. Revenue producing programs can include

- Providing an hors d'oeuvre and beverage selection for clubs and other groups that rent conference or meeting rooms
- Utilizing favorite recipes and excellent bakers to make and sell homemade bread, rolls, or pies to families and employees (If a baker is not available, the use of frozen dough products can still produce the aroma of fresh baked products throughout the facility. Consider establishment of a display case near the entrance of the facility to display baked-to-order goods or freshly baked items to create interest in the program.)
- Owning and supplying vending machines to use "leftover" sandwiches, soups, and desserts (A chief dietitian in a 200-bed hospital helped turn her department into a profit center by making a $2,000 profit monthly from vending machines. Although the influx of visitors and the number of employees may not be as great in a long-term care facility, profits can still be realized.)
- Offering gift certificates for a gourmet meal or a gift basket of fruit or sundries

to families (Sample gift ideas could be displayed and packaged per order, depending upon the item.)

- Participating in local "Meals on Wheels" or senior citizen meal programs (This service not only brings in immediate revenue but serves as a public relations/referral program for potential residents in the future.)
- Participating in local Headstart programs (One facility realized over $8,000 monthly by preparing the city's Headstart meals four days per week. With the additional revenue, another cook could be hired without affecting the budget.)
- Establishing an in-house meal program for senior citizen groups such as the "Golden Key" club (Again this service promotes both revenue and referrals.)

Is marketing really a key aspect of the foodservice department, one may ask? You bet it is! As the health care industry (especially long-term care facilities) continues to become more competitive, innovative and progressive services will need to be offered in order to "stay in the game." Foodservice can make a major contribution to the overall image and revenue-generating strategies of a long-term care facility.

REFERENCES

Beasly, Marjorie. 1989. Perspectives on renovation. *Food Management* 24:10.

Doyle, Bridgett. 1989. The dining environment and food intake of the elderly in long term care. *Food and Nutrition News* 61:1.

Edge, Marianne Smith. 1986. Nursing home foodservice takes on new look, purpose. *American Health Care Association Journal* 12:2.

Elkins, Trudy H. 1986. Retirement centers accent dining with style. *American Health Care Association Journal* 12:2.

Molt, Mary, Grace Shugart, and Maxine Wilson. 1986. *Food for fifty,* 7th ed. New York: John Wiley & Sons.

Smith, Sheldon L. 1986. Project hospitality brings adventure to eating. *American Health Care Association Journal* 12:2.

Stokes, Judy Ford. 1989. Revenue from Food Service? You Bet! *Provider* 15:7.

Unicare Health Facilities. 1985. *Dining service guide.* Milwaukee: Unicare Health Facilities Inc.

Appendix A

Sample Forms

NUTRITION ASSESSMENT OF TUBE-FED PATIENTS

Name: _____   Date: _____ Birthdate: _____

                              Physician: _____

Diagnosis: _____

_____

Diet Information   *Anthropometric Information*

Formula ordered: _____   Wt.: _____ Ht.: _____ Av. past

Additional fluid ordered: _____   wt.:_____

Total amount fluid received: _____   Ideal wt. range: _____

Formula as ordered provides: History of wt. loss: _____

Cal.: _____ Protein:_____   *BEE*

Iron: _____ Potassium: _____   Base cal.: ___ Activity factor: ___

% RDA's vit./min.:_____   Stress factor: _____

Nitrogen ratio:_____   Total cal. requirements: _____

                              Requirements: Fluid _____

                              Protein _____

Complications (check if apply)

_____ Gastric	_____ Respiratory	_____ Diabetes
residual	disease	_____ Skin
_____ Diarrhea	_____ Edema	breakdown
_____ Vomiting	_____ Poor skin	Other: _____
_____ Fever	turgor	
	_____ Blood	
	pressure	

Laboratory Values

Albumin _____	Na _____	Bun _____
Prealbumin _____	K+ _____	Creatinine _____
Total lymphocyte ct. _	TIBC _____	Other _____
Transferrin _____	Hemoglobin _____	Other _____
Glucose _____		

Additional Information/Comments

_____

_____

_____

_____

NUTRITION ASSESSMENT OF TUBE-FED PATIENTS (*Continued*)

Routine Drugs
_____
_____
_____
_____

Summary / Recommendations
_____
_____
_____
_____
_____

Date: _____   **Signature:** _____

NUTRITIONAL RECOMMENDATIONS FROM DIETITIAN'S CONSULTANT VISIT

New Admissions	Comments/Recommendations

Nutritional Reassessments

Continued

NUTRITIONAL RECOMMENDATIONS FROM DIETITIAN'S CONSULTANT VISIT (*Continued*)

Other Charts Reviewed _____

_____

_____

_____

_____

_____

Date of Visit _____

NUTRITION ASSESSMENT

Name: _____ Date: _____
Birthdate: _____ Religion: _____
Physician: _____ Diet Order: _____
Previous Residence: _____ Modification: _____
Diagnosis: _____

BACKGROUND DATA:

Vision _____ Nausea _____
Hearing _____ Food Allergies _____
Mental Status _____ Loss of Appetite _____
Communication _____ Compliance with Diet _____
Bowel Function _____ Skin Breakdown _____
Dentures _____ Altered Taste Acuity _____
Own Teeth _____ Distinct Food Preferences __
Condition Teeth/Dentures _____ Activity Level _____

WEIGHT   *LABS*   *BEE*

Present _____ Hgb. _____ Bun. _____ Base _____
Ideal _____ Hct. _____ Alb. _____ Activity Factor _
Height _____ Glucose _____ Chol. _____ Stress Factor ___
Avg. Past ____ Na. _____ Trigs. ____ Total Calories __
% Ideal _____ K+ _____ Other _____ Protein _____
% Loss _____ Other _____   Fluid _____

                MEDICATIONS   *INTAKE*

Diuretic _____ Vitamin _____   % Meals _____
KCL _____ Insulin _____   % Supplements ___

Continued

NUTRITION ASSESSMENT (*Continued*)

MEDICATIONS

Fe _____ Oral Hypoglycemic _____

B12 _____

Other medications with possible impact on nutrition status:

_____

_____

_____

_____

Ability to Feed Self _____

Hunger between Meals: _____

Other Pertinent Information:

Supplement Program _____

Snack in Room _____

Other Information: _____

PHYSICAL APPEARANCE

_____ Hair, dull, dry, sparce, shedding

_____ Eyes–cloudy, pale, dry, red

_____ Lips–swollen, red

_____ Gums–bleeding, abnormally red, swollen

_____ Tongue–swollen, fissured, magenta, coated smooth

_____ Mouth–pallor, vertical or lateral fissuring, ulcers

_____ Skin–dry, flakey, hyperpigmented "tenting", decubiti, ecchymosis, petechiae

_____ Edema

_____ Muscular system wasted

_____ Nails–spoon-shaped, brittle, ridged, white spots, splinter-type hemorrhages

_____ Face–dark skin, scaling, pallor

Food Preferences

Food Dislikes

SUMMARY:

Nutritional Problems Identified	Goal	Action	Department

DIETARY NUTRITIONAL ASSESSMENT

Name _____ Date _____ Room _____

Diet _____ Food allergies _____

Supplements _____ Eats in: _____ Room _____ Dining area _____

Diagnosis _____

Wt. on admission _____ Ht. _____ Ideal weight range _____

Birthdate _____ Sex _____ Physician _____

Degree of Self-Help

___ Tube feeding
___ No help needed
___ Needs some assistance (butter, bread, etc.)
___ Cut food in small pieces
___ Prepare condiments (cream, sugar, salt etc.)
___ Feeds self with fingers
___ Needs to be fed
___ Needs self-help feeding device: type _____
___ Needs encouragement to eat and/or to finish

Special Problems

___ None
___ Blind
___ Wears glasses
___ Deaf
___ Hearing aid
___ Poor hearing
___ Dentures
___ No problem
___ Ill-fitting
___ Won't wear
___ Few/no teeth
___ Difficulty chewing
___ Difficulty swallowing

___ Picky eater
___ Fragile skin
___ Pressure sores, stage _____
___ Edema
___ Catheter
___ Poor coordination
___ Confused/belligerent
___ Language barrier
___ Over-medication

Other: _____

Pertinent Lab Data

___ Glu on _____
  (N: 65–110 mg/dl)
___ Hgb on _____
  (N:men−16+/−2; women−14+/−2)
___ Hct on _____
  (N:men−47+/−5; women−42+/−5)
___ K+ on _____
  (N: 3.5–5.0 mEq/1)

Pertinent Meds and Supplements

Food supplement _____

Vitamin/mineral _____

Hypoglycemic agents: insulin/oral
  Type _____ amount _____
Laxative/stool softener _____

_____ Albumin on _____   Diuretic _____
(N: 3.5–5.5 gm/dl)
_____ BUN on _____   Potassium _____
(N: 10–20 mg/dl)

Other: _____   Other _____

Daily Requirement   *Form of Ambulation*

Kilocalories _____   _____ No Restriction   _____ Wheelchair

Protein _____   _____ Walker   _____ Nonambulatory

Fluid _____

Level of Awareness   *Appetite*

_____ Resident alert-information reliable   Good: 75–100%

_____ Resident somewhat confused—check information with family and/or nursing   Fair: 50–75%

_____ Resident unable to relate reliable information, all information obtained from family   Poor: Less than 50%

or nursing   _____ Other information _____

Dietary History/Food Habits

Former occupation _____   Food preferences: _____

Wt. problem: over/under _____ yrs.   Food dislikes _____

Resident admitted from: Home   Hospital   Other facility

Date: / / / / / / / / / / / /

Wt: / / / / / / / / / / / /

NOTES

_____

_____

_____

_____

Initiated by: _____   Date: _____

Completed by: _____   Date: _____

CONSULTANT DIETITIAN REPORT

Date _____

Facility _____   Consultant _____

Administrator _____   Registration number _____

Foodservice Manager _____   Time of visit _____

Return visit _____   Hours _____

I. Comments:

    A. Food Production/Service: Meal service observed _____

    B. Patient care/nutrition documentation:

    C. Sanitation and food handling techniques:

    D. Inservices:

    E. Management and staff development:

II. Recommendations:

III. Administrator's Response:

Signed by: _____   _____

             Consultant   Administrator

PRECONSULTATION FORM

To be completed by foodservice manager for consultant dietitian

A. Nutritional concerns:
1. List of new admissions since last consulting visit:
   Name   Date of admission   Diet order   Weight

2. Listing of residents with pressure sores:
   Name   Stage of pressure sore
                                (obtain from nursing)

3. Residents or family members requesting conference with dietitian:
   Name   Room number   Diet order   Topic

4. List of residents with recent weight loss (5 lb./mo.):
   Name   Current weight   Previous weight

5. Action taken on dietitian's previous recommendations by physicians/nursing.
   Name   Action taken

B. Administrative concerns:
1. Resident acceptance and suggestions for any revisions needed:
   Name   Suggestions

2. New diet orders received not covered by menu:
   Name   Diet order

3. Average food intake:

4. Nutritional supplements:

5. Food-related medications:

6. Food preferences/dislikes:

7. Current nutritional problems
   or recommendations:

8. Diet compliance:

DIETITIAN'S CHARTING RECORD

ROOM NO.	Resident's Name	DIET	HT	WEIGHTS											
				JAN	FEB	MAR	APRIL	MAY	JUNE	JULY	AUG	SEPT	OCT	NOV	DEC

SUBSTITUTION RECORD

Date	Meal	Item Added	Item Omitted	Reason for Change	Approved By

DIETARY DEPARTMENT INSERVICE TRAINING PROGRAM

Name of Representative		Title
Location of Program		Date/Time

Remarks

PRESENT FOR TRAINING

MONTHLY REPORT OF THE FOODSERVICE PAPER SUPPLIES

Month or period   year

A. Beginning inventory value $ _____
B. Costs of supplies/paper during the month
    (purchased and donated) $ _____
C. Value of supplies/paper available during the
    month (A + B = C) $ _____
D. Closing inventory value (Inventory value at
    end of month) $ _____
E. Cost of supplies/paper used during the month $ _____
    (C − D = E).
F. Total patient days for month   _____
G. Average cost per patient day (Divide E by F $ _____
    to get G)

MONTHLY REPORT OF THE FOODSERVICE CLEANING SUPPLIES

Month or period   year

A. Beginning inventory value $ _____
B. Cost of supplies/paper during the month
    (purchased & donated) $ _____
C. Value of supplies/paper available during the
    month (A +B =C) $ _____
D. Closing inventory value (Inventory value at
    end of month) $ _____
E. Cost of supplies/paper used during the month $ _____
    (C − D = E)
F. Total patient days for month   _____
G. Average cost per patient day (Divide E by F
    to get G) $ _____

Appendix B

Sample Four-Week Cycle Menu

Menu Planning for Week of _____

	SUNDAY	MONDAY	TUESDAY	WEDNESDAY	THURSDAY	FRIDAY	SATURDAY
B R E A K F A S T	Orange Juice Hot/Cold Cereal Poached Egg Toast/Mar./Jelly Milk 2%	Orange Juice Hot/Cold Cereal Scrambled Egg Bacon Strip Toast/Mar./Jelly Milk 2%	Orange Juice Hot/Cold Cereal Poached Egg Toast/Mar./Jelly Milk 2%	Orange Juice Hot/Cold Cereal Fried Egg Bacon Strip Toast/Mar./Jelly Milk 2%	Orange Juice Hot/Cold Cereal Toast/Mar./Jelly Scrambled Egg Milk 2%	Orange Juice Hot/Cold Cereal Pancakes/Mar./ Syrup Grilled Ham Slice Milk 2%	Orange Juice Hot/Cold Cereal Fried Egg Bacon Toast/Mar./Jelly Milk 2%
L U N C H	Roast Turkey/ Gravy Bread Dressing Seasoned Green Beans Bread/Mar. Pumpkin Pie/ Cranberry Sauce Garnish	Meat Loaf/Brown Gravy Creamed Escalloped Potatoes Parslied Carrots WW Bread/Mar. Raspberry Sherbet	Hungarian Pork Cutlet Sweet Potatoes or Acorn Squash Baked Tangy Cole Slaw Bread/Mar. Peanut Butter Bar Garnish: Tomato Wedge	Crumb Baked Chicken Seasoned Lima Beans Cauliflower Au Gratin Bread/Mar. Carrot Cake/ Frost Garnish: Cranberry Sauce/Lettuce	Beef Liver/ Onions Baked Potato Stewed Tomatoes Biscuit/Mar. Rice Pudding	Chicken Divan Seasoned Rice Perfection Salad/ Lettuce Bread/Mar. Strawberry Cake Garnish: Spiced Apple Ring	Beef/Vegetable Soup Sliced Cheese/ Crackers Carrot/Celery/ Pickles Purple Plum Delight
D I N N E R	Hot Beef & Cheese on Bun Lettuce/ Tomatoes/ Catsup Pea Salad Fresh Banana Homemade Cookie Milk 2%	Breaded Veal Cutlet Potatoes Parmesan Harvard Beets Bread/Mar. Homemade Peach Cobbler Milk 2% Garnish: Parsley Sprig	Hearty Beef Stew Marinated Tomato Wedge on Lettuce Leaf Cornbread/Mar. Spiced Apples Garnish: Parsley Sprig	Hot Roast Beef Sandwich Whipped Potatoes/ Gravy Scandinavian Vegetables Blushing Pear Halves/Lettuce Milk 2% Garnish: Kale Leaf	Hot Dog/Bun Mustard/Catsup/ Relish Tater Roundabouts Deviled Egg Half Fresh Citrus Sections Milk 2%	Sausage Egg Bake Hash Browns Toast/Mar. Apple Butter Fruit Cocktail/ Marshmallows Milk 2% Garnish: Tomato Wedge	BBQ Pork French Fries Creamy Cole Slaw Rye Bread/Mar. Sliced Peaches/ Topping Milk 2% Garnish: Parsley Sprig

Continued

Menu Planning for Week of _____

<table>
<tr><th></th><th>SUNDAY</th><th>MONDAY</th><th>TUESDAY</th><th>WEDNESDAY</th><th>THURSDAY</th><th>FRIDAY</th><th>SATURDAY</th></tr>
<tr>
<td>B
R
E
A
K
F
A
S
T</td>
<td>Orange Juice
Hot/Cold Cereal
Fried Egg
Bacon Strip
Toast/Mar./Jelly
Milk 2%</td>
<td>Orange Juice
Hot/Cold Cereal
Poached Egg
Toast/Mar./Jelly
Milk 2%</td>
<td>Orange Juice
Hot/Cold Cereal
Scrambled Egg
Bacon Strip
Toast/Mar./Jelly
Milk 2%</td>
<td>Orange Juice
Hot/Cold Cereal
Poached Egg
Toast/Mar./Jelly
Milk 2%</td>
<td>Orange Juice
Hot/Cold Cereal
Fried Egg
Sausage/Gravy
Biscuit/Mar.
Milk 2%</td>
<td>Orange Juice
Hot/Cold Cereal
Scrambled Egg
Toast/Mar./Jelly
Milk 2%</td>
<td>Orange Juice
Hot/Cold Cereal
Poached Egg
Toast/Mar./Jelly
Milk 2%</td>
</tr>
<tr>
<td>L
U
N
C
H</td>
<td>Yankee Pot
Roast
Whipped
Potatoes
Seasoned Carrots
Roll/Mar.
Cherry Pie
Garnish: Parsley
Sprig</td>
<td>Ham & Beans
Marinated
Tomatoes
Cornbread/Mar.
Oatmeal Cookie
Garnish: Onion
Slice</td>
<td>Pork Roast/
Brown Gravy
Parsley Boiled
Potatoes
Seasoned Green
Beans
Roll/Mar.
Strawberry Ice
Cream
Garnish: Tomato
Wedge</td>
<td>Salisbury Steak/
Mushroom
Gravy
Potatoes in
Jacket
Broccoli
Casserole
Bread/Mar.
Cranberry Sauce
Square</td>
<td>Chicken &
Noodles
Oriental
Vegetables
Pear Halves/
Shredded
Cheese
Roll/Mar.
Gingerbread/
Lemon Sauce
Garnish: Tomato
Wedge</td>
<td>Fried Fish Filet/
Tartar Sauce
Baked Beans
Marinated
Vegetable
Salad
Bread/Mar.
Pineapple/Orange
Sections
Cookie
Garnish: Lemon
Slice</td>
<td>Swiss Steak
Baked Potato
Broccoli Spears
Assorted Bread/
Mar.
Cherry Crisp
Garnish: Tomato
Wedge</td>
</tr>
<tr>
<td>D
I
N
N
E
R</td>
<td>Broccoli Cheese
Quiche
Garden Salad/
French
Dressing
French Bread/
Mar.
Citrus Fruit Cup
Milk 2%
Garnish: Sliced
Apple Ring</td>
<td>Crumb Baked
Veal
Oven Brown
Potatoes
Seasoned
Spinach/Egg
Assorted Bread/
Mar.
Peach Basket
Surprise
Milk 2%</td>
<td>Tuna Noodle
Casserole
Seasoned Green
Beans
Assorted Bread/
Mar.
Sunshine/Salad/
Snickerdoodles
Milk 2%
Garnish: Orange
Slice</td>
<td>Cream of Potato
Soup
Saltines
Grilled Italian
Cheese
Sandwich
Marinated
Carrots
Apple Crisp
Milk 2%</td>
<td>Shaved Ham on
Rye
Mustard/Dill
Pickle
Potato Chips
Vinaigrette, Cole
Slaw
Apricot Halves
Milk 2%</td>
<td>Steakhouse Stew
Seasoned Green
Beans
Biscuit/Mar.
Chocolate/Vanilla
Pudding
Milk 2%
Garnish: Tomato
Wedge</td>
<td>Sausage Links
Pancakes/Syrup
Garden Cottage
Cheese/
Lettuce
Baked Apples
Milk 2%
Garnish: Parsley
Sprig</td>
</tr>
</table>

	Day 1	Day 2	Day 3	Day 4	Day 5	Day 6	Day 7
BREAKFAST	Orange Juice Hot/Cold Cereal Fried Egg Bacon Strip Toast/Mar./Jelly Milk 2%	Orange Juice Hot/Cold Cereal Fried Egg Bacon Strip Toast/Mar./Jelly Milk 2%	Orange Juice Hot/Cold Cereal Scrambled Egg Toast/Mar./Jelly Milk 2%	Orange Juice Hot/Cold Cereal Poached Egg Toast/Mar./Jelly Milk 2%	Orange Juice Hot/Cold Cereal Fried Egg Bacon Strip Toast/Mar./Jelly Milk 2%	Orange Juice Hot/Cold Cereal Scrambled Egg Toast/Mar./Jelly Milk 2%	Orange Juice Hot/Cold Cereal Fried Egg Bacon Strip Toast/Mar./Jelly Milk 2%
LUNCH	Baked Pork Chop Whipped Potatoes/Gravy Seasoned Spinach/Egg Assorted Bread/Mar. Blushing Pears/Lettuce	Roast Pork Loin Potatoes in Jacket Seasoned Cabbage Assorted Bread/Mar. Tangy Fruit Dessert Garnish: Spiced Apple Ring	Veal Parmaesan Parsley Noodles Italian Mixed Vegetables Garlic Bread/Mar. Lemon Cream Pie	Pinto Beans/Sliced Ham Seasoned Greens Cornbread/Mar. Apricot Halves Garnish: Tomato Wedge	Beef Liver/Onions Scalloped Potatoes Peas/Mushroom Biscuit/Mar. Molded Red Hot Applesauce on Lettuce Leaf	Spaghetti/Meat Sauce Seasoned Green Beans Tossed Salad/Dressing Garlic Bread/Mar. Fruited Parfait Garnish: Parsley Sprig	Baked Veal/Brown Gravy Whipped Potatoes Marinated Carrots Assorted Bread/Mar. Blushing Pear Halves Garnish: Tomato Wedge
DINNER	Chicken Pot Pie Stewed Apples Cucumber Salad Assorted Bread/Mar. Rainbow Sherbet Milk 2% Garnish: Parsley Sprig	Savory Beef Hash Parslied Carrots Roll/Mar. Cheesecake/Strawberry Glaze Milk 2%	Sliced Turkey Whipped Potatoes/Gravy Seasoned Green Beans Assorted Bread/Mar. Sliced Peaches/Whipped Topping Milk 2% Garnish: Cranberry Sauce	Sloppy Joes/Bun Potato Wedges Tossed Salad/French Dressing Iced Cupcake Milk 2% Garnish: Parsley Sprig	Cheesy Hamburger Casserole Baked Potato Sunshine Salad Assorted Bread/Mar. Pumpkin Cake Milk 2% Garnish: Parsley Sprig	Cream of Broccoli Soup Egg Salad on WW Bread Potato Chips Ving. Cole Slaw Frosted Chocolate Cake Milk 2% Garnish: Tomato Wedge	Homemade Chili Saltine Crackers Cheese Slices Garden Salad/French Dressing Banana Pudding Milk 2% Garnish: Pickle Chips

Continued

Menu Planning for Week of _____

	SUNDAY	MONDAY	TUESDAY	WEDNESDAY	THURSDAY	FRIDAY	SATURDAY
B R E A K F A S T	Orange Juice Hot/Cold Cereal Sausage Pancakes/Mar./Syrup Milk 2%	Orange Juice Hot/Cold Cereal Fried Egg Bacon Strip Toast/Mar./Jelly Milk 2%	Orange Juice Hot/Cold Cereal Scrambled Egg Toast/Mar./Jelly Milk 2%	Orange Juice Hot/Cold Cereal Poached Egg Toast/Mar./Jelly Milk 2%	Orange Juice Hot/Cold Cereal Scrambled Egg Toast/Mar./Jelly Milk 2%	Orange Juice Hot/Cold Cereal French Toast/Mar./Syrup Bacon Strip Milk 2%	Orange Juice Hot/Cold Cereal Scrambled Egg Toast/Mar./Jelly Milk 2%
L U N C H	Oven-Fried Chicken Whipped Potatoes/Gravy Green Bean Casserole Ruby Red Fruit Mold/Lettuce Assorted Bread/Mar. Vanilla Ice Cream Garnish: Cranberry Slice	Roast Beef Oven Brown Potatoes/Carrots Roll/Mar. Frosted Lime Mold/Lettuce Peach Halves/Whipped Topping Garnish: Parsley Sprig	BBQ Chicken Seasoned Corn Broccoli Casserole Rye Bread/Mar. Pineapple Upsidedown Cake	Ham & Beans Stewed Tomatoes Cornbread/Mar. Apple Crumb Pie Garnish: Onion Slice	Beef Stroganoff Noodles Winter Mixed Vegetables Roll/Mar. Cherry Pie Garnish: Orange Slice	Breaded Fish Filet/Tartar Sauce Peas & Mushrooms Carrifruit Salad Assorted Bread/Mar. Nutmeg Top. Custard Garnish: Lemon Slice	Glazed Baked Ham Au Gratin Potatoes Peas & Pearl Onions Roll/Mar. Angel Cake/Fruit Glaze Garnish: Spiced Apple Ring
D I N N E R	Homemade Vegetable Soup Lunch Meat Subs/Bun Lettuce/Tomato Potato Chips Fresh Banana Milk 2%	Tuna Salad Sandwich on WW Bread Lettuce/Tomato Tater Tots Two-Bean Salad Strawberry Ice Cream Milk 2%	Beef/Vegetable Soup Crackers Pimento Cheese Sandwich Potato Chips Waldorf Salad/Lettuce Butterscotch Brownie Milk 2%	Chicken Livers Boiled Potatoes/Jackets Seasoned Green Beans Assorted Bread/Mar. Citrus Sections Milk 2%	Sliced Turkey on WW Bread Oven-Baked Beans Molded Vegetable Salad Orange Sherbet Milk 2% Garnish: Parsley Sprig	Sausage Gravy/Biscuit Deviled Egg Halves Seasoned Hominy Stewed Apples Milk 2% Garnish: Parsley Sprig	Cream of Tomato Soup/Crackers Cold Cuts/Cheese Sandwich Potato Salad Mixed Fruit Cup Milk 2% Garnish: Carrot/Celery Sticks

Appendix C

Sample Selective Menu

Breakfast

JUICES & FRUITS (Circle 1)
Orange Juice   Banana
Tomato Juice   Stewed Prunes
Cranberry Juice

CEREALS (Circle 1)
Creamy Oatmeal   Rice Crispies
Cornflakes   Cheerios
Raisin Bran

ENTRÉES (Circle 2)
Omelet   Sauteed Ham
Scrambled Egg   Bacon

BREADS (Circle 1)
White Toast   Whole Wheat Toast
Biscuit

Lunch

ENTRÉE (Circle 1)
Fresh Fruit Plate with Chicken
Salad or Cottage Cheese
Grilled Chicken Breast

SIDE DISHES (Circle 2)
Buttered Peas
Rice Pilaf
Turkish Carrots

DESSERTS (Circle 1)
Ice Cream
Chocolate Cream Pie
Chilled Sliced Peaches

BREADS (Circle 1)
White Bread   Dinner Roll
Wheat Bread   Crackers

Dinner

APPETIZER (Circle if desired)
Soup of the Day

ENTRÉE (Circle 1)
Beef Liver and Sautéed Onions
Baked Pork Tenderloin with Rosemary
Brown Sauce

SIDE DISHES (Circle 2)
Whipped Potatoes
Buttered Broccoli
Whole Kernal Corn

DESSERTS (Circle 1)
Tropical Fruit Salad
Strawberry Cream Dessert
Sherbert

BEVERAGES

Coffee	Skim Milk
Hot Tea	Hot Cocoa
2% Milk	Decaffeinated Coffee
Water	

CONDIMENTS

Cream	Honey
Jelly	Margarine
Lemon	

Salt
Pepper
Sugar

OR

CONTINENTAL BREAKFAST
Served in Room at 9 A.M.

Juice _____
Danish _____
Beverage _____

Name _____
Diet _____
Room Number _____

BEVERAGES

Coffee	Skim Milk
Iced Tea	Chilled Soft Drink
2% Milk	Diet Soft Drink
Water	Decaffeinated Coffee

CONDIMENTS

Cream	Lemon Wedge
Margarine	
Sugar Substitute	

Salt
Pepper
Sugar

Name _____
Diet _____
Room Number _____

BEVERAGES

Coffee	Skim Milk
Diet Soft Drink	Iced Tea
Chilled Soft Drink	2% Milk
Decaffeinated Coffee	Water

CONDIMENTS

Cream	Lemon Wedge
Margarine	
Sugar Substitute	

Salt
Pepper
Sugar

Name _____
Diet _____
Room Number _____

Breakfast	Lunch	Dinner

Breakfast

JUICE & FRUITS (Circle 1)

Orange Juice   Banana
Prune Juice   Broiled Grapefruit
Cranberry Juice   Half

CEREALS (Circle 1)

Creamy Oatmeal   Rice Crispies
Raisin Bran   Corn Flakes
Cheerios

ENTRÉES (Circle 2)

Omelet   Scrambled Egg
Sausage   Bacon
French Toast

BREADS (Circle 1)

White Toast   Whole Wheat Toast
Muffin   Biscuit

Lunch

ENTRÉE (Circle 1)

Shrimp Salad on Lettuce with
Avocado, Tomato, Cucumber,
and Black Olives
Roast Beef with Gravy

SIDE DISHES (Circle 2)

Corn on the Cob   Harvard Beets
Buttered New Potatoes

DESSERTS (Circle 1)

Ice Cream   Chilled Fruit
Cocktail

BREADS (Circle 1)

White Bread   Wheat Bread
Dinner Roll   Crackers

Dinner

APPETIZER (Circle if desired)
Soup of the Day

ENTRÉE (Circle 1)
Grilled Barbequed Pork Chop
Pan-fried Catfish Fillet

SIDE DISHES (Circle 2)
French Fries   Creamy Cole Slaw
Seasoned Greenbeans

DESSERTS (Circle 1)
Ice Cream   Rosy Pear Halves
Chocolate Almond Cheesecake

BREADS (Circle 1)
White Bread   Wheat Bread
Dinner Roll   Hush Puppies
Homemade Cornbread

BEVERAGES
Coffee   Skim Milk   Hot Tea
2% Milk   Hot Cocoa
Decaffeinated Coffee   Water

CONDIMENTS
Salt   Pepper   Sugar   Jelly
Cream   Lemon   Honey   Margarine

OR

CONTINENTAL BREAKFAST
Served in Room at 9 A.M.

Juice _____
Muffin _____
Beverage _____

Name _____

Diet _____

Room Number _____

BEVERAGES
Coffee   Iced Tea   Skim Milk   2% Milk
Chilled Soft Drink   Diet Soft Drink
Decaffeinated Coffee   Water

CONDIMENTS
Salt   Pepper   Sugar
Cream   Margarine
Sugar Substitute
Lemon Wedge

Name _____

Diet _____

Room Number _____

BEVERAGES
Coffee   Iced Tea   Skim Milk   2% Milk
Chilled Soft Drink   Diet Soft Drink
Decaffeinated Coffee   Water

CONDIMENTS
Salt   Sugar Substitute   Ketchup
Pepper   Lemon Wedge   Sugar
Cream   Tartar Sauce   Margarine

Name _____

Diet _____

Room Number _____

Breakfast

JUICES & FRUITS (Circle 1)
Orange Juice   Chilled Grapefruit Sections
Prune Juice   Banana
    Cranberry Juice

CEREALS (Circle 1)
Cream of Wheat   Raisin Bran
Oatmeal   Cornflakes
    Rice Crispies

ENTRÉES (Circle 2)
Scrambled Eggs   Omelet
Crisp Bacon
Sausage and Cream Gravy

BREADS (Circle 1)
White Toast   Homemade Biscuit
Whole Wheat Toast   Danish

Lunch

ENTRÉE (Circle 1)
Club Sandwich With Bacon,
Lettuce, Tomato, Turkey, Ham and
Mayonnaise
Oven Fried Chicken

SIDE DISHES (Circle 2)
Chilled Potato Salad   Sautéed Zucchini
        Peas and Carrots

DESSERTS (Circle 1)
Ice Cream   Chilled Apple Sauce
Homemade Chocolate Chip Cookies

BREADS (Circle 1)
White Bread   Dinner Roll
        Crackers

Dinner

APPETIZER (Circle if desired)
Soup of the Day

ENTRÉE (Circle 1)
Baked Orange Roughy
Apple Brandy Chicken with Apples
and Walnuts

SIDE DISHES (Circle 2)
        Broccoli with Cheese
Baked Potato
Steamed Cauliflower

DESSERTS (Circle 1)
Ice Cream
Strawberry Cream Dessert
Cherry Pie

BREADS (Circle 1)

BEVERAGES
Coffee Skim Milk 2% Milk
Hot Tea Hot Cocoa
Decaffeinated Coffee Water

CONDIMENTS
Salt Pepper Cream Lemon
Sugar Margarine Honey Jelly

OR

CONTINENTAL BREAKFAST
Served in Room at 9 A.M.

Juice _____
Danish _____
Beverage _____

Name _____
Diet _____
Room Number _____

Whole Wheat Bread

BEVERAGES
Coffee Iced Tea 2% Milk Skim Milk
Chilled Soft Drink Diet Soft Drink Water
Decaffeinated Coffee Water

CONDIMENTS
Salt Pepper Cream Sugar
Margarine Lemon Wedge
Sugar Substitute

Name _____
Diet _____
Room Number _____

White Bread   Whole Wheat Bread
Dinner Roll   Crackers

BEVERAGE
Coffee Iced Tea Skim Milk 2% Milk
Chilled Soft Drink Diet Soft Drink
Decaffeinated Coffee Water

CONDIMENTS
Salt Pepper Cream Sugar Margarine
Lemon Wedge Sugar Substitute Tartar Sauce

Name _____
Diet _____
Room Number _____

Breakfast   Lunch   Dinner

Breakfast

JUICES & FRUITS (Circle 1)
Orange Juice   Fresh Orange
Prune Juice   Banana
         Cranberry Juice

CEREALS (Circle 1)
Creamy Oatmeal   Raisin Bran
Cornflakes   Rice Crispies
         Cheerios

ENTRÉES (Circle 1 or 2)
         Cheese Omelet
         Crisp Bacon
Scrambled Egg with Diced Ham

BREADS (Circle 1)
White Toast   Biscuit

Lunch

ENTRÉE (Circle 1)
Chicken Salad Sandwich with Avocado, Lettuce
         and Tomato
Grilled Hamburger (Choose Bun Below)

SIDE DISHES (Circle 2)
Lima Beans   Steak Fries
Sliced Fresh Tomatoes on Leaf Lettuce

DESSERTS (Circle 1)
Ice Cream   Banana Pudding
         Angel Food Cake

BREADS (Circle 1)
White Bread   Whole Wheat Bread
Dinner Roll   Crackers
         Bun

Dinner

APPETIZER (Circle if desired)
         Soup of the Day

ENTRÉE (Circle 1)
         Fettucini Roberto
Spinach Pasta, Sauteed with Prosciutto and Ham
A Creamy Parmesan Cheese Sauce
Roast Turkey with Gravy

SIDE DISHES (Circle 2)
Cornbread Dressing   Glazed Carrots
         Steamed Asparagus

DESSERTS (Circle 1)
         Ice Cream
         Apple Pie
         Fresh Cantaloupe

Whole Wheat Toast

BEVERAGES

Coffee Decaffeinated Coffee Water
Hot Tea 2% Milk Skim Milk
Hot Cocoa

OR

CONTINENTAL BREAKFAST
Served in Room at 9 A.M.

Juice _____
Cinnamon Raisin Biscuit _____
Beverage _____

Name _____
Diet _____
Room Number _____

BEVERAGES

Coffee Iced Tea Skim Milk 2% Milk
Chilled Soft Drink Diet Soft Drink Water
Decaffeinated Coffee

CONDIMENTS

Salt Pepper Sugar Cream
Ketchup Margarine Lemon Wedge
Mayonnaise Sugar Substitute Mustard

Name _____
Diet _____
Room Number _____

BREADS (Circle 1)

White Bread Whole Wheat Bread
Dinner Roll Crackers

BEVERAGES

Coffee Iced Tea 2% Milk Skim Milk
Chilled Soft Drink Diet Soft Drink
Decaffeinated Coffee Water

CONDIMENTS

Salt Pepper Cream Sugar
Sugar Substitute Margarine
Lemon Wedge

Name _____
Diet _____
Room Number _____

Breakfast

JUICES & FRUITS (Circle 1)
Orange Juice   Chilled Grapefruit Wedges
Prune Juice   Cranberry Juice
                Banana

CEREALS (Circle 1)
Creamy Oatmeal   Raisin Bran
Cornflakes   Rice Crispies
        Cheerios

ENTRÉES (Circle 1 or 2)
Scrambled Egg   Omelet
Crisp Bacon   Sausage
        French Toast

BREADS (Circle 1)
White Toast   Whole Wheat Toast
Homemade Biscuit   Danish

Lunch

ENTRÉE (Circle 1)
Benedict Arnold-
Scrambled Eggs & Canadian Bacon on a
Toasted English Muffin Topped with
Creamy Hollandaise Sauce
Salmon Croquettes

SIDE DISHES (Circle 2)
Steamed Broccoli   Scalloped Tomatoes
Buttered New Potatoes

DESSERTS (Circle 1)
Ice Cream
Lemon Meringue Pie

BREADS (Circle 1)
White Bread   Whole Wheat Toast
Dinner Roll   Crackers

Dinner

APPETIZER (Circle if desired)
Soup of the Day

ENTRÉE (Circle 1)
Grilled Chicken Dijonnaise
Marinated Boneless Chicken Breast with
Dijon Mustard Sauce
Honey Glazed Ham

SIDE DISHES (Circle 2)
Spinach Soufflé   Julienne Beets
        Wild Rice

DESSERTS (Circle 1)
Ice Cream   Sherbert
Cherry Delight

BREADS (Circle 1)
White Bread   Whole Wheat Bread

BEVERAGE
Coffee   Skim Milk   2% Milk
Hot Tea   Hot Cocoa   Decaffeinated Coffee
Water

CONDIMENTS
Salt   Pepper   Sugar   Cream
Jelly   Margarine   Lemon   Honey
Maple Syrup

OR

CONTINENTAL BREAKFAST
Served in Room at 9 A.M.

Juice _____
Danish _____
Beverage _____

Name _____
Diet _____
Room Number _____

BEVERAGES
Coffee   Iced Tea   Skim Milk   2% Milk
Decaffeinated Coffee   Water
Chilled Soft Drink   Diet Soft Drink

CONDIMENTS
Salt   Pepper   Sugar
Cream   Sugar Substitute
Margarine
Lemon Wedge

Name _____
Diet _____
Room Number _____

Homemade   Crackers
Muffin

BEVERAGES
Coffee   Iced Tea   Skim Milk   2% Milk
Decaffeinated Coffee   Water
Chilled Soft Drink   Diet Soft Drink

CONDIMENTS
Salt   Pepper   Sugar   Cream
Margarine   Sugar Substitute
Lemon Wedge

Name _____
Diet _____
Room Number _____

Breakfast

JUICES & FRUITS (Circle 1)
Orange Juice   Stewed Prunes
Prune Juice   Banana
        Cranberry Juice

CEREALS (Circle 1)
Creamy Oatmeal   Raisin Bran
Cornflakes   Cheerios
   Rice Crispies

ENTRÉES (Circle 1 or 2)
Scrambled Eggs   Crisp Bacon
Omelet   Sausage
    Cheese Melt

BREADS (Circle 1)
White Toast   Homemade Biscuit
Wheat Toast   Danish

Lunch

ENTRÉES (Circle 1)
Grilled Ham & Cheese
Sautéed Chicken Livers with Cream Gravy

SIDE DISHES (Circle 2)
Whipped Potatoes   Seasoned
     Greenbeans
     Creamy Succotash

DESSERTS (Circle 1)
     Ice Cream
     Chilled Fruit Cup

BREADS (Circle 1)
White Bread   Dinner Roll
     Whole Wheat Bread
          Crackers

Dinner

APPETIZER (Circle if desired)
     Soup of the Day

ENTRÉES (Circle 1)
Deep Fried Chicken Strips
     Orange Pork Chop

SIDE DISHES (Circle 2)
Cheese Grits   Buttered Peas
Buttered Turnip Greens

DESSERTS (Circle 1)
     Ice Cream
Chocolate Pudding with Whipped Topping
          Chilled Apricots

BREADS (Circle 1)
White Bread   Dinner Roll

314

Menu 1

BEVERAGES

Coffee   Skim Milk   Hot Tea
Decaffeinated Coffee   2% Milk
Water   Hot Cocoa

CONDIMENTS

Salt   Pepper   Jelly
Sugar   Margarine   Lemon
Cream   Honey

OR

CONTINENTAL BREAKFAST
Served in Room at 9 A.M.

Juice _____
Danish _____
Beverage _____

Name _____
Diet _____
Room Number _____

Menu 2

BEVERAGES

Coffee   Skim Milk   Iced
Tea   Water   2% Milk
Decaffeinated Coffee   Diet Soft Drink
Chilled Soft Drink

CONDIMENTS

Sugar
Salt   Pepper   Cream
Margarine   Sugar Substitute
Lemon Wedge

Name _____
Diet _____
Room Number _____

Menu 3

Whole Wheat   Crackers
Bread

BEVERAGES

Skim Milk   Iced Tea
Decaffeinated Coffee
Coffee   Chilled Soft Drink
2% Milk
Water   Diet Soft Drink

CONDIMENTS

Pepper   Sugar   Cream
Salt   Margarine
Sugar Substitute
Lemon Wedge

Name _____
Diet _____
Room Number _____

Breakfast

JUICES & FRUITS (Circle 1)
Orange Juice   Chilled Grapefruit Half
Prune Juice   Banana
Cranberry Juice

CEREALS (Circle 1)
Creamy Oatmeal   Raisin Bran
Cornflakes   Rice Krispies   Cheerios

ENTRÉES (Circle 1 or 2)
Scrambled Eggs   Crisp Bacon
Omelet   Sausage
French Toast

BREADS (Circle 1)
White Toast   Homemade Biscuit
Wheat Toast   Danish

Lunch

ENTRÉES (Circle 1)
Baked Meatloaf
Tuna Melt—Fresh Tuna Salad on Toasted
English Muffin Topped with Melted Cheese
(Select Muffin Below)

SIDE DISHES (Circle 2)
Corn Pudding   Country Cabbage
Tomatoes & Zucchini

DESSERTS (Circle 1)
Ice Cream
Chilled Applesauce

BREADS (Circle 1)
White Bread   Dinner Roll
Whole Wheat Bread   Crackers
Toasted English Muffin

Dinner

APPETIZERS (Circle if desired)
Soup of the Day
Sliced Tomatoes Vinaigrette

ENTRÉES (Circle 1)
Baked Flounder
Salisbury Steak

SIDE DISHES (Circle 2)
Duchess Potatoes
Seasoned Greenbeans
Buttered Carrots

DESSERTS (Circle 1)
Ice Cream
Chocolate Almond Cheesecake
Tropical Fruit Salad

BEVERAGES

Coffee   Skim Milk
Hot Tea   Hot Cocoa
2% Milk   Decaffeinated Coffee
Water

CONDIMENTS

Salt   Pepper   Sugar   Maple Syrup
Cream   Jelly   Lemon   Honey
Sugar Substitute   Margarine

OR

CONTINENTAL BREAKFAST
Served in Room at 9 A.M.

Juice _____
Danish _____
Beverage _____

Name _____

Diet _____

Room Number _____

BEVERAGES

Coffee   Skim Milk
Iced Tea   Chilled Soft Drink
2% Milk   Diet Soft Drink
Decaffeinated Coffee   Water

CONDIMENTS

Salt   Sugar Substitute   Pepper
Cream   Sugar   Margarine
Lemon Wedge

Name _____

Diet _____

Room Number _____

BREADS (Circle 1)

White Bread   Dinner Roll
Whole Wheat Bread   Crackers

BEVERAGES

Coffee   Skim Milk
Iced Tea   Chilled Soft Drink
2% Milk   Diet Soft Drink
Decaffeinated Coffee   Water

CONDIMENTS

Salt   Sugar Substitute   Pepper
Cream   Sugar   Margarine
Lemon Wedge   Tartar Sauce

Name _____

Diet _____

Room Number _____

Appendix D

Sample Modified Menu

	Portion Size	Regular	Puréed	DIABETIC CALORIE RESTRICTED	1000	1200	1500	1800	2000	Low Sodium	2 GM Sodium	Low Fat	Low Cholesterol	High Fiber	Private
B	4 oz.	Juice			------	------	----→	8 oz	8 oz						
R	#16	Egg (1)			------	------	----→	#8	#8	LS	LS	Egg Beaters	--------→		
E	6 oz.	Oatmeal	Ground		X	X	4 oz.	4 oz.	4 oz.					Branflakes	
A	1	Toast			1	1	1	2	2					WW	
K	1 ea.	Marg., Jelly		Diet Jelly	No Marg.	1	1	1	1						
F	8 oz.	Milk—2%		Skim 4 oz.	------			----→	8 oz						
A															
S															
T															
N	3 oz.	Fried Chicken	Pureed Baked Chicken	Baked					⟩		LS	Baked	Baked		
O	#8	Rice Pilaf							⟩	LS	LS	LF	LF		
O	#8	Bu Mixed Vegetables							⟩	LS	LS	LF	LF		
N	1	Biscuit	Breadcrumbs		X	1	1	1	2		Bread	Bread	Bread		
	1	Margarine			X	X	X	1	X						
	1/8 pie	Cream Cheese Pie		Diet Peaches						Peaches	Peaches	Peaches	Peaches		

Continued

Portion Size	Regular	Puréed	DIABETIC CALORIE RESTRICTED	1000	1200	1500	1800	2000	Low Sodium	2 GM Sodium	Low Fat	Low Cholesterol	High Fiber	Private
8 oz.	Milk—2%		Skim 4 oz.	----				→		Omit	Skim	Skim		
	Tomato Wedge		Juice		X	X	X	4 oz.						
3 oz.	Ham Roll						X	→		Baked Pork Chop --------→				
#8	Noodles Alfredo		Plain Noodles	----				→	LS	Plain --------→	LF	LF		
#8	Diced Beets			----				→	LS	LS				
1	Bread	Breadcrumbs		X	1	2	2	2					WW	
1	Margarine			X	X	X	1	1						
#12	Sherbert		Diet Pears											
8 oz.	Milk—2%		Skim Milk				----→	8 oz			Skim	Skim		
	Parsley													
			Skim Milk	X				----→						
			Diet Pudding	X	X	1/2 c	1/2 c	1/2 c						

NIGHTS / HS (meal section markers)

* 1. Thaw ground beef for Monday

Mechanical Soft - Grind Meats

Appendix E

Sample Dietary Inservices

DIETARY INSERVICE: LABORATORY INTERPRETATION IN THE ELDERLY

I. Physiological aging
   A. Affects all physiological processes
   B. Aging is accumulative
   C. Distinction between normal attrition of body function and loss of function due to the onset of disease (important point)
II. Normal age-related physiological changes
   A. Cardiovascular system
      1. Cardiac output decrease of 1 percent per year after the third decade
      2. Progressive increase in blood pressure after the first decade
      3. Increase in arteriosclerosis by 30 percent from age 20 to 70
   B. Renal system
      1. Kidney size and weight decrease of 30 percent from age 30 to 80
      2. Decline by 30 percent in number of glomeruli from age 40 to 65
      3. Age-related decrease in creatinine clearance
      4. Age-related increase in BUN
   C. Glucose control
      1. Decrease in the number and function of beta cells of pancreas
      2. Insulin secreted as proinsulin, a nonactive precursor of insulin
      3. Increase in glucose intolerance
      4. Decrease in renal tubular reabsorption of glucose—glycosuria more pronounced
   D. Musculoskeletal system
      1. Loss of muscle cell mass
      2. Decreased protein stores
      3. Indirect decrease of creatinine
III. Lab error
   A. Spoiled specimen
   B. Incorrect sampling
   C. Incomplete sampling
   D. Faulty reagents
   E. Human error
   F. Diet
   G. Drugs
      1. Alteration
      2. Interference
   H. Procedures/trauma
IV. Electrolytes
   A. Sodium
      1. General
         a. 132–145 mEq/l
         b. Major cation of extracellular fluid

  c. Intake required to prevent depletion 50 mEq/day (3 g NaCl)

 2. Hyponatremia

  a. Decrease in sodium in relation to water

  b. Decrease in sodium intake

  c. Loss of sodium-rich body fluids

   i. Sweat

   ii. Vomitus

   iii. Diarrhea

  d. Diseases with edema

   i. Renal failure

   ii. Congestive heart failure

   iii. Cirrhosis

 3. Hypernatremia

  a. Increases in sodium in relation to water

  b. Diseases

   i. Diabetes insipidus

   ii. Cushing syndrome

   iii. Stress

  c. Drugs

   i. Sodium salts of antibiotics

   ii. Steroids

   iii. Phenylbutazone

   iv. Methyldopa

B. Potassium

 1. General

  a. 3.5–4.5 mEq/l

  b. Major intracellular cation

  c. Total body stores = 3,500 mEq 70 kg—man

  d. Extracellular fluid contains only 50 mEq

 2. Hypokalemia

  a. Decreased dietary intake

  b. Increased urinary losses

   i. Diuretics

   ii. Steroids

   iii. Large sodium intake

  c. G.I. losses

  d. Cellular entry

   i. Insulin/glucose

   ii. Alkalosis

   iii. Treatment for megaloblastic anemia

 3. Hyperkalemia

  a. Increased intake

   i. Food

   ii. Blood products

          b. Internal bleeding
          c. Impaired excretion
          d. Drugs
               i. Spironolactone
              ii. K salts of drugs
             iii. Salt substitutes
     4. Errors in potassium blood samples: Errors in blood sample
        collection and analysis show increase K levels, whereas de-
        creased K levels are generally correct
V. Chem 12
     A. Calcium
          1. 8.5–10.5 mg percent
          2. 45–50 percent protein bound (inactive)
          3. Corrected calcium for hypoalbuminemia—Ca − meas. alb. + 4
     B. Phosphate
          1. 2.8–4.5 mg percent
          2. Hypophosphatemia
               a. Nutritional recovery producing ATP
               b. Alcohol withdrawal
               c. Malabsorption
               d. Phosphate-bonding antacids (aluminum)
               e. Nephrotoxic drug exposure
     C. Blood urea nitrogen (BUN)
          1. 10–26 mg percent
          2. Protein + amino acids + ammonia + urea
          3. Uses
               a. Renal function—filtered by glomeuli and reabsorbed by tu-
                  bules
               b. Liver function
               c. G.I. bleeding—amount of protein
               d. Nutrition—protein wasting
               e. CHF/shock—perfusion to kidneys
     D. Albumin
          1. 3.5–5.0 gm percent
          2. Drug carrier
          3. Hypoalbuminemia
               a. Malnutrition
               b. Chronic liver damage
               c. Chronic disease
               d. Loss from body
                    i. Bleeding
                   ii. Burns
                  iii. Pyelonephritis
     E. Liver Enzymes
          1. LDH

    a. 100–225 mu/ml
    b. Liver, heart, and muscle
  2. SGOT
    a. 7–40 mu/ml
    b. Liver, heart, and muscle
  3. Alkaline phosphatase
    a. 30–115 mu/ml
    b. Liver and bone
VI. Hematological system (no such thing as anemia of old age)
  A. Reasons of anemia
    1. Number of diseases
    2. Number of drugs
    3. Nutritional deficiencies
    4. Hgb may be 1–2 g percent less in elderly
  B. Laboratory diagnosis of anemia
    1. RBC, hgb, hct will be decreased
    2. Retic count may be increased
    3. Mean corpuscular volume (mcv)
      a. Normal—blood loss
      b. Increase—B_{12} or folic acid deficiency
      c. Decrease—iron deficiency
    4. Mean corpuscular hemoglobin
      a. Normal—blood loss
      b. Increase—B_{12} or folic acid deficiency
      c. Decrease—iron deficiency

REFERENCE

Wagner, John. 1984. *Laboratory interpretation in the elderly.* Indiana Consultant Dietitians in Health Care Facilities. January 1984.

Quiz

T F 1. The aging process affects all physiological processess.
T F 2. A decrease in glucose intolerance occurs with the aging process.
T F 3. Hypokalemia may be related to increased urinary losses (for example from diuretics) or decreased dietary intake of potassium.
T F 4. Hgb may be 1–2 g percent more in an elderly person than in a 45-year-old person.
T F 5. Blood urea nitrogen (BUN) values can detect liver function complications as well as renal function complications.
      6. Name two reasons why anemia may occur in the elderly.
      7. The normal albumin level is _____ g percent, but hypoalbuminemia may occur due to _____ (name one).
      8. Name two areas that may cause lab error.

DIETARY INSERVICE: INFECTION CONTROL—
FOOD AND CHEMICAL POISONING

I. Introduction
  A. The nursing home works toward the best sanitary conditions, cleanliness and healthful conditions.
  B. The elderly population have less resistance to disease than younger people.
II. Bacteria or germs that can cause serious illness
  A. Salmonella bacteria
    1. Causes food infections. Symptoms are violent flulike illness that occur 12–24 hours after eating.
    2. Salmonella is spread by contaminated utensils; for example, using a utensil for one product and then using it in a different product without washing and sanitizing the utensil. It is also spread by work surfaces not cleaned before reuse, unwashed hands, by flies, and in meat and poultry if not thoroughly cooked.
  B. Botulinum bacteria
    1. Causes botulism. Symptoms are headaches, dizziness, failure to breathe, and even death.
    2. Botulism can be found in improperly canned foods. Cans that are bulged or dented or have broken seals have the potential for causing botulism.
  C. Staphylococcus or "staph" bacteria
    1. Causes food poisoning. Symptoms are violent flulike illness 12–30 hours after eating.
    2. Staph is spread by persons with boils, infected sores, or unwashed hands.
  D. Perfringens bacteria
    1. Causes cramps and/or diarrhea about 12 hours after eating.
    2. Perfringens can be found in food that has been precooked, inadequately cooked, and then inadequately reheated. For example, roast pork may be cooked a day ahead of serving, cooled at room temperature and put in the refrigerator, and reheated the next day before serving but not at a high enough temperature to kill the bacteria.
III. Conditions that promote bacterial growth
  A. Foods such as custards, dairy products, meats, and warmed-over foods provide *food* and *moisture* for bacteria to multiply.
  B. Bacteria grows well at *room temperature*. Never leave food out while you are on break. Bacterial growth slows down if the temperature is below 45°F or above 140°F.
IV. How to prevent food poisoning
  A. Wash utensils, pots, and pans in hot soapy water, rinse in hot water, sanitize, then air dry completely. Water left on pans is a good place for bacteria to grow.

B. Keep fingers out of glasses and dishes.
C. Silverware and serving utensils should be picked up by the handles.
D. Try to avoid touching hair, face, or mouth while working.
E. Wash hands thoroughly following use of the restroom, coughing, sneezing, blowing your nose, or smoking a cigarette.
F. Wear a hairnet and a clean uniform and apron. Change the apron during the day if needed.
G. If you are sick stay home.

V. Chemical Poisoning
A. Pesticides are used to keep insects and plant diseases from harming food. All fresh fruits and vegetables should be washed before preparation.
B. Detergents, drying agents, and sanitizers should not come in contact with food.
  1. Chemicals should be stored away from food.
  2. Chemicals should be labeled for identification (in case of accidental poisoning and with directions for use).
  3. Poisonous metals: poisoning can result when high-acid foods such as tomatoes are stored or prepared in copper, brass, galvanized, or gray enamelware. Lead-based products should never be used in foodservice areas.

REFERENCES

National Institute for the Foodservice Industry. 1978. *Applied foodservice sanitation*, 31–45.
American Hospital Association. 1981. *Food service manual for health care institutions*, 78–80.
Channing L. Bete Co. 1973 *About food germs*.
Channing L. Bete Co. 1967. *48 Ways to foil food infections*.

Quiz

T F 1. If you are vomiting, have diarrhea, and feel as if you have the flu, you may have food poisoning.
T F 2. It is all right to touch the rim of a glass when serving a resident.
T F 3. Food eaten from a bulging can can be deadly.
T F 4. Germs grow best above 140° F.
T F 5. Water left on a pan or utensil is a good place for bacteria to grow.
T F 6. You do not need to wash your hands after smoking a cigarette.
T F 7. It is not necessary to wash tomatoes before serving.
T F 8. Never store chemicals and food together.
T F 9. Food samples need to be kept for 48 hours for testing purposes by the state board of health.

DIETARY INSERVICE: THE IMPORTANCE OF FIBER IN THE DIET

I. Definition of fiber
   A. The components of food that are resistant to digestion in the gastro-intestinal tract
   B. Other terms used for fiber
      1. Roughage
      2. Residue
      3. Crude fiber
   C. Good sources of fiber
      1. Whole grain breads and cereals
      2. Fresh fruits and vegetables
      3. Dried fruits and vegetables
      4. Nuts
   D. Reasons for low fiber in today's diet
      1. In "refined foods" most of the fiber has been removed from grains through milling.
      2. Fiber is also reduced by peeling or cooking fruits and vegetables.
II. Effect of fiber on bowel habits
   A. Dietary fiber has a great capacity to hold water, giving bulk and softness to the stool.
   B. The stools are then able to pass through the intestinal tract more easily and quickly, resulting in less strain and pressure on the bowel.
III. Alleged benefits of fiber in the diet
   A. Constipation and hemorrhoids
      1. Incidence
         a. Constipation is very common especially among the elderly.
         b. Hemorrhoids are present in one-half the people over 50.
      2. Fiber gives bulk and softness to stool, reducing strain and preventing constipation and hemorrhoids.
   B. Diverticular Disease
      1. Incidence
         a. Relatively uncommon 50 years ago
         b. Now affects 50 percent of all over age 40
         c. Almost unknown in countries on high-fiber diets
      2. Disease as related to fiber
         a. Diverticulosis is a condition in which out-pouchings develop in weak areas of the bowel wall.
         b. This condition may result from a low-fiber diet, which makes the intestinal contents hard and firm and causes difficulty in moving the intestinal contents along. High-pressure points result.
   C. Colon cancer: Some health professionals believe that with the more rapid movement of the feces that occurs with a high-fiber diet, bowel

tissues are less likely to be exposed to toxins and cancer-causing substances.

   D. Possible benefits of a high-fiber diet
       1. Decreased incidence of obesity
          a. A high-fiber diet is generally low in fat and therefore calories.
          b. A high-fiber diet could reduce food consumption because of an increased feeling of fullness.
       2. Heart disease
          a. Since the transit time in the bowel is shortened, there is a decreased absorption of dietary cholesterol.
          b. High-fiber plant foods contain no animal fat.
       3. Diabetes: Blood sugar levels of patients taking insulin were significantly lower on a high-fiber diet than on a low-fiber diet.

REFERENCES

Owen, Lois J., James C. Rose, Dorothy J. Wrase, and Ardelle Revland, 1979. *Dietary lesson plans for health care facilities.* Rochester, N.Y.: Learning Resources Dept., Rochester Methodist Hospital.

The Institute of Food Technologists' Expert Panel on Food Safety and Nutrition and the Committee on Public Information. 1979. Dietary fiber. *Contemporary Nutrition,* 4:9 (Nutrition Dept., General Mills, Minneapolis).

Quiz

T F 1. Most fiber in the diet is digestible in the gastrointestinal tract.

T F 2. The terms "residue" and "fiber" have different definitions.

T F 3. Constipation can be relieved by following a high-fiber diet.

T F 4. Over 50 percent of those over 50 years old have hemorrhoids.

T F 5. You are less likely to be overweight if your diet is high in fiber.

T F 6. A person with diverticulosis could benefit from a diet low in fiber.

T F 7. Blood sugar levels of diabetic residents taking insulin were significantly lower on a high-fiber versus a low-fiber diet.

       8. Circle the foods high in fiber:

a. White bread	f. Raw cabbage, lettuce, etc.
b. Wheat bread	g. Green beans
c. Bran flakes	h. Bananas
d. Tomato juice	i. Red potatoes in jackets
e. Mashed potatoes	j. Fresh fruits

DIETARY INSERVICE: NUTRITIONAL NEEDS OF THE GERIATRIC RESIDENT

I. Introduction
    A. Reasons nutritional requirements change with age
        1. Alteration in the amount of physical activity
        2. A change in the weight and body composition (increased percentage of fat)
        3. Decrease in muscular efficiency (including the heart, lungs, liver and kidney)
        4. Decrease in nutrient absorption
        5. Chronic diseases
        6. Malabsorption or malutilization of nutrients (can also be caused by drugs): gradual loss of calcium from bones, 1/2 percent each year; up to 30–40 percent loss of calcium by age 65.
        7. Longer time required for digestion
        8. Decreased elasticity of digestive tract, causing heartburn
    B. Diets which lead to development of nutritional deficiency are
        1. Monotonous
        2. Low in food energy
        3. Restrictive
        4. Low in nutrient–calorie ratio

II. Nutrient changes in the elderly
    A. Calories
        1. Energy allowances for persons over 50 decrease proportionally due to a decrease in basal metabolic rate, activity level, and increased proportion of body fat. Basal metabolism decreases by 2 percent each decade; by age 65 it may be 60 percent lower.
        2. Energy allowances cannot be based strictly on chronological age, since the rates of decrease vary widely among individuals.
    B. Protein
        1. Researchers have had conflicting ideas regarding increased or decreased protein needs for the elderly.
            a. Some say lower protein intake is needed because of the diminished ability of the kidneys. By age 70, 50 percent of nephrons in the kidney are lost.
            b. Others think increased protein intake is needed because of a decreased ability to digest protein.
        2. Recent research shows healthy elderly persons require similar amounts of protein to a younger adult. The usual protein requirement is 0.8 g/kg body weight.
    C. Vitamins and minerals
        1. Current evidence reports that for most elderly subjects, the vitamin and mineral requirements remain the same as for young adults.

2. Due to decreased caloric requirement, foods high in nutrient–calorie ratio should be consumed.
3. Vitamins and minerals most likely to be deficient
   a. Fat-soluble vitamins (A, D, E, K), because of a reduction in pancreatic function
   b. Calcium, because of decreased absorption and the possible role of calcium deficiency in the development of osteoporosis (Average intake is 400 mg; RDA is 800 mg; 1000–1500 mg;—the amount supplied by 3–4 cups of milk—are now recommended). Vitamin D intake is important for calcium metabolism.
   c. Iron because of low intake and excessive losses resulting from conditions such as GI bleeding, diverticular disease, and colon cancer
   d. Other possible deficiencies resulting from excessive aspirin intake, including niacin, vitamin B_{12}, and folic acid

D. Fiber
1. There is not an RDA for fiber.
2. High-fiber diets aid in elimination.
3. In countries where diets include significant amounts of fiber, diseases such as colon cancer, diverticulosis, and gallstones are less prevalent.
4. These diseases as well as constipation are more common in the elderly.
5. Therefore, a moderate fiber intake for the elderly seems appropriate.

III. Conclusion
A. More research needs to be conducted to determine the nutrient needs of the elderly.
B. Chronic diseases and medications can alter nutrient absorption, metabolism, and excretion and therefore, increase the nutrient requirement.
C. Factors affecting nutritional requirements are individual and should be carefully assessed.

REFERENCES

Ross Laboratories. 1982. *Aging and nutrition,* 15–16. Columbus, Ohio: Ross Laboratories.
Roe, Daphne A. 1983. *Geriatric nutrition,* 64–67, 83, 110. Englewood Cliffs, N.J.: Prentice-Hall, Inc.

Suggested Activities

1. Have participants identify foods with a high nutrient–calorie ratio by using the National Dairy Nutrient Comparison Cards.

2. Have a contest to see which student can think of the most foods containing each nutrient.
3. Have participants write down everything they ate and drank yesterday. Have them compare this to the Basic Four Food Groups.

Suggested Handouts

1. Copy of the RDAs
2. Examples of nutrient composition tables

Quiz

1. Name one reason that nutritional requirements change with age.

2. A restrictive diet can contribute to nutritional deficiencies.
   True _____
   False _____
3. Change in activity level is one of the reasons why the elderly may need fewer calories.
   True _____
   False _____
4. A diet high in _____ may help with constipation.
5. Name one vitamin or mineral that is likely to be deficient in the elderly's diet.

DIETARY INSERVICE:TECHNIQUES TO IMPROVE FOOD CONSUMPTION

I. Evaluation and Planning
   A. Determine whether the resident is receiving an appetite stimulant.
   B. Determine whether the diet order is too strict to expect adequate consumption.
   C. Honor food preferences and obtain a complete list of likes and dislikes.
      1. Talk with the resident and his or her family about food preferences.
      2. Talk with the nursing staff about food preferences.
   D. Develop a meal pattern to suit the resident's food preferences.
      1. Provide large servings at breakfast if the resident is a big breakfast eater.
      2. Provide a sandwich at 10:00 P.M. if the resident is awake at night.
      3. Provide three small meals at 10:00, 2:00, and 8:00 if the resident has typically eaten small frequent meals.
   E. Investigate the resident's readiness before mealtime.
      1. Is the resident awake at least 30 minutes before mealtime?
      2. Is proper mouth care given in the A.M.?
      3. Is there proper positioning of the resident at mealtime?
   F. If there is any difficulty chewing or swallowing the food, request a change in the diet order and/or request dysphagia evaluation for suggestions.
II. Mealtime
   A. Proper positioning is a must: the hips should be in alignment with the shoulders.
   B. Placing a cracker or piece of bread in the hand sometimes helps to remind the resident that it is mealtime.
   C. For those who refuse to open their mouths, stroking the side of the mouth may stimulate an opening response.
   D. Stroking the throat in a downward motion will remind the resident to swallow.
   E. If a resident has suffered a stroke to the right side, place food in the mouth on the left side.
   F. Use self-help feeding devices with instructions given for the proper use to the resident and staff. When a plate guard is used, nursing aides must remember if the resident pushes or pulls the food for proper plate guard placement.
III. Feeding the cancer patient
   A. Preferences are varied and it is difficult to obtain a complete list of likes and dislikes because many times the thought of food is nauseating to the resident. There are a few consistent patterns to take into consideration:
      1. Do not provide double servings or large servings unless re-

quested. Often a large amount of food can depress whatever appetite is present.

2. Encourage the staff to remove the plate cover before entering the patient's room because the odor of food, especially combined odors, may be nauseating to the resident.

3. Sweets generally are not preferred but a carbonated beverage such as ginger ale may be accepted. Encourage residents to have nursing contact the dietitian/dietary manager when they feel like talking about their food preferences. Provide them with a list of food items available upon request at any time.

4. Of all flavors preferred, black walnut seems to be the one most requested. Some commercial supplements may not be available in this flavor. However, try an artificial flavoring in fortified milk or instant breakfast without the added sugar to determine acceptance.

5. Encourage family support and the bringing of the resident's favorite food items.

6. If there are dietary restrictions, try to eliminate them. Remember that with the cancer resident weight gain is not a feasible goal, but minimizing weight loss is the desired goal.

IV. State regulations related to feeding:

Surveyors will observe if residents consume 75 percent or more of the food offered and if not try to find out why. They look to determine if the proper consistency of diet was ordered or requested, if the food is acceptable in flavor and temperature, if the resident's food preferences are being followed, if nursing is offering a menu substitution, and if proper positioning and mouth care are in place.

Remember, it is your responsibility to address residents' behaviors through the use of care plans. For example, if you have a resident who normally eats in a position that does not allow for adequate food intake but refuses to be positioned, your care plan must address this problem and you must document the approaches and attempts you have made to correct it. If a resident normally eats only 50 percent of the food offered and is maintaining an appropriate weight, again this fact must be documented. Indicate in your notes the comments or explanations provided to the resident and the resident's responses.

V. Suggested activities

A. Have employees try to drink water with their head tilted back as far as possible, then tilted back slightly, and finally tilted forward slightly to see which way is easiest to swallow liquids.

B. Have employees feed each other. After the feeding takes place, ask the employee who was being fed what was right or wrong with the feeding. Was the feeding too fast? Was there conversation? Was the food seasoned? Was attention given to proper positioning?

Quiz

1. List 3 ways to increase a resident's food consumption.
2. List 2 items state surveyors will look for during mealtime to assure that state regulations are being followed.
3. List two special techniques in feeding the cancer patient.
4. Define proper positioning of a resident for mealtime.

Answer Sheet for Quiz

1. Ways to increase a resident's food consumption: (1) Assure proper positioning; (2) request a multi-vitamin supplement, (3) prepare resident for a meal by proper mouth care and by waking him or her up at least 15 minutes before breakfast; (4) place a piece of bread in the hand; (5) consult with the speech therapist if the physician approves.
2. State inspectors will be looking for several items during mealtime to assure that state regulations are being followed: The offer of meal replacements if less than 75 percent of the food is consumed; proper tray pass; proper positioning; and honoring of food preferences.
3. Special techniques in feeding the cancer patient: Avoid large servings unless desired by the resident, avoid food and other odors; capitalize on those times the resident will eat.
4. Proper positioning of a resident for mealtime: Feet on the floor, hips in alignment with shoulders; If the resident is fed in bed, knees should be slightly bent, hips in alignment with shoulders, and the patient sitting in at least a 45° angle.

DIETARY INSERVICE: WORK SIMPLIFICATION

I. Definition: Work simplification is the process of making a job easier. It is the organized use of common sense to find easier and better ways of doing work.
   A. Higher quality product
   B. Increased efficiency
II. Steps in work simplification
   A. Select the job to be improved.
   B. Make a detailed breakdown of the job.
   C. Challenge each operation and detail.
   D. Work out a better method of doing the job.
      1. Eliminate
      2. Combine
      3. Rearrange
      4. Simplify
   E. Apply the new method.
III. Principles
   A. Make rhythmic and smooth flowing motions such as overlapping, figure eight stroke, and circular motion.
      1. Spreading frosting on a cake
      2. Sandwich making
      3. Stirring
      4. Slicing or chopping vegetables using a French knife
      5. Floor mopping
   B. Make both hands productive at the same time.
      1. The motion of the two hands should be symmetrical and simultaneous.
      2. Productivity is doubled in specific tasks.
         a. Making grilled cheese sandwiches
         b. Breading chicken pieces
   C. Make hand and body motions few, short, and simple.
      1. When it is possible to accomplish a task by using a hand motion, it is inefficient to use the whole arm.
      2. When it is possible to accomplish a task by an arm motion, it is inefficient to use a reach that requires the whole body to move or turn.
   D. Maintain comfortable working positions and conditions.
      1. Worktable height
      2. Good lighting
      3. Noise and vibration
      4. Ventilation
   E. Locate materials for an efficient sequence of motions.
      1. Tray line setup
      2. Dishwashing techniques
      3. Wrapping silverware
   F. Use the best available equipment for the job.

        1. Steamer
          a. Boil eggs
          b. Cook eggs for salads—remove shells before cooking
        2. Lakeside carts
        3. Bins with wheels
        4. Slicer
          a. Slice tomatoes
          b. Slice cucumbers
        5. Pastry bag
          a. Deviled eggs
          b. Stuffed fruits and vegetables
    G. Locate activity in normal work areas when possible (within range of motion).
    H. Store materials in an orderly manner.
IV. Evaluate Methods and Costs

Quiz

T F   1. Work simplification means to make a job easier while sacrificing some product quality.

T F   2. The quickest method to make sandwiches for 50 residents is to assemble them individually.

T F   3. Before making a change to simplify a job, a detailed breakdown of the present system must be evaluated.

T F   4. The most efficient way to boil eggs is in the steamer.

T F   5. Vegetables such as onions, tomatoes, or cucumbers must be sliced with either a French knife or food processor. The slicer is inappropriate.

T F   6. Always use a lakeside cart to "collect" all items needed in the storeroom prior to a meal.

T F   7. It is okay to chop onions using a paring knife.

T F   8. It is unrealistic to make both hands productive at the same time such as in sandwich making.

T F   9. It is best to mop the floor by utilizing smooth flowing motions.

T F 10. Making hand and body motions few, short, and simple is an important principle of work simplification.

DIETARY INSERVICE: THERAPEUTIC DIETS AND RATIONALE FOR USE

Several different types of therapeutic diets are used in health care facilities. We will discuss the general principles of each and what conditions will warrant their use.

1. *Regular diet:* Provides all the nutrients needed for individuals in a day's time. There are no restrictions on this diet. It is used for patients who have no special dietary needs.
2. *Soft/mechanical soft diet:* Provides foods that are soft in consistency, easily digested, and easy to chew. Meats are usually ground. Used for patients who have difficulty in chewing or swallowing, whose dentures do not fit well, or who do not have dentures or teeth. Also used as the final stage for the postoperative patient before resuming a regular diet.
3. *Bland diet:* Rarely prescribed anymore. The main items restricted on this diet are chili powder, black and red pepper, and caffeine. Other items restricted would be those that cause distress to the individual. Used for patients who need to avoid irritation to the digestive tract (ulcer and colitis patients).
4. *Low residue/fiber:* Seldom used. Provides foods low in fiber/bulk. It omits foods that are difficult to digest. Used in patients with rectal diseases where the lower digestive tract needs to be spared.
5. *High fiber:* Provides any foods high in fiber, such as bran, fruits, and vegetables. Used in patients with diverticulosis, irritable bowel syndrome, and constipation.
6. *Clear liquid/full liquid:* Clear liquid diet allows broth, ginger ale, and certain fruit juices. Full liquid diet allows those foods that are liquid at body temperature such as liquids, ice cream, gelatin, etc. Used in patients who are having short-term digestive problems, such as nausea/vomiting. Also used as progressive diets after surgery.
7. *High calorie:* Provides nutritious foods that are high in calories such as ice cream and milkshakes. Used for patients who are malnourished or underweight.
8. *Low calorie:* Provides a limited caloric intake. Restricts fats, desserts, etc. Used for patients who are overweight.
9. *Diabetic:* Provides a balanced intake of carbohydrates, protein, and fats. Used to help control blood sugars in diabetics.
10. *High protein:* Includes extra amounts of high-protein foods, such as meat, fish, cheese, milk, and eggs. Used in patients who have pressure sores or other skin problems. Also helps in growth and repair of tissues wasted by disease.
11. *Low protein:* Limits foods that are high in protein. Used primarily in patients with kidney disease and diseases of the liver.
12. *Low fat:* Limits foods high in fat, such as butter, cream, fats, and eggs. Used in diseases where there is difficulty with digestion of fats, as with gallbladder, cardiovascular, and liver diseases.

13. *Low cholesterol:* Low in eggs, whole milk, certain fats; some restrictions on meats. Used when blood cholesterol levels are high.
14. *Low sodium:* No salt allowed in cooking or at the table; restrictions on foods high in sodium. Used in patients who have fluid retention or certain heart or kidney conditions.
15. *Tube feeding:* A commercial formula is given to the patient through some type of feeding tube. Used in patients who are unable to swallow or to tolerate oral feeding, or who cannot maintain an adequate oral intake.

Quiz

1. Name one spice that is restricted on a bland diet.
2. If a person were having gallbladder attacks, what type of diet would probably be needed?
3. If you had a patient that was below ideal body weight, what type of diet would you suggest?
4. Name one food that would be served often on a high-protein diet.
5. If you had been having frequent nausea and vomiting, what diet would you follow for a few days?
6. Are there any restrictions on a regular diet?
7. Name one food that is high in sodium.

DIETARY INSERVICE: EFFECTIVE USE OF LEFTOVERS

I. Introduction
   A. An excessive quantity of food left at the end of a meal is usually due to overproduction.
   B. The most effective approach to leftovers is not to overproduce.
      1. Follow recipes
      2. Follow production sheets
      3. Use correct portion sizes
II. Activity
   A. Ask employees how they use leftovers.
      1. Bread, crackers, and pasta
      2. Cakes and cookies
      3. Eggs
      4. Poultry
      5. Meat
      6. Vegetables
      7. Fruits
   B. Compare answers with handout A.
III. Storage of leftovers
   A. Label, date, cover, and refrigerate leftovers immediately.
   B. If leftovers are to be served hot, heat to an internal temperature of at least 160°F.
   C. Leftovers can be stored under refrigeration for 48 hours depending on the facility's policy.
   D. Leftovers can be frozen for an extended period of time (see handout B).
IV. Recommendations
   A. Whenever possible, wrap portions individually rather than several together.
   B. Wrap in clear plastic food wrap and then with aluminum foil for double protection against freezer burn.
   C. Note if product (meat) is cooked or raw.
   D. When layered items are to be frozen, separate each layer with waxed paper to insure easy separation upon thawing.

Handout A: Effective Use of Leftovers

Starred items can be used as diabetic nourishment.

Breads, crackers, pasta
   Bread crumbs for toppings
   Cracker crumbs for toppings
   Croutons for soup accompaniment
   Stuffing (dressing)
   Bread pudding

French toast
Rice custard
Soup with rice, spaghetti, or noodles
Casseroles with rice, spaghetti, or noodles

Cakes and cookies

Selective dessert cart
Freeze until next menu cycle
HS snack
Crumb cookies
Trifle
Cake and cookie crumbs in place of graham cracker crumbs
Cake in place of bread in bread pudding

Eggs

Wedges of hard-boiled eggs for garnish
Deviled eggs
Potato salad
Egg salad, chicken salad, tuna salad*

Meats

Sliced for meat sandwiches*
Ground or cubed for meat salad sandwiches*
Ground for meat sauce, stuffed peppers, chili, cabbage rolls, and so on
Cubed for beef tips or stew
Bar-B-Q meat sandwiches
In soups
Frozen and used as meat alternate

Poultry

Sliced for sandwiches*
Ground or cubed for salad sandwiches*
Soups
Frozen and used as meat alternate
Cubed for casseroles

Vegetables

Frozen and used as vegetable alternate
Frozen and used in combination with other vegetables for "mixed vegetables"
Soups
Stews
Casseroles
Salads
Garnish
Potatoes (hash browns, lyonnaise potatoes, duchess potatoes, potato salad)
Tomatoes (sauces, meatloaf, chili, salads, garnish)

Fruits

Selective dessert cart

Fruit alternate
Garnish
Cobblers
Muffins and quick breads
Fruit salad or fruit cup
Gelatin salads

Handout B: Freezer Storage Times[a]

Product	Months at 0° F
Poultry	
Chicken (whole or quartered)	10
Chicken livers	3
Cooked poultry	6
Turkey, duck, goose	6
Fish	
Fillets and steaks (cod, flounder, haddock, sole)	6
Fillets and steaks (perch, salmon, "fatty fish")	2.5
Breaded fish or seafood	3
Clams	3
Cooked fish or seafood	3
Crab	10
Lobster tails	3
Scallops	3
Shrimp, raw only	12
Beef/veal	
Beef (roast only)	6–12
Veal (roast only)	6–9
Beef (ground meat only)	2–3
Veal (ground meat only)	2–3
Pork	
Roast (fresh, unsmoked)	3–6
Chops (fresh, unsmoked)	2–3
Cubed or ground (fresh, unsmoked)	1 to 2
Bacon and ham (smoked, cured)	1 Max.
Frankfurters and luncheon meats (freezing not recommended— emulsion may be broken and product will "weep")	
Sausage, bulk and link (freezing alters flavor of this product)	1 to 2

[a]All storage times are for uncooked meat unless noted otherwise.

Quiz

1. Name one way to avoid leftovers.
2. What is the correct storage procedure for leftovers in the refrigerator and freezer?

3. What is the length of time leftovers can be stored under refrigeration?
4. If you have two cups of green beans left after a meal is served, what should you do with the beans?
5. If you have three pork cutlets left after meal service, what should you do?
6. How would you use the following?
    a. Broken cookies
    b. Leftover cornbread or biscuits
    c. 5 servings of cake
    d. Stale bread
    e. 1/2 can of fruit

DIETARY INSERVICE: KEEPING A CHILD HEALTHY AND HAPPY

I. Need for a healthy diet

Children of any age need nutrients and calories for proper growth. Adults eat to maintain weight and repair tissues while children eat to add new tissues and to grow. Food gives nutrients and energy for their changing bodies. As a general rule, children do not need weight reduction diets which may deprive them of essential nutrients. Children have small stomachs and cannot eat large quantities at one time. Therefore, they need meals with nutritious foods and healthy snacks in between meals.

II. Daily food needs of growing children (refer to handout A)

III. Tips on meals and snacks for young children

    A. Try to serve meals at the same time each day.

    B. Introduce new foods in small amounts, one at a time. Do not be surprised if the child plays with the food, is reluctant to try new foods, and rebels if forced to eat. Most children go through these periods. Include well-liked foods in the same meal with new or less popular ones. Do not force or bribe a child to eat.

    C. Snacks are not always bad. The important thing is for snacks to be nutritious, not "empty calorie" foods.

    D. If you are concerned with nutritional deficiencies in your child's diet try to monitor food intake over a period of time. Usually the deficiencies in the diet on one day are made up on another day.

    E. Children may get into a "food jag," wanting to eat a certain food every chance they get. It typically occurs among toddlers. As long as the food is nutritious and the jag does not last long, there is nothing to worry about.

    F. Children's appetites may suddenly decrease around the age of two because of a slowing in their growth. As growth slows so do energy requirements.

    G. Children involved in meal preparation are more enthusiastic about eating and trying new foods (see handout B).

IV. Special problems

    A. Overweight

        1. Do not drastically cut food intake.

        2. Encourage the child to eat favorite high-fat, "empty calorie" foods less often.

        3. Avoid using food as a reward.

        4. Encourage more physical activities.

    B. Underweight

        1. Never force eating. Tension at mealtime has negative results.

        2. Serve your child small portions. Many children prefer to eat frequent meals instead of just three a day.

        3. Offer a variety of foods. Do not be afraid to serve foods that are high in fat and calories, including whole milk and cheese.

Handout A: Daily Food Needs of Growing Children[a]

	Average Serving Size	
Food Group	1–3 Years	4–10 Years
Milk (4 servings each day)		
Milk	3/4–1 1/2 cups	3/4–1 cup
Cheese	1 oz.	3/4–1 1/2 oz.
Yogurt	1/2 cup	3/4–1 cup
Meat (2 or more servings each day)		
Meat, Fish, Poultry	2–3 tbsp.	2–3 oz.
Eggs	1 whole	1 whole
Peanut butter	1–2 tbsp.	2–3 tbsp.
Luncheon meat	1 slice	2 slices
Vegetables, fruits (4 or more servings each day)		
Orange, tomato juice	1/2 cup	1/2–1 cup
Strawberries	3/4 cup	1 cup
Broccoli, spinach, carrots	1/4 cup	1/4 cup
Cantaloupe	1/4 fruit	1/4–1/2 fruit
Potato	1/4–1/2	1/2–1
Apple, banana	1/4–1/2	1/2–1
Breads and cereals (4 or more servings each day)		
Bread	1/2–1 slice	1–2 slices
Dry cereal (unsweetened)	1/2–3/4 cup	1 cup
Cooked cereal, rice, pasta	2–4 tbsp.	1/2 cup

[a]Adequate calories are essential to growth. Toddlers (2–3 years) should be eating 1,000–1,300 calories a day, while children 4–10 years old should be eating 1,700–2,100 calories a day. The calories should come from a variety of foods, because no single food contains all the essential nutrients.

Handout B: Involving Children in Meal Preparation

Children involved in meal preparation develop a more active interest in food. They can accomplish many different tasks when working one-on-one with an adult in the kitchen. Activities that children can do successfully at various ages are listed below. Having patience and time to spend is the key to success.

If you would like to involve children in food preparation, be sure to

- Supervise all activities
- Match the task to the child's capabilities
- Provide detailed instructions, demonstrations, and time for practice
- Repeat instructions before a child begins to perform a task

- Incorporate cleanup as part of each job
- Have children stand on sturdy stools when necessary to perform some tasks

Food Preparation Activities

Two- and three-year olds
    Wash vegetables
    Shuck corn
    Snap beans
    Unload dishwasher
    Wipe table
    Put toast in toaster
    Tear lettuce
    Shape burgers and meatballs
    Peel bananas (if the top is cut)
    Place things in the trash
    Clear own place setting
Three- and four-year olds
    Break eggs into a bowl
    Measure and mix ingredients
    Open packages
    Knead and shape dough
    Turn pancakes and grilled foods with help
    Pour cereal, milk, and water
    Make sandwiches
    Toss salads
    "Wash" baking utensils (water play)
Five-year olds
    Make cakes and cookies using baking mixes
    Use blenders or hand mixers with close supervision
    Set and clear the table
    Load the dishwasher
    Make pancakes, French toast, scrambled eggs, hot cereal, and rice with close supervision

Quiz

1. As a general rule, children do not need weight reduction diets.
    _____ True
    _____ False
2. What is a "food jag"?
3. Name two ways to promote weight loss for an overweight child.
4. Name two ways to promote weight gain in an underweight child.
5. Toddlers (2–3 years) need approximately _____ calories per day while children 4–10 years old need __ calories per day.

DIETARY INSERVICE: QUALITY ASSURANCE IN FOOD PREPARATION

The ultimate test of quality control system in a foodservice operation is the acceptance or rejection of foods by the resident. Plate waste should be routinely noted as trays come back. Residents should be visited at mealtimes to check for consumption and any problems they may have. Negative comments should be followed up to determine whether they are valid and then necessary changes made. Reducing plate waste is an excellent way to reduce food cost as well as to satisfy residents.

Quality Assurance Criteria

I. Food appearance
   A. The appropriate color for each item
   B. A pleasant variety of food color combinations
   C. Attractive garnishes
   D. Variety in the shape and size of food items
   E. Adequate portion sizes and correct utensils
   F. Food is neatly prepared and served (for example, sandwich filling should not hang out, and cobbler filling should not drip on the side of the bowl.

II. Food taste
   A. Pleasant flavor combinations
   B. Characteristic taste of food items preserved
   C. Adequate seasoning (when diet allows)
   D. No undesirable or off-flavors
   E. Pleasing aroma
   F. Proper temperature

III. Food texture
   A. Proper texture for each item; neither overcooked nor undercooked (especially vegetables)
   B. Variety of textures
   C. Suitable moisture content
   D. Meat texture: not tough or stringy (Meat should be prepared by the correct cooking method. When a less tender cut of meat is used, cook with a moist heat method.)
   E. Texture suitable for resident's specific diet orders

IV. Food safety
   A. Proper hot serving temperature is maintained: minimum 140°F.
   B. Proper cold serving temperature is maintained: liquids 35°F, foods 45°F.
   C. Foods are prepared and portioned using utensils or disposable gloves to avoid contamination by employees' hands.
   D. Clean spoons or forks instead of preparation utensils are used for tasting food products.

E. Special care is used in handling clean dishes and utensils to prevent contamination.

F. Unused raw ingredients or cooked leftover foods are refrigerated promptly and used within 24–48 hours, or frozen immediately.

G. Single use utensils and containers are not reused.

H. Employees' clothing and personal hygiene meet established standards.

V. Tray appearance

A. Tray size is adequate; overcrowding is avoided.

B. The specified setup is used.

C. Each item is correctly placed on the tray and arranged for eating convenience.

D. Dishes and flatware are in good condition.

E. Food is neatly served, with no spills.

F. Separate dishes are used for foods that contain liquid.

VI. Tray accuracy

A. All food items specified on the menu are present on the tray; the preparation method is as specified on the menu or recipe. Recipes are followed correctly.

B. The food on the tray is allowed on the resident's diet.

C. Correct utensils are provided on the tray.

Quiz

T F 1. Overcooking and cooking in too much liquid are the two most common errors of vegetable cookery.

T F 2. Once a product has been made following a recipe, there is no need to use the recipe next time the product is made.

T F 3. "Portion control" means "serving the correct and specified amount of a prepared item."

T F 4. Plate waste is a good indicator of food acceptance.

T F 5. Spills on a tray should always be wiped up before the tray is sent out to the resident.

6. Hot foods must be served at a temperature greater than_____.

7. Name one way that you can be sure that juices are served at the correct temperature.

8. Name one method used to tenderize meat.

DIETARY INSERVICE: FACTS AND FADS—
WEIGHT CONTROL DIETS

I. Administer pre-test.
II. Discuss pre-test questions.
   1. Weight is usually kept off if lost slowly. With rapid weight loss, much is fluid loss and weight is usually put back on.
   2. Neither fat nor any other nutrient should ever be eliminated from the diet. There are essential fatty acids found in fats that are necessary to bodily functions.
   3. Any type of fat has the same calorie content: 1 g fat = 9 kcal.
   4. One g carbohydrate = 4 kcal and 1 g protein = 4 kcal.
   5. "Diet" foods are not necessarily lower in calories. There are many types of diet foods designed for different kinds of diets, such as salt-restricted diets and low-fat diets, as well as calorie-restricted diets.
   6. Toasting bread does not change calories. The only way calorie content would be affected is if something is added prior to toasting.
   7. Children who gain an excessive amount of weight in the first year of life tend to develop additional fat cells that they can never lose. These babies tend to retain this extra fat in adulthood.
   8. Again, weight is more apt to be kept off, if lost slowly.
   9. Exercise helps with weight loss by raising your metabolic rate, allowing calories to be burned faster.
   10. One lb. of fat represents the intake of 3,500 kcal; therefore, to lose 1 lb./week, you must reduce your intake by 500 kcal/day (3,500 kcal/week).
   11. Again, no nutrient should to be eliminated completely from the diet. (Starches are complete or complex carbohydrates needed by the body.)
   12. Gelatin is often considered a "diet" food, but it is only "empty calories." 1/2 cup = 100 calories.
   13. Both pork and beef have approximately the same number of kcals if both are lean cuts and trimmed of fat.
   14. The fat-soluble vitamins (A, D, E, and K) can be toxic in excessive amounts. Excess water-soluble vitamins are excreted in the urine.
   15. One oz. of meat prepared in a low-calorie way such as by broiling or baking contains about as many calories as a slice of bread.
   16. Meal skipping usually causes you to eat excessive amounts at the next meal or to snack between meals.
   17. High-protein foods and fruits do have calories. Protein foods contain protein and fat. Fruits contain carbohydrates.
   18. You can lose fat and gain muscle and the scales may show a weight gain because muscle weighs more than fat.
   19. Honey, like white sugar, is high in carbohydrates and calories. One tablespoon of honey contains 64 kcal and 1 tablespoon of sugar contains 46 kcal.

20. Again, gelatin is high in calories and contains minimal nutrients. 1/2 cup gelatin = 100 calories.

Facts and Fads—Weight Control Diets Pre-test

T F 1. Quick reducing diets are the best way to lose weight.
T F 2. When on a reducing diet, never eat fat.
T F 3. Margarine and butter have the same calorie content.
T F 4. Carbohydrates are more fattening than protein.
T F 5. "Dietetic" foods are always lower in calories than their regular food counterparts.
T F 6. Toast has fewer calories than untoasted bread.
T F 7. The best time to start weight watching is in childhood.
T F 8. Losing 1–2 lb. a week over several months is better than going on a "crash" diet.
T F 9. Exercise is no help in weight control; it just makes you hungry.
T F 10. One lb. of body fat represents the storage of 3,500 calories.
T F 11. One of the best ways to lose weight is to cut as much sugar and starch out of your diet as possible.
T F 12. A cup of gelatin dessert contains about 200 calories, more than the average serving of ice cream.
T F 13. Pork is more fattening than beef.
T F 14. A well-balanced daily diet supplies the necessary amounts of most vitamins and minerals, and scientific data have proven that excesses of some vitamins can be very toxic.
T F 15. One oz. of meat contains about the same number of calories as a slice of bread.
T F 16. Meal skipping is a good way to lose weight.
T F 17. High-protein foods and fruits have no calories.
T F 18. You can lose fat while the scales stay the same.
T F 19. Honey can be used on a diabetic diet, because it is a natural sugar.
T F 20. One-third cup of gelatin contains almost the same number of calories as a slice of bread.

DIETARY INSERVICE: SAFETY FIRST

Objectives

1. To understand how good safety precautions help prevent accidents
2. To become familiar with good safety procedures
3. To know what to do in case of an accident

Introduction

Every person has the right to work under safe conditions. In 1970 the Occupational Safety and Health Act was passed to guarantee that right to every working American. This act is often referred to as OSHA.

Good safety practices are important in preventing accidents in institutional kitchens.

Safety Points

There are three important points to consider when we speak of employee safety:

1. Safe equipment to use
2. Knowledge of correct safety precautions
3. The practice of good safety precautions

To know good safety measures is not enough. They must be practiced. If an accident does happen it should be reported immediately to the person in charge.

Accidents

What are some types of accidents that can occur in the kitchen?

1. Falls
2. Burns
3. Cuts
4. Backstrain from lifting

Which one of these do you think is the most common in institutional kitchens? Falls occur most often in institutional kitchens.

Falls

The most common causes of falls are

1. Wet floors
2. Spills on floors
3. Small items or clutter on floors

Falling can easily be avoided. As a matter of fact, it has been found that 90 percent of all accidents can be avoided. Safety is everyone's business and everyone's right.

If there has been a fall, do not move the person. He or she may have a broken bone. Get professional help.

Burns

Burns are another hazard in the kitchen. Stoves, ovens, and grills should be turned off as soon as they are no longer needed. The handles of pots and pans on the stove should be turned away from the front of the stove. Otherwise, they may be knocked over.

Towels should never be used to remove hot pans from the stove or oven. Dry potholders should be used.

If there is a burn, do you know what to do? Cold water or ice should be placed on the burn immediately. Never place butter on a burn.

Cuts

Cuts can also happen easily. It is important always to use safety guards on the food slicer. Never put your fingers near the blade of the food slicer. Always unplug the slicer when you are finished with it. It should be cleaned very carefully and never taken apart but put in the sink for someone to wash.

Knives should never be put in the sink. It is very easy for someone to put a hand in the sink without knowing a knife is there and receive a cut.

Tampers should be used to push food through the food grinder—never hands or spoon handles.

Never put your hands near the garbage disposal. If the garbage disposal should become jammed, turn it off and notify the supervisor.

If someone does receive a cut, the bleeding must be stopped as soon as possible. Pressure should be applied to the cut with a bandage, clean cloth, or even your finger if necessary.

Backstrain

Backstrain can happen very easily. Never lift items that are too heavy. There is a proper way to lift. Do you know what it is?

If an employee can demonstrate the correct lifting method, ask that person to demonstrate.

You should always use your leg muscles to pick up anything that is heavy. Stand with your legs slightly apart and your knees bent. You should never use your back muscles—they are not strong enough.

Back strain is very serious and may take a long time to heal. Never try to lift anything that you know is too heavy. Ask someone for help.

Safety Tips

Safety is everyone's responsibility. Here are some tips to remember:

1. Keep electrical cords in good working order; if frayed, notify your supervisor.
2. Carry knives with the point downward.
3. Always use a cutting board.
4. Report broken equipment to your supervisor immediately.
5. Wear shoes with rubber soles and closed toes.
6. Sweep up broken china and glass immediately.
7. Keep floors free of debris.
8. Wipe up spills immediately.
9. Report any unsafe conditions to your supervisor.

It is your responsibility to help make your kitchen a safe environment to work in!

Quiz

Mrs. Lane is 49 years old. She is a cook at the Goldenbriar Nursing Home. She likes her job very much and has worked at the nursing home for 12 years. She is friendly with all the patients and staff.

Bill Waters is the night maintenance man at Goldenbriar. He is 22 and works part time while he attends college.

One afternoon, while Mrs. Lane was making gravy for the evening meal, she accidentally spilled some of it on the stove and floor. She had been very busy all afternoon and was behind schedule. She took the gravy pot off the stove when the phone rang in the office.

Off she ran to answer the phone, being careful not to step on the gravy on the floor. Meanwhile, Bill Waters had reported to the kitchen to start work and noticed the gas burner on. Bill went over to the stove to turn off the flame. Not seeing the spilled gravy on the floor, he slipped and fell. He had a great deal of pain in his back. Mrs. Lane heard a scream and ran out of the office to see what was wrong. She found Bill lying on the floor and in pain.

1. If you were Mrs. Lane, what would you do when you found Bill Waters?
2. Why did this accident happen?
3. How could this accident have been avoided?
4. Could other accidents also have happened because of this incident?

DIETARY INSERVICE: PRESENTING MEALS WITH FLAIR

I. Definition of *garnish*: "An edible ornament that is added to a dish to make food more satisfying to the eye and palate."
II. Reasons for garnishing
    A. The ultimate goal of cooking is to present foods that have as much eye appeal as taste appeal. There's an old saying, "That which is pleasing to the eye is also pleasing to the appetite."
    B. The appeal of foods depends greatly upon presentation. Garnishing adds to food presentation.
    C. Garnishing gives food that finished look.
III. Criteria for garnishes
    A. Simplicity may create more eye appeal than elaborate garnishes.
    B. Garnishes should add contrast in color and shape.
    C. A garnish should be relative to the size of the food it garnishes.
    D. A good garnish complements the flavor and texture of the food it garnishes.
    E. Freshness in appearance is essential.
IV. Criteria for good plate presentation
    A. Attractiveness in plate presentation can be gained by using good arrangement and food combinations.
    B. Cutting sandwiches into varied shapes can add interest.
    C. Different shaped glasses used in plate presentation add variety.
    D. Foods in liquids are best served in separate dishes and then placed on the plate.
    E. Bread and butter plates should be used to serve breads or bread should be placed in bread bags. This prevents bread from absorbing liquids of other foods resulting in an unacceptable product.
    F. Recipes and plate presentation guides are designed to aid staff in serving food attractively.
V. Activities: Use food pictures from magazines to illustrate the criteria for garnishment and plate presentation.

Quiz

1. What is a garnish?
2. Name one reason for garnishing.
3. The arrangement of the food on the plate is an important part of eye appeal.
    _____ True
    _____ False
4. What is a good way to serve bread to prevent it from absorbing liquids from the plate?
5. Garnishes should add contrast in _____

DIETARY INSERVICE: MENU SUBSTITUTIONS

I. Definition
II. Desirability of avoiding substitutions
  A. Change is a cause of change
  B. Decreased control
    1. Nutrition
    2. Costs
    3. Purchasing
III. Reasons for substitutions (Ask class to classify reasons as good or poor and note on blackboard.)
  A. Good reasons
    1. Patient preference
    2. Holiday/special meal
    3. Delivery failure
  B. Poor reasons
    1. Product sales
    2. Errors
      a. Preparation
      b. Purchasing
      c. Quantity determinations
IV. Procedures
  A. Change the posted menu copy face or affix the change to the menu.
  B. Keep a permanent record of the change and the reason for it. (Show an example of Menu Substitution Form.)
  C. Outline staff responsibilities.
V. Importance of equivalence
  A. Explain handout A, Equivalent Menu Substitutions.
  B. Discuss examples of equivalent sustitutions.

Handout A: Equivalent Menu Substitutions

The following is a list of suggested substitutions for menu items, should the need arise. The items within each category contain approximately the same food value as other items in the category. This list has been provided for the convenience of the dietary manager. It is to be utilized only when absolutely necessary because menus have been carefully developed and approved according to nutritional values and in coordination with color, taste, and texture combinations.

Protein Entrées

The average protein serving generally is 2–3 oz., which is about the size of a dollar bill and a quarter of an inch thick. A combination of any two or three items, or a double or triple amount of the quantity listed, should be substituted to equal the amount of food value in 2–3 oz. of the original protein entrée.

Substitution	Amount	Substitution	Amount
Beef, Pork	1 oz.	Frankfurter	1
Poultry	1 oz.	Egg	1
Bacon	4 strips	Salmon, tuna	1/4 cup
Pork sausage	1 oz.	Cheddar or American cheese	1 oz.
Liver, lamb	1 oz.		
Fish	1 oz.	Cottage cheese	1/4 cup
Cold cuts	1 thin slice	Peanut butter	2 tablespoons

Vegetables

All calculations are based on the standard half-cup serving, unless indicated otherwise.

1. Collard greens, mustard greens, spinach, turnip greens, kale, broccoli, carrots, sweet potatoes, winter squash, pumpkin (vegetables are excellent sources of vitamin A)
2. Broccoli, tomatoes (1 cup), brussels sprouts, mustard greens (vitamin C source)
3. Cabbage, cauliflower, sauerkraut, green pepper
4. Asparagus, green beans, okra (similiar nonstarchy vegetables)
5. Cabbage, lettuce, cucumber, tomatoes (cold vegetable/salad substitutes)

Fruits

1. Cantaloupe, apricots
2. Peaches, prunes, blueberries, strawberries, raspberries, blackberries
3. Bananas, plums, pears, figs, raisins
4. Tangerines (1 cup), oranges, grapefruit, cantaloupe, strawberries
5. Applesauce, honeydew melon
6. Pineapple, cherries

Starches

1. Cereal (cooked), cereal (dry: flaked or puffed)
2. Bread, biscuits, muffins, cornbread, graham crackers, saltines, soda crackers
3. Rice, corn, pasta, baked beans (no pork), potatoes (Irish, baked, mashed, sweet, or yams)

Dairy

Cheddar or American cheese	1 1/2 oz.
Swiss cheese	1 oz.

Cottage cheese	1 1/3 cups
Ice cream	1 1/2 cups

Quiz

1. Is substitution a desirable practice?
2. What is a good reason for making a menu substitution?
   _____ Patient preference
   _____ Product sale
3. What is a poor reason for making a menu substitution?
   _____ Error in preparation or purchasing
   _____ Holiday/special meal
4. Where should a menu substitution be noted?
5. If a resident does not like the 2-oz. roast beef entrée or if you run out of roast beef, which of the following would be an equivalent substitution?
   _____ 1/4 cup cottage cheese or tuna
   _____ 2 hard-boiled eggs

DIETARY INSERVICE: CALCIUM AND ITS SOURCES

I. Introduction

Of the approximately 1,200 g of calcium in the adult body, 99 percent is combined as salts that give hardness to bones and teeth. Body need is a major factor governing the amount of calcium absorbed. Healthy adults receiving a diet that meets the recommended allowances absorb approximately 40 percent of their dietary calcium. Bone is the principal reserve of calcium and phosphorus in the body. Bones are continuously remodeled and reshaped. About 700 mg of calcium enter and leave the bone each day in the adult.

II. Factors affecting absorption
   A. Vitamin D deficiency seriously impairs the absorption of calcium.
   B. Emotional stress impairs calcium absorption.

III. Excretion

Calcium excretion is increased as protein intake is increased. Thus high-protein diets in patients with osteoporosis, weight reduction diets, and other clinical situations could lead to a negative calcium balance.

IV. Sources

Dairy products, excluding butter, account for 3/4 of calcium in the American diet. One cup of milk (in any form) contains 288 mg calcium.

V. RDAs for calcium
   A. Males 51+ years old = 800 mg
   B. Females 51+ years old = 800 mg

VI. Foods other than milk containing 130 mg or more calcium

Food	Amount		Calcium
Cheese, cottage uncreamed	1	cup	131
Tuna and noodles	5	oz.	132
Broccoli, cooked cuts	1	cup	136
Beans, pork, and tomato sauce	1	cup	138
Raisins	8	oz.	141
Cream cheese	1	cup	144
Beet greens, cooked	1	cup	144
Pie, custard, 1/6	1	piece	146
Ensure Plus, supplement	1	cup	150
McDonald's Big Mac	1		157
Pancake, 6 in.	1		157
Broccoli, cooked stalks	1		158
Soup, cream of tomato	1	cup	159
Cheese spread, American	1	oz.	160
Beans, pork and sweet	1	cup	161
Soup, cream of potato	1	cup	166
Tapioca pudding	1	cup	173
Soup, cream of chicken	1	cup	180
Sugar, brown	1	cup	187

Bread, white	8	oz.	191
Ice cream	1	cup	194
Turnip greens	1	cup	195
Cheese, cottage, small-curd	1	cup	197
Cheese, American, pasteurized process	1	oz.	198
Ice milk	1	cup	204
Rhubarb, frozen, cooked	1	cup	211
Cheese, cheddar	1	lb.	213
McDonald's hot fudge sundae	1		215
McDonald's 1/4 lb. cheeseburger	1		219
McDonald's Egg McMuffin	1		226
Spinach, frozen, cooked	1	cup	232
Pimento cheese spread	2.66	tablespoons	238
Spinach, canned	1	cup	242
Ice cream, soft serve	1	cup	253
Beans, dry, pinto	1	cup	257
Beans, dry, great northern	1	cup	259
Cheese, Swiss	1	oz.	262
Pudding, chocolate	1	cup	265
Almonds, slivered	1	cup	269
White sauce	1	cup	288
Bread pudding	1	cup	289
Yogurt	1	cup	294
Hot cocoa	1	cup	295
Buttermilk	1	cup	296
Custard, baked	1	cup	297
Potatoes, scalloped	1	cup	311
McDonald's chocolate shake	1		320
McDonald's strawberry shake	1		322
McDonald's vanilla shake	1		329
Macaroni and cheese	1	cup	362

Quiz

T   F   1. An adult over 50 years requires 4 cups of milk daily.
T   F   2. Chocolate flavored milk is not a good source of calcium.

Assume you cannot tolerate more than 1/2 cup milk daily. Using the foods listed above, write a day's menu that would bring your total daily intake to 800 mg of calcium.

DIETARY INSERVICE: MODIFICATIONS FOR CANCER TREATMENT THROUGH DIET

I. Introduction

We are now seeing more cancer patients in skilled nursing facilities, making us more aware of problems associated with these patients.

Nutritional care is a very important part of cancer treatment because chemotherapy, surgery, and the disease itself often cause the patient's appetite to change, and as a result malnutrition can occur. The dietitian's role is to find various ways to make food more attractive and acceptable, as well as to educate staff and patients on the importance of optimum nutrition intake.

Since each cancer patient is different, one needs to know what part of the body is affected in order to anticipate any difficulty in chewing or swallowing, probable degree of absorption, and other problems that may arise.

Visiting with the patient offers a chance to explore food preferences and to educate the patient on the importance of nutrition to therapy. Nutritional assessment of the patient and close monitoring of intake are also important. By following these principles one can improve the quality of life for the patient.

II. Problems associated with cancer that may cause inadequate nutrient consumption
   A. Anorexia (loss of appetite)
   B. Alteration of taste and smell
   C. Early satiety and a feeling of fullness
   D. Difficulty in chewing and swallowing
   E. Anxiety and pain

III. Therapy problems that may affect appetite
   A. Chemotherapy
      1. Nausea, vomiting, diarrhea, or constipation
      2. Mucositis, stomititis, gingivitis, and glossitis
      3. Malabsorption
      4. Anorexia
   B. Radiation therapy: dryness of mouth and loss of taste

IV. Problems which may be experienced and possible solutions
   A. Anorexia
      1. Serve small, frequent, nutritious meals.
      2. Merchandise trays: Create color and variety.
      3. Present a pleasant, relaxed atmosphere.
      4. Offer a glass of wine to help stimulate the appetite (check with the physician).
      5. Offer high-protein, high-calorie supplements.
      6. Encourage adequate food intake (the patient should not be forced to eat).
      7. Suggest a small amount of exercise before meals.
      8. Offer nourishing snacks for nibbling.
      9. Check for food preferences.

      10. Help patients understand that food and nutrition are a large part of their therapy.

B. Nausea and vomiting

    1. Provide small frequent meals (if tolerated).

    2. Caution patients to eat and drink slowly.

    3. Offer carbonated beverages, popsicles, Jello, and clear liquids to replace fluid loss.

    4. Offer dry toast and crackers.

    5. Prepare cold plates and sandwiches. Cold foods may be tolerated since these lack the aroma that may cause nausea.

    6. Offer salty foods such as broth and tart foods such as lemon to some patients with nausea.

C. Loss of taste

    1. Provide frequent, small meals.

    2. Prepare what the patient likes if possible.

    3. Utilize a nutritional supplement.

D. Alterations of taste and smell

    1. Offer acid foods to stimulate taste buds.

    2. Appeal to the senses of smell and sight.

    3. Utilize a nutritional supplement.

    4. Offer a drink before meals. Drinking liquids such as tea, gingerale, or water may eliminate the strange taste in the mouth.

E. Difficulty in chewing or swallowing

    1. Try a soft or puréed diet.

    2. Make foods moist by adding butter, sauces, and gravies.

    3. Grind meat with sauces or gravy.

    4. Avoid dry foods such as toast, crackers, or potato chips.

    5. Use a blender if necessary.

F. Early satiety and feeling of fullness

    1. Offer smaller meals more often.

    2. Keep snack foods available.

    3. Encourage the patient to chew slowly.

    4. Avoid gas-forming or greasy foods.

    5. Offer beverages that have optimum nutrition (milkshakes and nutritional supplements).

G. Glossitis, gingivitis, mucositis, and stomatitis:

    1. Offer prescribed diet as tolerated.

    2. Avoid salty foods, which may burn.

    3. Avoid rough, raw, acid, or spicy foods.

H. Constipation

    1. Increase fiber in the menu.

    2. Encourage the patient to chew food well.

    3. Increase fluids.

    4. Offer hot liquids to stimulate bowel activity.

    5. Suggest light exercise (if possible).

REFERENCE

Pratt, Mana. 1985. Modifications for cancer treatment through diet. *Indiana Consultant Dietitians in Health Care Facilities* (July).

Quiz

1. Match the following terms with their correct meaning:

a. Nausea	1. Satisfaction, especially with food/full
b. Anorexia	2. Loss of appetite
c. Gingivitis	3. Inadequate uptake of nutrients
d. Satiety	4. Unpleasant sensation usually preceding vomiting
e. Malabsorption	5. Inflammation of the gums

2. List three ways to increase cancer patients' intake.
3. List two ways to help control nausea.
4. What types of diet modifications might you make if the patient complained of inflamed gums, tongue, and mucous membranes?

DIETARY INSERVICE: CALORIES DO COUNT IN WEIGHT CONTROL

I. Introduction
    A. Explain the purpose of weight control.
    B. Explain that weight control is a matter of energy balance.
    C. Explain that healthy eating requires planning.
II. Calories and food groups
    A. Explain the terms "calorie" and "food group."
    B. Explain in general the calories in each food group.
    C. Explain how to reduce calories from each food group by choosing foods wisely and preparing them properly.
        1. Vegetables and fruits
            a. Vegetables
                i. Steam or cook vegetables in a small amount of water. Do not deep fry.
                ii. Stir-fry vegetables in a small amount of cooking oil or use nonstick cooking spray.
                iii. Season with herbs, spices, lemon, onion, vinegar, or "Butter Buds."
                iv. Potatoes are allowed. A medium baked one has only 100 calories.
            b. Fruits
                i. Use fresh or frozen, packed without sugar or in light syrup; or canned, packed in water, juice, or light syrup.
                ii. Compare labels for calories. Remember each teaspoon of sugar adds 15 calories.
        2. Breads and cereals
            a. Breads
                i. Breads do not have to be omitted from a reducing diet.
                ii. Choose carefully. Whole grains add variety and nutrients. Using thin-sliced bread saves 20 or more calories per slice.
                iii. Use cornbread sparingly. It has over 100 calories per 1-1/2-in. square.
                iv. Tortilla shells are in this group. Calories vary but some are as low as 50 calories each. Read labels.
                v. Pastas add variety. Watch serving sizes.
                vi. Use rice cakes for open-faced sandwiches or snacks. Rice cakes are only 35 calories each.
            b. Cereals
                i. Buy unsweetened products such as Cheerios, Shredded Wheat, Puffed Wheat, or Puffed Rice. Use artificial sweetener instead of sugar.
                ii. Avoid granola cereals, or choose those without added items.

      iii. Buy regular oatmeal (quick-cooking or old fashioned). Avoid instant oatmeal mixes wtih fruit or high calorie additives.

3. Milk and cheese
   a. Use low-fat or skim dairy products.
   b. Choose plain yogurt and add your own fruit. Use yogurt instead of sour cream in dips.
   c. Use neufchatel cheese instead of cream cheese.
4. Meat, poultry, fish, and beans
   a. Buy cuts with little fat marbling.
   b. Trim visible fat. Remove poultry skin prior to cooking.
   c. Use luncheon meats sparingly
   d. Bake, broil, grill, stew, or stir-fry.
   e. Cook soups and stews ahead and skim excess fat.
   f. Use water-packed tuna—200 calories per 6.5-oz. can.
   g. Use canned mackerel and salmon for low calories and high calcium content.
5. Fats and oils
   a. Reduce fat in recipes by 1/3 in sauces, puddings, and quick breads.
   b. Salad dressings
      i. Use lemon juice or vinegar instead of commercial dressings.
      ii. Use light versions and reduce calories by 1/3.
      iii. Make your own with a vinegar, tomato juice, or low-fat yogurt base.
   c. Sour cream (25 calories per tablespoon compared to 100 calories for butter)
   d. Butter or margarine
      i. Use sparingly.
      ii. Use diet margarine and save 50 calories per tablespoon compared to regular margarine and butter.
6. Miscellaneous
   a. Use club soda or seltzer for no-calorie beverages.
   b. Use artificial sweeteners in place of sugar in uncooked foods and artificially sweetened products such as puddings and gelatins.
   c. To whiten coffee use nonfat dry milk powder.
   d. Use plain popcorn as a snack.
   e. Reduce sugar in recipes by 1/3 in fruit drinks, puddings, and some cakes and cookies.

III. Light, reduced-calorie, and low-calorie foods
    A. Reduced-calorie foods are required to have 1/3 fewer calories than the standard product.

    B. Low-calorie foods are limited to a maximum of 40 calories per serving or 4 calories per gram.

    C. Light foods have no set definition. Some are lower in fats, others are lower in sugar, and some are lower in fats and sugars; all are generally lower in calories.

    D. Look at labels of such items as reduced-calorie salad dressings, light cheeses, and canned fruits. Compare these labels with labels on regular products. Also compare appearance, flavor, consistency, and cost in addition to nutrient content and calories.

IV. Menu planning with fewer calories

    A. Explain that 1,200 calories is a good baseline and can be used for an adult female to lose 1 lb. per week. Adult males need about 1,800 calories.

    B. Discuss two sample 1,200-calorie reducing diets.

        1. Ask how further calories could be cut from the 1,200 calorie diet plan.

        2. Ask how calories could be added to supply 1,800 calories for adult males.

V. Reducing calories in recipes

    A. Use a macaroni and cheese recipe as an example.

        1. Make substitutions in the recipe.

            a. Use diet margarine.

            b. Use skim or low-fat milk.

            c. Use only egg whites instead of whole eggs.

        2. Use light ingredients.

            a. Skim milk

            b. Diet margarine

Quiz

1. What is energy balance?
2. How does weight gain occur?
3. List six methods to reduce calories in food preparation.
4. List four ways to save calories when shopping for food.

DIETARY INSERVICE: PRESSURE SORES

I. Define pressure sores and discuss how they form.
   A. A pressure sore is an open sore of the skin or membrane resulting from prolonged pressure, which interferes with blood circulation to the skin.
   B. If not cared for, a pressure sore can progress to an open wound that is difficult to treat and can lead to infection and death.

II. Discuss the prevalence of pressure sores and the costs involved.
   A. They are common among long-term care patients.
   B. Care involves time-consuming procedures such as frequent turnings and constant monitoring by nursing.
   C. Treatments can cost facilities close to $10,000 per year.

III. Discuss ways to reduce the occurrence of pressure sores.
   A. Evaluating all residents on admission who are at risk of developing pressure sores can help facilities take preventative steps to reduce their occurrence.
   B. Residents at risk are immobile, bedfast, and incontinent, and suffer from poor nutrition and low fluid intake.

IV. Discuss ways to treat pressure sores should they occur.
   A. Provide a nutritionally adequate diet—approximately 2,000 calories or more including 100 g of protein.
      1. Increase protein and calories in the diet.
         a. Provide double portions of meat, poultry, fish, or beans.
         b. Offer between meal nourishments.
            i. High-protein milk drink
            ii. Fortified milk
            iii. Fortified pudding
         c. Provide large portions of milk on trays or substitute fortified milk for regular milk with meals.
         d. Request a high-protein diet order.
      2. Assure adequate vitamin intake.
         a. Increase vitamin C for maintenance and repair of body tissue.
         b. Request a multivitamin supplement with zinc from the physician. Zinc deficiency tends to impair healing. Zinc increases taste awareness and may increase food intake.
      3. Add variety to foods consumed, to supply needed vitamins and minerals.
      4. Make meals appealing and attractive.
      5. Honor likes and dislikes (get to know the resident).
      6. Supply extra fluids on trays.
      7. Watch plate waste and replace those meals not eaten.

Quiz

1. What is a pressure sore?
2. Why are pressure sores dangerous for residents to develop?
3. Why are pressure sores a concern to health care facilities?
4. Name four ways to treat pressure sores with nutrition intervention.

Appendix F

Enteral Complete Formulas

Standard	Calories/ml	Protein g/1,000 ml	Features
Isocal	1.06	34.2	300 m0sm/kg
Precision Isotonic Diet	1.0	29	"
Osmolite	1.06	37.2	"
Osmolite HN	1.06	44.4	"
Renu	1.0	35	"
Travasorb MCT (powder)	1.0	49.3	"
Compleat, modified	1.07	43.00	"
Entrition	1.0	35	"
Vitaneed	1.0	35	"
Glucerna	1.0	41.25	"
Ensure	1.06	37.2	Standard
Compleat (regular)[a]	1.07	43	"
Travasorb (liquid)	1.06	35	"
Travasorb Standard	1.0	30	"
Vital HN	1.0	41.7	"
Sustacal	1.0	61	"
Resource Instant Crystals	1.06	37.2	"
Meritene Liquid[a]	0.96	57	"
Meritene (powder)[a]	1.0	69	
Travasorb HN	1.0	45	"
Precision High Nitrogen Diet	1.05	43.9	"
Ensure HN	1.06	44.4	"
Isotein HN	1.2	68	"
Sustacal Powder[a]	1.33	77	"
Sustacal HC	1.5	61	"
Ensure Plus	1.5	54.9	"
Ensure Plus HN	1.5	62.6	"
Travasorb MCT Liquid Diet	1.5	74	"
Traumacal/Fulfil	1.5	82.5	"
Sustagen	1.7	111.5	"
Isocal HCN	2.0	75	"
Two Cal HN	2.0	83.4	"
Magnacal	2.0	70	"

[a] Contains lactose.

Appendix G

Nutrition Formulas with Special Features

	Calories/ ml	Protein g/1,000 ml	Features
Stresstein	1.2	70	44% BCAA
Hepatic Aid II	1.1	44.1	46% BCAA
Travasorb Hepatic	1.1	28.6	50% BCAA
Traum-Aid HBC	1.0	56	50% BCAA
Vivonex T.E.N.	1.0	38	33% BCAA
Amin-Aid	2.0	19.4	Free AA
Travasorb Renal	1.35	22.9	Free AA
Pulmocare	1.5	62.6	High fat, low chol.
Enrich	1.1	39.7	Dietary fiber
Jevity	1.06	44.4	"
Criticare HN	1.06	38	Elemental
Vivonex High Nitrogen	1.0	46	"
Vivonex Standard	1.0	20.4	"
Vital HN	1.0	41.7	"
Citrotein	0.66	41	CL egg white solid
Precision LR Diet	1.1	26	"
Ross SLD	0.82	37.5	"

Appendix H

Examples of Dietary Problems, Needs, and Solutions

ETIOLOGIES OF SOME COMMON DIETARY PROBLEMS

1. Dissatisfaction with dietary restrictions
2. Inability to chew food
3. Low activity level
4. Fatigue
5. Nausea
6. Vomiting
7. Poor dentition
8. Impaired arm/hand mobility
9. Impaired arm/hand strength
10. Unhappiness about admission to the facility
11. Inability to cut food into small pieces
12. Rapid eating; failure to chew food properly
13. Improperly fitting or broken dentures
14. Sore mouth
15. Sore throat
16. Cognitive impairment
17. Gastrointestinal distress
18. Difficulty swallowing
19. Edentulousness
20. Short attention span
21. Difficulty chewing meat
22. Noncompliance with prescribed diet
23. Noncompliance resulting from eating food from other residents' trays
24. Refusal to eat
25. Altered taste sensation

EXAMPLES OF PROBLEMS AND NEEDS THAT CAN BE IDENTIFIED BY THE DIETARY DEPARTMENT

1. Inability or refusal to eat
2. Significant weight loss or gain
3. Weight below or above IBW
4. Routine refusal of foods containing vital nutrients
5. Pressure sores
6. Low hemoglobin or hematocrit
7. Inability to make wants known because of difficulty in speaking, hearing, or seeing
8. Medications causing possible food/drug interactions
9. Patients who are immobile or bedfast
10. Constipation, prolonged or recurring
11. Acute illness or infection
12. Post-surgical or post-burn state
13. Excessive snacking between meals
14. Inability to chew foods of regular consistency
15. Consumption of less than _____ percent of meals
16. Aspirates food easily
17. Inability to eat without assistance
18. Consumption of food from other residents' trays
19. Dysphagia
20. Complaints of hunger
21. Elevated or erratic blood sugar levels
22. Protein depletion: muscle wasting, low serum protein levels
23. Nausea and vomiting
24. Nutrient-depleting medication
25. Inadequate nutrient intake
26. Chronic infection
27. Postinjury requirements

EXAMPLES OF COMMON NUTRITIONAL GOALS

1. Have a hemoglobin level within the normal range by _____.
2. Have an iron level within the normal range by _____.
3. Have a blood sugar level within the normal range by _____.
4. Maintain current weight range of _____ by_____.
5. Not show signs of fluid volume overload, such as frothy sputum, high blood pressure, and weight gain by _____.
6. Lose at least _____ lbs. by _____.
7. Have a serum protein level within the normal range by _____.
8. Follow the therapeutic diet as ordered by _____.
9. Accept supplemental diet by _____.
10. Gain at least _____ lb. by _____.

11. Maintain stable weight by _____.
12. Show signs of adequate hydration by _____.
13. Have bowel movements of normal consistency by _____.
14. Have bowel movements 3 times per week by _____.
15. Be free of pressure sores by _____.
16. Reduce pressure sores to stage _____ by _____.
17. Come to dining room for meals _____ times a day by _____.

EXAMPLES OF COMMON APPROACHES TO DIETARY PROBLEMS AND NEEDS

1. Allow the resident extra time to eat.
2. Ask the family to limit the amount of food brought in to the resident.
3. Ask the family to limit the types of food brought in to the resident.
4. Give a consistency of food to the resident that is easily swallowed.
5. Give supplemental nourishment between meals (specify frequency, type, and amount).
6. Hand feed the resident.
7. Use appropriate devices to assist the resident to eat independently (specify).
8. Elevate the head of the bed at least _____ degrees for eating.
9. Elevate the head of the bed at least _____ degrees for at least _____ hours after meals.
10. Elevate the head of the bed at least _____ degrees at all times.
11. Keep the resident up in a chair for _____ after meals.
12. Monitor the abdomen for distention (specify frequency).
13. Monitor intervals between bowel movements.
14. Monitor the resident's intake.
15. Offer small meals _____ times per day.
16. Offer large servings of food.
17. Offer second helpings of food.
18. Offer preferred foods.
19. Offer substitutes for uneaten foods.
20. Ask the family to bring preferred foods to the resident.
21. Feed slowly.
22. Stimulate swallowing with a spoon or by stroking the throat.
23. Adjust the calorie level upward to _____ calories per day.
24. Adjust the calorie level downward to _____ calories per day.
25. Allow the resident ample time to eat.
26. Offer a between-meal supplement _____ times per day.
27. Provide a diabetic diet, as ordered by the physician.
28. Determine the resident's ideal body weight.
29. Eliminate concentrated sweets and refined sugars from the diet.
30. Eliminate food causing adverse symptoms.
31. Offer foods of high biological protein value.

32. Praise the resident's attempts to follow the diet.
33. Prompt the resident to eat at least one bite of each food served at a meal.
34. Offer high-protein snacks _____ times per day.
35. Encourage the resident to eat independently.
36. Monitor the resident during meals.
37. Place the resident at a table with other residents' trays out of reach.
38. Determine the resident's food preferences and dislikes.
39. Refer to the occupational therapist for evaluation and recommendations.
40. Assist the resident to eat after he or she becomes fatigued.
41. Ensure that dentures are in place.
42. Offer liquids every hour.
43. Advance the diet as tolerated by the resident.
44. Encourage or remind the resident to eat slowly and chew food thoroughly.
45. Remind the resident to eat.
46. Refer to the dentist for evaluation and recommendations.
47. Instruct the resident concerning dietary restrictions.
48. Instruct the family concerning dietary restrictions.
49. Attempt to have the resident drink at least _____ glasses of fluid per day.
50. Monitor blood sugar levels (frequency or date).
51. Monitor the hemoglobin level (frequency or date).
52. Monitor the blood iron level (frequency or date).
53. Monitor the ferritin level (frequency or date).
54. Monitor for signs of dehydration, such as skin turgor and dry mouth (frequency).
55. Monitor intake and output.
56. Monitor blood pressure (frequency).
57. Monitor weight.
58. Monitor the serum protein level (frequency or date).
59. Monitor dietary compliance by the resident.
60. Monitor dietary regime compliance by the family.
61. Calculate calorie and protein intake for _____ days.
62. Maintain present food intake.
63. Avoid the resident's food dislikes.
64. Evaluate the insulin dosage with present caloric intake.
65. Evaluate oral hypoglycemic agent dosage with present caloric intake.

Index